STRATEGIC CONTRACTING

CONTRACTING

for

Health
Systems

and

Services

STRATEGIC CONTRACTING

for
Health
Systems
and
Services

Jean Perrot and
Eric de Roodenbeke, editors

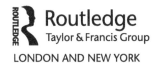

Routledge
Taylor & Francis Group

LONDON AND NEW YORK

First published 2012 by Transaction Publishers

Published 2017 by Routledge
2 Park Square, Milton Park, Abingdon, Oxon OX14 4RN
711 Third Avenue, New York, NY 10017, USA

Routledge is an imprint of the Taylor & Francis Group, an informa business

Library of Congress Catalog Number: 2011002427

Library of Congress Cataloging-in-Publication Data

Strategic contracting for health systems and services / [edited by] Jean Perrot and Eric de Roodenbeke.
    p. ; cm.
Includes bibliographical references.
ISBN 978-1-4128-1499-7 (alk. paper)
    1. Health services administration. 2. Contracting out. I. Perrot, Jean. II. Roodenbeke, Éric de, 1956- [DNLM: 1. Contract Services—organization & administration. 2. Health Care Sector—economics. 3. Delivery of Health Care—organization & administration. 4. Public-Private Sector Partnerships—economics. W 74.1]

RA971.S79 2011
362.1068—dc22

                                    2011002427

ISBN 13: 978-1-4128-1499-7 (hbk)
ISBN 13: 978-1-4128-1500-0 (pbk)

Strategic Contracting for Health Systems and Services

Foreword

Health systems in low- and middle-income countries, following the trend in high-income countries, are getting increasingly complex with an increasing number of diversified health system actors: the central Ministry of Health and the autonomous institutions attached to it; lower levels of government and local authorities in a decentralized context; other parts of the central government either providing or financing health services, such as the military or police; profit driven or not-for-profit private service providers or funders including the spectrum of NGOs; and, finally, health insurance institutions which have taken an increasingly prominent role in health financing. In this context, managing relationships between these different actors becomes a vital element for health system performance. On one hand the specific public good elements related to many aspects of health and the well known market failures particularly relating to information pose limits to the optimization of these relationships through the markets. On the other hand technocratic regulation has often been linked to waste and maladapted measures that do not encourage quality, efficiency and equity.

Contracting is a tool and a strategy that can increase health system performance by building on one type of market mechanism while recognizing the specific public good nature of health with the associated market failures. Even though the formalization of a contractual arrangement most naturally passes through a contract, the concept of contracting is much wider than a written contract. Contracting is a process and an approach that lead the health sector actors to define the modalities of their relationships and the results they want to attain. The growing attention focused on performance incentives is something that links to this approach. Monitoring and evaluating these type of relationships is the key to their success. Performance incentives, which sometimes are implemented in the form of Performance Based Contracting schemes, but which, in the low- and middle-income country contexts, are more commonly known as Performance/Results Based Financing schemes, follow the same basic logic of reorganizing, through incentives and through an agreement on objectives and rewards, the relationship between different actors in order to make them work towards specified public health goals. This book will have a specific chapter on supply side performance incentives that will further explore their use in health systems.

If taken at its face value, contracting can seem to be simple. But in reality this is not the case, making strategic decisions about when to contract and how to conduct a contractual process requires specific capacities and know-how which often are still lacking among some of the important health system actors. For example, when contracting is constructed around performance incentives, questions related to the choice of indicators and methods to monitor attainment or the way the provider bonuses are calculated are only two of the issues that need to be examined carefully. It is, therefore, important for countries seeking to implement some for of contracting approach in health to have information on the objectives, approaches, modalities and the instruments of contracting and what has worked and not worked in other settings - this is the objective of this book which relies both on conceptual guidance and on lessons learned from concrete experiences.

The diversity of possibilities for contracting makes it a very interesting but complicated subject. The purpose for contractual relationships varies. For a better understanding this book proposes a typology based on three common purposes of contractual relationships: 1) Delegation of responsibility; 2) Act of purchase; 3) Cooperation. The modalities of implementing contractual arrangements vary as well. In some contexts, formal negotiations and market based methods such as an open call for bids open up the possibility of competition, while elsewhere the contractual relationship can based on informal agreements between partners that know each other already - e.g. between a central ministry of health and lower levels of government. This book covers this diversity of contracting while underlining that each country and each situation is different and that contextual factors such as social norms or administrative set-up will need to be taken into account.

In order to be effective contracting needs to be subject to some type of framework at the country level. Uncoordinated development of contracting will undermine a systemic approach to achieving health systems goals which is the basis of an effective health system. The question of regulating contracting will be an important dimension covered by the book. One of the challenges is to tie contracting to the government's stewardship function. The elaboration of a national policy on contracting is an element that brings us closer to this objective by defining the rationale for and "raison d'être" of contacting and the modalities of its implementation. This means that the government, so often criticized, still has an essential but a new role that puts it in charge of regulating the use of contracting in order to increase efficiency and equity in the health system.

A lot of international attention has recently focused on examples of the successful use of contracting, leading to pressure for its increased use. Some of the successes are undeniable, but as for any approach that comes with positive results, there is a danger of turning it into a fad leading to its inappropriate use. Even though contracting should always be viewed as one of the various options for increasing efficiency and/or equity, it is also important to evaluate its operational feasibility and the associated costs. The level of existing capacities for managing and monitoring a contractual arrangement should also be considered before opting to follow this approach.

It is hoped that this book will allow all the health sector actors to gain a broad understanding of the different dimensions of contracting in health systems and instruments related to it. The book facilitates the sharing of a common language which is essential in any contractual process. It provides the information that can guide different actors to gain the most from it. For those who are already engaged in a contractual process, the book will provide new perspectives that can guide them to go further or to rationalize the use of the instruments that they have chosen.

In several countries, especially in Africa, reaching the Millennium Development Goals will need additional efforts and new approaches to financing or delivering health services might be appropriate; the evidence presented in this book suggests there is a role for contracting as a tool and a strategy to support these efforts. The World Health Report for 2010: *Health Systems Financing: the Path to Universal Coverage* argues that in order to get closer to universal coverage countries need to find ways to use their existing resources, and any additional resources that become available, more efficiently and equitably. The Report for example makes the case for moving towards suitable provider payment methods and towards strategic purchasing in order to create efficiencies. Contracting, including the performance incentives that might be linked to it, is a tool and a strategy that can carry those objectives.

David Evans
Director, Health Systems Financing,
World Health Organization, Geneva, Switzerland

Introduction

Jean Perrot &
Eric de Roodenbeke

"To find a form of association which will defend and protect with the whole common force the person and property of each associate, and in which each individual, while uniting himself with all, may still obey himself alone, and remain as free as before. This is the fundamental problem of which the social contract provides the solution."

"Each one of us puts his person and all his power in common under the supreme direction of the general will; in body we receive each member as an indivisible part of the whole."

Jean-Jacques Rousseau, *The Social Contract*, Book I, Chapter VI, 1762.

The commitments which bind us to the social body are obligatory only because they are mutual, and their nature is such that, in fulfilling them, one cannot work for others without also working for oneself."

Jean-Jacques Rousseau, *The Social Contract,* Book II, Chapter IV, 1762.

"A contract is an agreement by which one or several persons bind themselves, towards one or several persons, to transfer, to do or not to do something."

French Civil Code, Article 1101.

"Agreements lawfully entered into constitute the law for those who have made them."

French Civil Code, Article 1134.

"Economics come closer to being a 'science of contracts' than a 'science of choice'."

James Buchanan, *A Contractarian Paradigm for Applying Economic Theory*, American Economic Review, May 1975.

Today, everyone knows that a young woman in a developing country, because she has been to primary school, has every chance of having healthier children. In the same way, using clean water helps avoid many diarrhoeal diseases that are harmful to health, especially that of young children. A broad range of health determinants are outside the scope of the health system.

However, there is a consensus that health systems have also played an important role in increasing life expectancy. The World Bank's annual report of 1993 highlighted investment in health care as an important component of human development. Dr G.H. Brundtland, the then Director-General of WHO, stated, "when I became Director-General in 1998, one of my prime concerns was that health systems development should become increasingly central to the work of the WHO."[1]

Yet for a long time, efforts to strengthen health systems focused solely on the public sector and health programmes overseen by public bodies. Because health is not an ordinary good, it is logically a prerogative of the State. In the years that followed the Alma-Ata Declaration, responsibility lay with States to take the necessary action to meet the objective "Health for All by the Year 2000". The private sector was thus sidelined; in countries such as Ethiopia, Greece (in the case of hospitals), Mozambique and the United Republic of Tanzania it was even banned, as it still is in Cuba. But at the same time, some private-sector stakeholders readily adapted themselves to this special situation and did not wish to become part of a structured health system, fearing that they would lose their room for manoeuvre and have to comply with requirements that curtailed their activities.

This state of compartmentalization, which persists in some health systems, has nevertheless evolved considerably in recent years for two main reasons:

- The concept of the welfare state, long the basis for state action in the health and other social sectors (namely education), has shown its limitations. The subsequent acknowledgment of the private sector led, in the early 1990s, to advocacy of privatization of all or part of the public health sector;

- We are witnessing profound changes in two areas. First, the stakeholders involved in the heath sector are increasing in number and diversifying as a result of the development of the private sector and a process of democratisation and decentralization that is conducive to the emergence of civil society and organized and accountable territorial bodies. Second, these developments are paralleled by greater differentiation of functions: the various stakeholders are increasingly specializing in particular areas of the health system (service delivery, procurement, management, financing, and regulation).

Public and private sectors that exist in isolation are less and less representative of reality. The implementation of national health policies in general, and the delivery of health services in particular, is increasingly complex. The interdependence of health stakeholders becomes more conspicuous with the increased complexity of delivery systems as these respond to changing demand. There is a compelling need to forge relationships, and such relationships are in fact emerging and proliferating in developed countries and, more recently, in developing countries. They may be informal. But they are increasingly organized and structured: **contracting is a tool that helps to create interrelations between partners with potentially different status and responsibilities.**

The health-care system cannot be likened to a traditional administrative organization governed by procedures and hierarchical rules, nor to a market governed by a price system. It is composed of networks of interdependent stakeholders. It should therefore be understood as a set of relationships that bind together the various stakeholders of the system. Their status, be it public or private, makes little difference: what matters are their goals and objectives, and finding ways to create resulting synergies.

It is also essential that these relations should be formalized to avoid the risk of conflict arising from different interpretations of the role and mission of each party. The contracting process is a solution to the inherent problems of a system that interconnects a number of stakeholders.

Formalization is an essential aspect of the contracting process

A contract may thus be moral or legal and exist either orally or in writing. In societies where transactional systems are becoming more and more complex in terms of practicalities and because of the increasing number of stakeholders involved, the formalization of moral contracts would appear essential to enable the transactional system to operate as smoothly as possible. Formalization imposes a duty on each entity to clarify its objectives and how it intends to meet them. It also helps to characterize the nature of the transactions that occur within an organization, and between it and other stakeholders in the system. It is these elements that help to improve efficiency because they fix a goal for the organization's activity, which takes into consideration aspects that go beyond the producer's interests alone.

Contracting is more than the formalization of business transactions

A formalized contract is not an agreement that focuses exclusively on market transactions. Approaching a contract in this way considerably reduces the scope of this instrument, which is meant to formalize exchange mechanisms, i.e. all types of transactions that exist between stakeholders from different entities. Such transactions do not always give rise to a form of remuneration and, where they do, the remuneration does not necessarily follow market logic. This is because the contracting process can be formalized by a series of reciprocal actions tending towards mutually agreed goals. When resources go hand in hand with the signature of a contract, this can be a useful means of performing an activity that involves essential public goods.

A contract is not just an act of legal significance

It is important to bear in mind that contracting goes beyond the concept of a commercial contract based on a legal instrument and a system of legal arbitration. Contracting should therefore be understood as the formalization of relationships between entities. When this is embodied in a contract that has a legal force, the contract is the expression of a legal mechanism. But a contract can also be moral in nature, in which case it falls within the social sphere.

Intra- and extra-institutional operation is based on relationships between stakeholders in a transactional system, whether mercantile or otherwise. It would thus be wrong to think that only legal contracts have consequences. All procedures devised to codify activities that involve a number of stakeholders could fit this pattern, so long as the stakeholders concerned were directly involved in framing them through a process of negotiation.

The performance of an institution is based on optimizing the production process and matching this process to demand. Such optimization can only be achieved by minimizing the factors that interfere with the institution's activities. Formalizing a moral contract enables uncertainties to be minimized by specifying what each party can expect from the other. This facilitates transactions in a climate of trust by limiting uncertainties about the activities of the other parties. Thus moral contracts formalized in writing or agreed tacitly play a decisive role in the structure of institutions. The consequences of breaching this type of contract are just as serious as breaching contracts that are subject to legal oversight.

In situations where a given authority regulates the system, various means can be brought to bear to punish those who do not honour their commitments: the revocation of the right to practise, or the discontinuation of a subsidy, may have a greater impact than a court sanction. Sanctions aside, the loss of trust leads to a loss of credibility and engenders new strategies between stakeholders. These strategies could heavily penalize the party that did not respect the terms of the contract: everything then depends on the power relations and/or the degree of dependency between the parties to the contract. Furthermore, the content of such a contract will be much better internalized than any bureaucratic procedure. The nature and complexity of these relationships will weigh heavily when deciding whether contracting should be preferred to other ways of organizing relations between stakeholders.

Thus, a stakeholder in a health system could develop contractual relations with all its partners. The latter are not, however, all in the same position in relation to the

11

stakeholder. Classifying contracts vertically or horizontally makes it easier to identify the nature of the relationship:

- Vertical: contracting between two stakeholders at different levels. It is interesting to refer to the economic theory of agency here. When the stakeholder concerned is the "principal" we may speak of vertical upstream contracting. When the stakeholder is the "agent" we may speak of downstream contracting.

- Horizontal: contracting between stakeholders at the same level. The theory of agency is of no help here because a hierarchical dependency relationship no longer applies. It is a partnership of mutual dependency. In economic theory we would refer to it as the cooperative game theory.

However, we will also see that this node of contracts cannot exist without a regulatory body.

The State, i.e. the public authorities,[2] thus retains an active role in the health sector, not through its traditional function of direct provision or financing but through its general administrative, governance, steering and stewardship duties in the health-care system.

The ultimate purpose of this tool should never be forgotten. Stakeholders entering into a contractual relationship thus need to reconcile the individual interests they wish to advance via the contractual relationship with a collective quest to improve the performance of the health-care system. This is why the regulatory function entrusted to the public authorities plays a key role in ensuring that the public interest is not derailed.

At this stage, it is important to avoid two misunderstandings:

Some people consider contracting as the first step towards privatisation. In the eyes of its supporters, contracting signals the disengagement of the State, and is initially expressed in contracting arrangements with the private sector. The private sector then performs the activities that used to be undertaken by public bodies. Sooner or later, this process will result in the privatization of these activities; contracting is therefore supposedly the Trojan horse of privatization of the public sector. The approach outlined in this book does not support this reasoning. On the contrary, contracting must be thought of as a process that facilitates coordination among stakeholders. Whether they belong to the public or the private sector is ultimately of little importance. Contracting respects the identity of each stakeholder; it is only interested in establishing the relationship between them.

Some consider contracting to be merely a management tool for reducing health costs, a means whereby a budget manager seeks to purchase better services at lower cost. While financial considerations are indeed often reflected in contractual arrangements, they are not always the key component. It is to be observed, moreover, that contracting is especially unwelcome when its stated goal is to reduce health spending; it then becomes a lightning rod for the criticisms of those who view it as a means to shrink budgets, eliminate jobs or close down health facilities.

These two perspectives do a disservice to contracting, making it out to be a tool of economic liberalism and its excesses. In contrast, as we shall explain, contracting is part of the search for an alternative that lies somewhere between the consignment of health care to the private sector, which obeys only the laws of the market, and the administration of health care by a domineering central State.

The concept of privatization

Privatization is a concept that at first sight appears simple. According to the dictionary definition, privatization involves the transfer of ownership of an entity from the public to the private sector, its opposite being nationalization.

In everyday parlance, this is the sole meaning of privatization, and as such contracting cannot be understood as a form of privatization. This is because privatization involves a transfer of ownership whereas contracting builds on the existing situation, with the stakeholders already present, and seeks to establish relationships among them. Privatization is an institutional arrangement whereas contracting is concerned with relationships.

However, in specialist literature on State reform, privatization is defined more broadly: it is understood as the adoption of a management model that draws on the rules of the market. According to the theories of D. Rondinelli and M. Iacono,[3] this type of privatization can be achieved in several ways:

– By transferring ownership:[4] like a public enterprise whose ownership is transferred to the private sector, the ownership of certain public entities (hospitals, health centres, laboratories, drug distribution services, etc.) is transferred to the private sector. Some authors describe this as State "divestment"[5] since the entity's assets are transferred in whole or in part.

– By ensuring that public entities adopt private-sector managerial practices, while maintaining public-sector ownership: eliminating arbitrary subsidies and public monopolies, according autonomous status, and permitting the outsourcing of certain tasks and the drawing up of employment contracts outside the public administration. The public entity adopts private-sector managerial techniques and becomes an independent enterprise within a larger entity constituting an administration.

– By entrusting the management of public entities to the private sector, while maintaining public-sector ownership, also known as management by delegation.

– By purchasing services from private providers, whether or not they operate from health facilities, while maintaining control over public funding.

– By replacing the public sector with the private sector: in this case ownership is private and will remain so, but the private entity substitutes for the public stakeholder that previously carried out the task.

In each of the five cases above, we can therefore say that the health system would be more privatized in the sense that it would operate more in line with the rules of the market.

However, certain strategies may limit privatization: for example, ensuring that the private sector cooperates with the public sector: in this case ownership is private and will remain so, but the entity agrees to act in accordance with national health policy. This could be described as greater state control.

There are thus three factors to consider in assessing privatization:

– Ownership of the entity: typically, privatization is the transfer of ownership from the public to the private sector.

– Management of the entity: the entity is managed according to the rules of the market and private enterprise. In other words (i) users are treated as clients, (ii) services are determined by client demand, (iii) the production process is designed to respond to demand, and cost control is a major concern. The management must therefore abandon the model of administrative hierarchies to achieve a degree of independence.

– Missions or objectives of the entity: Are service providers entirely free to choose their terms of reference (economic liberalism) or does the State have a say in defining them (through contracting or regulations) and consequently influencing which products are produced and how?

The following table summarizes the above points:

Evaluation criteria *Reform*	*Ownership*	*Management*	*Terms of reference*
Transfer ownership	**Transition from public to private**	Owing to the transfer of ownership, management becomes private	**Economic liberalism** *or* **State intervention through contracting or regulations**
Grant autonomy to public entities	Status quo (public)	**Operates more in line with the rules of the market**	Quasi-status quo (public)
Delegate management of public entities	Status quo (public)	**Transition from public to private**	Quasi-status quo (public)
Substitute private for public	Status quo (private)	**Substitute private stakeholders for public stakeholders**	Quasi-status quo (public)
NB: Areas most affected by privatization indicated in bold.			

As an example, let us examine the case of a public hospital under private management. The effects of this decision, classified according to the three evaluation criteria above, are schematically illustrated as follows:

Degree of privatization

	0%	100%
Ownership		
Management of inputs		
Mission		

In this example, the hospital is publicly owned but management of inputs is delegated entirely (by contract) to a private stakeholder. The hospital's mission, although globally remaining in line with public objectives, may also include private objectives (e.g. accepting that the introduction of cost recovery will entail a loss in equality of access for users).

The contracting process opens up new perspectives for analysing how organizations function

The methodology outlined in this work illustrates how the contracting process makes it easier to recast the relationships among organizational stakeholders. In view of the number of areas and organizations considered, the contracting process is universally applicable. Likewise, it is not based on a monolithic structure of the State. This universality is particularly important because it allows the performance of an organization to be improved without initially calling the existing system into question. This approach is important in a context where the globalization of exchanges can bring about standardization of practice. The wonder of humanity stems from diversity, which is a major source of progress.

The contracting process shifts the debate over organizational performance away from the nature of organizations and onto the efficacy of relations. It has been abundantly demonstrated that very diverse organizations can achieve high levels of performance if their operating environment ensures that the organizations' goals are consistent with modes of regulation. Occasionally heated debates tend to contrast the supposedly efficient private sector and the supposedly inefficient public sector, but performance in fact depends on an organization's analytical outlook. A given organization's economic efficiency can have a considerable social cost, the consequences of which will only be felt later on and by other organizations. Historically a perfect example of this has been the environmental and health consequences of contrasting structures of industrial production, whether capitalist businesses (the Bhopal disaster) or organizations in centrally planned economies (Chernobyl).

15

Contracting presupposes that all stakeholders will enter into a dialogue in which everyone can state their opinions. Yet it would be naïve to believe that all stakeholders will come to an understanding as a matter of course. Health system stakeholders do not necessarily share the same objectives, and they may adopt opposing strategies where their interests diverge, but by pursuing dialogue they can clarify organizational strategy while ultimately leaving responsibility for intervention to a regulatory authority.

In this book the authors would like to convey the following five fundamental messages:

1. **Contracting may involve all stakeholders** seeking to improve public health: stakeholders in the public sector (the Ministry of Health and its decentralized services and independent entities, e.g. agencies, hospitals) administrative units (municipalities, autonomous regions), communities, private-sector stakeholders (clinics, private practitioners, local NGOs, commercial enterprises), financing institutions (public or private, voluntary or mandatory), and development partners. They are all affected by contracting, without exception. Irrespective of whether they are public or private, what matters is their degree of independence in carrying out their activities.

2. **Contracting may involve all functions** in a health system: Naturally, non-medical services (maintenance, catering, security, management, training) and health services (whether delivered through health facilities or otherwise) spring to mind first of all, but contracting may also involve the production of health-related items (for example: insecticide-impregnated bednets, rehydration salts, etc.), health financing (through insurance institutions), and financial and technical support. In principle, none of these roles lies outside the scope of contracting and there is no reason to prioritize one over another.

3. **Contracting often relies on a pragmatic approach:** contractual arrangements are devised as tools enabling the individual interests of existing stakeholders to be reconciled. From this perspective, contracting is insufficient to safeguard the general interest, even though it may guarantee a better use of resources. Therefore, in order to make a significant impact on health system performance, a systemic approach must be adopted. Such an approach involves establishing a contracting policy, which can be drawn up for the national health system as a whole or for each of its components: priority health interventions (for example, integrated management of childhood illnesses), a specific health problem (tuberculosis or malaria control), a particular segment of the population (people living with HIV/AIDS), other health system functions (risk-sharing system,

drug distribution) or a specific geographic area (organization of a health district). The various contractual arrangements established among the stakeholders are the operational result of a collective and concerted strategy, more or less formalized, for example through framework agreements or target contracts. Where contracting is governed by a contracting policy, it becomes a strategic option for improving health system performance. It represents genuine and lasting partnerships rather than simply a relationship between contracting parties.

4. **The State must assume an indispensable regulatory role** in addition to possible direct involvement in specific contractual relations. This involvement can no doubt contribute to improving health system performance, but States are also aware of the limits of their direct involvement and they gauge the importance of the contribution of all other stakeholders (whether from the public sector, for example decentralized administrative regions, or the various branches of the private sector or the general public). This regulation of contractual relations is consistent with the development of State reforms currently ongoing in many countries. The role of the State is reconsidered, albeit not reduced; its functions tend increasingly towards safeguarding the general interest rather than delivering or funding services. Specifically, the Ministry of Health should endeavour to perform a stewardship function. It follows that the State should regulate contractual relations in such a way that they contribute to the general interest and improve health system performance.

5. **Contracting should be evaluated against its objective.** Nowadays, contracting experiments are of such recent date that we lack sufficient hindsight to assess the impact of contracting on system performance. But this aspect should constantly be borne in mind by the authorities advocating contracting. Only when enough proof exists of the benefits of contracting will we be able to view it as an essential tool for the organization of health services.

The goal of this work is to examine the potential of contracting, but also to highlight its limits, the prerequisites for its use and the conditions for its success. The work is intended mainly for decision-makers at national and local level in developing countries: Ministries of Health and local authorities, NGOs and private operators, health financing entities and development partners.

It is neither a theoretical work, nor a manual or guide. Neither is it a comparative analysis of experiments. It is something in between and no doubt closer to a treatise. It is upstream of the action. The goal is to assist anyone interested in contracting to act and react professionally.

The structure of the document gives rise to a certain number of redundancies. The authors chose this option because it allows the user to read the book entry by entry and obtain a coherent overview without having to peruse the entire book. Thus, stakeholders who wish better to understand and exploit the potential of contracting in their respective fields might focus on the chapter that specifically interests them, and if need be, expand their knowledge by referring to other sections of the book. This approach is also designed to make it easier to use the book in conjunction with training sessions organized in response to the growing interest in health-care contracting.

This book was drafted by a number of authors from various backgrounds, predominately from institutions in the United Nations system: mainly the World Health Organization (WHO) but also the International Labour Organization (ILO) and the World Bank. Academics and Health Ministry officials also made contributions. The book was therefore principally drafted from an institutional angle. It was coordinated by Jean Perrot, an economist at WHO who has been working on this subject for more than 10 years, and by Eric de Roodenbeke, an economist who has held various positions at the French Ministry of Cooperation, the World Bank and WHO before becoming Director General of the International Hospital Federation.

A book similar to this one was published in French, entitled, "La contractualisation dans le secteur de la santé: pour une utilisation efficace et appropriée", by Jean Perrot and Eric de Roodenbeke (eds.), Karthala, 2005. Some chapters from this work have been translated with certain modifications; some chapters were substantially rewritten prior to translation; others were deleted or are completely new, such as the chapter on performance incentives, which were not yet an issue when the French version was written. Most of the chapters were written in French and then translated. While the English translation is of high quality, there are inevitably some turns of phrase reflecting the original French and the French mindset.

Notes

[1] The World Health Report 2000 - Health Systems: Improving Performance. Message from the Director-General.

[2] For ease of reference it is important to define what is meant by the following frequently used terms:
Entity: a group of people sharing common objectives. This is the broadest term, used in reference to organized activities that could be performed by a unit in an organization, a territorial unit (State, region, commune, etc.) or an international organization.

18

Institution: a formal group pursuing objectives delegated to it by a regulatory body.

Organization: any group of varying status pursuing a set of self-imposed or externally imposed goals.

Public authorities: institutions with regulatory terms of reference whose mandate is legitimized by virtue of their position within a national system.

[3] Rondinelli, D and M. Iacono. 1996. *Strategic management of privatization: a framework for planning and implementation. Public Administration and Development* 16:247-263.

[4] Ownership of an entity and ownership of infrastructure are distinct concepts. Ownership of infrastructure implies developed sites (buildings) and undeveloped sites (land and principal investments). Ownership of an entity implies a legally autonomous economic unit, organized to produce goods or services. Consider the example of a hospital: let us say that the entity is an NGO that operates the hospital enterprise. The enterprise may or may not own the hospital buildings (which could, for example, belong to another NGO). What matters here is the ownership of the entity and not the infrastructure. This distinction is clear for shops that differentiate goodwill from tangible assets or private physicians who differentiate their surgery from their patients: where a transfer of ownership takes place these items are kept separate.

[5] Savas, E. S. 1989. A Taxonomy of Privatization Strategies. *Policy Studies Journal* 18, no. 2:343-355.

Part I

Chapter 1

Emergence of contracting in the health sector

Jean Perrot

INTRODUCTION

People's health has improved considerably in the course of the twentieth century. Proof of this is the spectacular increase in life expectancy; barely half a century ago it was no more than 48 years whereas today the global average figure is 66 years. Numerous determinants have certainly contributed to this; broad sectors of the population have seen their income increase, better working conditions have made life less harsh and dangerous, food has become healthier and individual and collective hygiene have improved. Moreover, the higher level of education, especially that of women, has led to a better understanding of health issues. In addition, medical knowledge and practices as well as methods of treatment have made great strides in recent decades. Finally, the organization of health systems, which broadly developed during the nineteenth century, has made it possible to coordinate efforts, notably under the aegis of States favouring conventional universalism, in other words free access to all types of care for all.

Nonetheless, despite all these efforts, the performance of health systems is still very often unsatisfactory. As the World Health Report 2000 *"Health Systems: Improving Performance"*, points out *"these failings result in very large numbers of preventable deaths and disabilities in each country; in unnecessary suffering; in injustice, inequality and denial of basic rights of individuals. The impact is most severe on the poor, who are driven deeper into poverty by lack of financial protection against ill-health"*.[1]

It is true that in recent years, health systems' organization has undergone a considerable evolution. One factor which has unquestionably contributed to these changes has been the mitigation of rivalry between the public and private sectors in all spheres of economic, social and political life. In an effort to make up for the inadequate performance of their health systems, most countries have undertaken reforms. Political decision-makers have several choices: deconcentration allows more authority to be vested in local Ministry of Health officials; administrative decentralization is a means of transferring responsibility for health to a local authority; autonomy for public providers is designed to endow health facilities with self-government, within the public sector, based on legal status; separation of funding bodies from service providers allows the introduction of competition between providers, whether public or private; the broadening of the range of possibilities for health financing, through risk pooling and insurance mechanisms, makes possible the emergence of an actor charged by its members with negotiating access to care; privatization, at least in the conventional sense, involves transfer of ownership from the public to the private sector; development of the private sector is a strategy option for political decision-makers wishing to withdraw from the provision or funding of health services.

The institutional reshuffles described above do not always yield the expected outcomes. The different actors continue to operate in isolation without seeking appropriate synergies. Moreover, the organization of health care provision still relies largely on hierarchical power, in other words on a vertical commandment method that does not favour a collaborative approach.

There is a new way of getting around these inconveniences. The actors can try to break away from their isolation and establish concerted activities in order to better respond to the needs and demands of communities. The relationships that they establish can rely on different modalities: coordination; exchange of information, and elaboration of joint principles of intervention (joint declarations, charters, etc.).These moral commitments have however their limits. In order to overcome these limits, these relationships are increasingly based on contractual arrangements which formalize the understanding between the mutually engaging actors.

The first section of this chapter will highlight the fact that the long lasting compartmentalization of health systems into private and public sectors no longer reflects the reality; the diversification of actors and functions in health systems inevitably leads to interactions. The concrete forms of these interactions and the difficulties in establishing them will need to be examined. The second section will focus on the fact that the actors are becoming increasingly aware of the evolutions in management methods. These two sections will lead us to the main point of this chapter: Contacting has not come out of nowhere; it is the consequence of different evolutions that have occurred, at an uneven global pace, in all the current societies.

1. INSTITUTIONAL EVOLUTIONS IN HEALTH SYSTEMS

1.1   The rationale underlying public sector - private sector compartmentalization

Until the end of the 1970s, in many developing countries the organization of health systems was relatively simple and could be summarized as follows. It involved two actors: on the one hand, a public system that was entirely organized by the central State which enacted laws, norms and regulations, laid down health policy and ran health facilities that were financed by public revenue and public assistance, and on the other a private system, either for-profit or run by the churches, and which operated independently and in complete autarky. [2] As a rule these two worlds live in separate   worlds. In line with the then prevailing welfare state rationale, most of these countries opted for a free and State-run health service. It is true that during the period the different private sectors developed, although in a compartmentalized fashion and almost without the State knowing.

This welfare state philosophy came to an end at the beginning of the 1980s.The Governments of the developing countries found themselves forced to address profound financial crises as a result of which virtually all of them introduced restrictions and/or reforms. The situation of the public facilities deteriorated inexorably. States long endeavoured to resist the deterioration and they would not or could not admit their failure. Shortages gradually and insidiously became the norm. There were even those who claimed they will manage the shortage: whatever the case, on learns to deal with it and to "muddle through".

A more manifest desire for "active privatisation" (to use J. Muschell's expression)[3] then emerged; this evolution was characterized by Governments, often urged on by development partners, encouraging the emergence of private actors. However, In the developing countries, transfer of ownership, in the strict sense of privatization, was still the exception. In these countries the privatization mainly manifested itself through the expansion of NGO operated health facilities (in particular non-denominational NGOs) and through the development of private clinics and private practice.

Nevertheless, both these periods were heavily marked by rigid compartmentalization of the efforts of health actors, with each of them setting up its activities in its own separate universe. Neither of them knew, or occasionally even wanted to know, what the other was doing. But at the same time, as each of them wanted to extend its sphere of influence, we also witnessed rivalry or clashes: installation of a new public health centre in the vicinity of an existing private centre; failure of a private practitioner to refer patients to the public hospital, etc. The consequences in terms of inefficacy within the health system could be dramatic for populations.

1.2   Recent trends

For some ten years now, it has been possible to observe a marked evolution in the organization of health systems. This is no doubt largely attributable to the disappearance of the public–private ideological confrontation. We have witnessed far-reaching reshuffles which have taken two directions. On the one hand, the number of actors involved in health has increased and become more diversified under the dual pull of private sector development and of democratization and decentralization, fostering the emergence of a civil society and of structured and responsible local authorities. On the other hand, this trend has gone hand in hand with sharper separation of roles; the different actors have increasingly specialized in a particular health system function (provision, procurement of services, management, financing and regulation, ...).

The diversification of actors

A situation in which the public sector, represented solely by the Ministry of Health, and the private sector, whether for profit or denominational, ignore or clash with one another to provide health services is increasingly remote from reality.

Internal institutional arrangements[4]

Historically, it has to be borne in mind that such reshufflings have taken place within the health system and among the sector's actors. Thus, recent years have been marked by two far-reaching changes which have resulted from the diversification of the ways in which public services are managed:

- *Deconcentration*: the heavily centralized administration which has long prevailed is gradually being replaced by a deconcentrated administration to which authority is delegated. Deconcentration within the health sector has essentially developed through the health districts. If it is to be effective, this system as a whole requires a certain degree of autonomy. It receives this via an action of deconcentration in which the central authority delegates some of its responsibilities to the health district. This new institutional arrangement obviously permits more effective management as it takes better into account the local circumstances. However, such autonomy is considerably limited if it the administrative unit does not have a proper legal personality, which alone will enable it fully to participate in contractual relations with its partners.

- *Autonomy*: while understanding that a health services production unit operating along traditional administrative management lines acts as a check on the efficacy of such facilities, but at the same time appreciating the undesirability of privatizing the facility or entrusting its management to a private institution, the Ministry of Health may opt to endow it with a status that permits greater autonomy. While remaining part of the public sector, the health facility possesses legal personality to perform a public service mission together with administrative and financial autonomy. There are two essential elements to this status: i) the public establishment is able to exercise all the rights attached to legal personality, in particular the right to sign contracts (for its day-to-day

25

running it need no longer follow the conventional administrative channels and is able directly to contract service providers: contracts for maintenance services, for catering or for laundry services), and ii) autonomy does not signify independence: the public establishment is subject to supervision and to the stewardship of the State (or a local authority). This autonomous status currently extends to various types of health service: first and foremost to hospitals, but also to agencies responsible for procurement and distribution of medicines and to training schools. The autonomy conferred by the status of a legal person (under public law) may nevertheless be limited by the very substance of its statutes and internal regulations, for example: The personnel of a public establishment are generally national or local civil servants; this means that the civil service salary scale applies directly to them. Likewise, the establishment of posts, transfers and the replacement of staff are decided by the civil service, leaving little leeway for the public establishment to develop a suitable human resources policy. The budget is heavily dependent on appropriations from the State; this means that in a developing country, only a small part of a hospital's budget is covered by payments from patients and is heavily dependent on State grants. In all cases in which this liberty is tightly restricted, there is a risk that autonomy will be a mere illusion and that the central State will continue to exert the full sway of its authority. In order to mitigate this, it is important to limit, via the statutes and internal regulations of the new corporate entity, the possibility for the State to intervene on an ad-hoc basis in the day-to-day running of the public establishment. This autonomous status may also be considered for the administrative function at the local level. As in the case of the regional hospital agencies in France or the Health Authorities in England, district or regional agencies are set up; although they possess public status, they enjoy greater managerial authority. These entities nevertheless possess legal personality and a board of management.[5] Autonomy should allow them the possibility not only to take responsibility for day-to-day management, but also to decide on their policy.

The interference of partners outside the health sector: external Institutional arrangements

The diversification of actors in health systems has also involved the integration of stakeholders that previously were operating outside the health sector.

- *Populations [communities]:* during the first half of the twentieth century, modern medicine was marked by the growing role of hospitals as a tool for improving people's health. The welfare State represented an ideal; as long as economic growth was assured, all countries would be able to provide technically effective health services. Health professionals determined peoples' needs using objective criteria based on the progress made by medicine[6] and generally using technically advanced health facilities such as hospitals. In such circumstances, the involvement of populations was virtually non-existent; the population relied on health professionals and trusted them to offer the best possible response to their health problems. Failing this, they fell back on traditional medicine. However, in the early 1960s, this idyllic vision was called into question, first of all on economic grounds, but also because people do not always react as health professionals would like them to: they wait too long before coming to consultation, fail to comply with instructions concerning treatment and neglect prevention. The trend then gradually turns: people's involvement has to cease being passive and become active. This approach was vindicated by the Alma Ata Declaration on Primary Health Care of 1978, which takes the view that populations are capable of identifying their needs and also of helping to resolve their problems. While this view is now accepted by all, a difference of opinion has emerged over how it translates into operational terms. A joint WHO-UNICEF committee has declared that "There are considerable benefits in organizing health services so that ownership resides with those for whom they are intended. Ideally, provision of health services should be under the supervision and management of the community itself". Even if there are few actual examples of communities supervising and controlling the provision of health services, the Bamako Initiative enabled communities to become involved in the management of health facilities. Through the management committees, communities become involved in the operation of primary care facilities. In most countries that have adopted the Bamako Initiative, instruments reflecting this have been drafted. However, it is worth noting that in most cases, the communities possess no specific status; such situations might be described as semi-institutional arrangements. Besides, the strategy is not so much one of seeking out partners as of involving communities in the actual running of the health facility. Consequently, it is not part of the rationale of setting up independent entities capable of negotiating and signing contracts.

- *Administrative decentralization* marks a new and far-reaching change in the evolution of health systems. This new external institutional arrangement - the creation of local authorities - may be characterized as follows:

    - It signals the appearance of an actor from outside the realm of health. Local authorities are elected bodies whose traditional activities are more concerned with civil status, order, roads, communication and the organization of social and festive events. However, its involvement in social sectors (education of health) is new and these bodies have little relevant expertise (with the exception of large towns).

– Responsibility for health and/or health facilities is devolved to them. This is an important distinction. In some countries the emphasis is mainly on health related administration, in this case, local authorities are responsibly for ensuring that health policy is implemented as well as possible. In other countries, the main focus is on the transfer of public health facilities to the local authorities which are required to ensure their proper management;

- *Institutions specialized in risk-sharing*: necessary as it undoubtedly is, direct payment for health services has limitations which are now well recognized, in particular as regards to access and equity. For a time, it was believed that these shortcomings could be overcome by risk sharing within and by health facilities. However, here again the facts have to be faced; health facilities, particularly in the developing countries, do not have the capacities to play this role. As a result, specialized institutions that go under different names: insurance and micro-insurance, community-based insurance, mutual health insurance systems; have come into being. These actors perform neither of the two functions referred to above (provision and management) yet their importance within the sector is increasing. On account of their considerable financial resources, which are more and more important to the operation of health facilities, they are capable of influencing the organization of the health sector. As the State is no longer capable of carrying the financial burden of the health sector, it accepts *de facto* the emergence of new actors who, in exchange for their funding, will negotiate their participation. These institutional arrangements are thus often a reflection of the State's financial withdrawal.

Separation of functions

Whereas in the past, a health actor simultaneously played all parts, the trend within contemporary health systems is towards greater specialization:

- *Separation of the financing of health services from their provision*: for many years, these two essential roles were played simultaneously by health actors: naturally, the first to come to mind is the State which, through its health facilities, offers generally free health services to the population. Nevertheless, the same is true of health facilities run by charitable organizations. In the developing countries, the practice of cost recovery -in Africa, the Bamako initiative- was to set in motion the separation of these two functions. However, in its conventional form, cost recovery is practised by health facilities themselves, without the establishment of a body specifically responsible for

28

organizing the funding. The emergence of prepayment systems led to the emergence of legally distinct entities specifically responsible for organizing health financing. However, at the same time, this separation has entailed the need for relations between these actors, in the form of contractual arrangements. In England, this Provider -Purchaser split is one of the cornerstones of the health system reform[7] initiated by Mrs Thatcher when she was Prime Minister; its corollary has been the creation of virtual markets between these actors.

- *Separation of ownership of capital from the managerial function*: in the commonest organization structures, the owner also performs the management function; he directs the establishment because he is its owner. As a result of the emergence of legislation conferring legal personality on public-sector establishments, the notion of Board of Management emerged, with a dual implication. First of all, there was now an internal entity in health facilities that was responsible for defining the establishment's policy orientations, overseeing its management and deciding what actions to undertake.[8] Moreover, this body, whose members may come from all horizons (users' associations, the population, municipal authorities, and the establishment's staff)[9] is not responsible either for the management or for the day-to-day running of the health establishment, which are entrusted to a team of specialists (executive management).[10]

- *Highlighting the capacity of the State to regulate relations between the health system stakeholders*; We need to remember that there are two channels through which the public administration may execute the tasks for which it is responsible: the public service, which is a service activity of general interest, and administrative policing, which is imposed on the private activities which it regulates. For many years, the State focused on producing and financing health services. Its gradual withdrawal from these two functions compelled it to re-examine its role.[11] As Musgrove observes, [12] it is not actually a question of State withdrawal but of selective commitment: careful use must be made of the provision and financing functions, which must target specific objectives, and there must be a focus on developing regulatory instruments. It is possible to exercise this regulatory role in different ways: for example, by means of accreditation mechanisms making it possible to identify health actors who align their actions with national health policy or by laying down a legal framework within which health actors may negotiate and draw up legal contracts.

This gradual transformation of the roles and status of traditional actors and the emergence of new ones has occasionally taken place spontaneously; for example, the growing importance of NGOs was not, at least initially, the result of a deliberate decision. However, it was also amplified by the health system reform programmes introduced by countries, frequently with the support of their development partners. The emphasis was then placed on institutional reform as a prerequisite for any improvement in health systems performance. Institutions with better defined objectives, enjoying greater autonomy and acting in greater proximity to populations should be the guarantee of greater efficacy. These health system reforms are part of a broader trend of New Public Management.[13]

The assumption is that institutional reshuffling is a prerequisite for improving health systems performance. As already discussed, several options are open to political decision-makers:

- deconcentration vests greater responsibility in local Ministry of Health officials; thus, in this setting, the district chief medical officer will no longer require prior authorization from the Ministry to implement certain activities;

- administrative decentralization allows some responsibility for health to be transferred to a local authority; for example, the State may decide that towns rather than the Ministry of Health will be responsible for running public health centres;

- autonomy for public providers is intended to assign, within the public sector, to some health facilities autonomy based on a legal status;

- separation of funding bodies from providers makes it possible to introduce competition between health providers, whether in the public or private sector;

- broadening the range of health funding options, through risk-sharing arrangements, makes possible the emergence of an actor, whose members (the population) have charged it with negotiating access to care;

- privatization, at least in the conventional sense, entails a transfer of ownership from the public to the private sector;

- development of the private sector may represent a strategy for political decision-makers wanting, by this means, to withdraw from providing or funding health care.

As a rule, these institutional reshuffling policies go hand in hand with regulatory measures; in order to mitigate the undesirable effects of these measures which, in one way or another, entail greater "privatization" of the health system, political decision-makers are generally inclined to accompany them with control and support measures based either on tighter control or incentives.

The evolution that has reshaped health systems in recent years has naturally taken different forms in different countries, but the general trend is clearly pointing towards a multiplication and a diversification of actors and towards a specialization of their roles in health systems. The gradual transformations of roles and statuses of the traditional actors and the rise of new ones, of which some are external to the health sector (health financing institutions, decentralized territorial administrations), have made it more complex to organize a health system. This complexity will require cooperation and dialogue in order to build and maintain interactions between the actors - new and old. Thus, the development of these new interactions is not a fashion phenomena but a consequence of the reconstitutions that have taken place in health systems.

2. GROWING AWARENESS OF CHANGES

Different actors are getting increasingly aware of changes which are occurring both inside and outside the health sector; these changes will induce modifications in the ways the actors operate and organize themselves.

2.1   Becoming aware of ones limits

For a very long time, the different actors believed that less an organization was dependant of others better it was off. Self-sufficiency was seen as a sign of strength. A car maker was supposed to design its models, produce the parts, assemble them and commercialise the final product. To avoid being dependant of others, the car maker could acquire, if necessary, a steel plant or build a railway in order to transport its products. Analogically, a hospital had to produce all the intermediary services: laundry, maintenance, gardening, catering, etc; but also laboratory exams and radiology. In the past, it often had even its own vegetable garden.

Progressively, all the actors became aware of their limits and they realized that they were not necessarily the most effective in operating certain functions. The notion of "core business" was gradually introduced; this concept underlines that an actor is defined by the specificity of its function. So, the specificity of a hospital is defined by the specialized health care services that it provides; other functions are not specific to it and one could assume that other actors will provide them more effectively.

Analogically, the specificity of the administration is linked with its "general administrative" functions : defining policy, planning, supervision, monitoring. On the other hand, the provision function is not specific to it and consequently it is conceivable that others fulfil this function. As the actors become aware of their limits, different structural changes occur:

- *Delegation of responsibility:* after assessing the situation an actor esteems that there are other actors, with more adequate capacities, that can better fulfil a given function. The first actor then entrusts the fulfilment of the function to a second actor, who will act on the behalf of the first actor. We shall discuss further the forms that these delegations of responsibility can take;

- *Outsourcing or externalization:* after assessing the situation, the actor can esteem that there are certain activities which do not belong to its core business and which it does not provide effectively. It will then find another actor who will be remunerated for fulfilling the function;

- *Service purchasing:* the actor reckons that it lacks the needed capacities for producing a given health service. In this case it will purchase the service from another actor who is willing to sell.

As emphasized earlier, this evolution is not specific to the health sector. But for a long time the health sector esteemed that its specificity ("health is not a common commodity") induced organizational methods that could not follow general trends. Today, these specificities are often considered as being less important and consequently the organizational evolutions in the health sector are aligned with those in other sectors.

Reconsidering the hierarchical model

The way in which the supply of health services is organized is broadly based on hierarchical authority, on a vertical command structure, which is not conducive to participation by all.

According to some historians specialized in government activities [14,15], we are currently in a water shedding moment where we are leaving behind the "commanding government" and witnessing the rise of a "partnership government".

The impersonal and coercive commanding government acting through traditional legal and regulatory channels is increasingly less adapted to the modern complex societies. The current crisis of "governability" reveals the inefficacity of these traditional governing methods. Laws, decrees and rules, implemented through an authoritarian and bureaucratic organization, were without doubt suitable tools in a certain period of time. Today this form of government is giving increasingly disappointing results and it is thus because of pragmatic necessity, and not because of ideological choice, that the forms of new public management have been developing.

32

The partnership government: The modern State no longer acts unilaterally from top to bottom, it accepts negotiations with its environing social actors. Modern law has to give more importance to general "game rules" or "negotiated law"[16] (flexible, reflexive, responsive ...); it has to liberate itself from the logic of regulating and imposing and turn towards establishing (open) frameworks for negotiations. The new governing rationale turns to delegation and to coordinating the type of networks defined by Williamson (1979)[17] and Kettl (1993)[18]. The modern administration is thus a cooperative administration that uses negotiations as a standard modality of action. Laws are more often implemented through contracts and less often through unilaterally imposing decrees. This has led to situations where a framework law in addition to pointing out the field of negotiations has also imposed a deadline upon the negotiating actors for reaching a contractual arrangement (for example, a French act from 1996 requires that all the hospitals have to sign an agreement with the government).

Considering the situation described below, the hierarchical model seems to be less and less appropriate. The reasons for this are clear:

- *When* the health system actors are independent - which is increasingly the case - vertical command and control is obviously no longer possible since these independent actors are not hierarchically positioned. For example, the public administration can control a private health facility to some extent (on respecting laws and regulations, on respecting deontology) and it can also, ex ante, implement control through a mechanism for authorization to practice, but it can not intervene in the everyday running of the private health facility. The public administration can for example advocate for an outreach strategy of immunization for children, but it can not impose it to a private health facility.

- Even when a hierarchical linkage exists, command and control through hierarchical means is often proven to be ineffective. For example, the classical conception of a health district is based on this principle of hierarchical commandment. In reality, hierarchical commandment between the central administration and the local administration (region or health district) usually gives unsatisfying results. Deconcentration is often proposed as a solution to this situation, but contracting has also been used increasingly in recent years in order to improve the effectiveness of the relationship between different levels of the public administration.

As we can see, the development of contracting has its origins also in this evolution of organizational arrangements. The health sector is in this case following an evolution that is not specific to it. The partnership government, using contracting as a tool, is developing in all the different sectors of activity. It is developing inside the administration but also in the markets: business management methods are giving more emphasis to concepts such as participation, collaboration and empowerment - these are preferred to unilateral hierarchical authority.

Recognizing the need to build alliances

Progressively, the actors become aware that it is in their interest to build alliances. In stead of staying alone and doing everything itself - like a welfare state that is solely responsible for providing the services and the goods for the population - the actors will consider themselves stronger if they pool their efforts. Adding up competencies and synergizing each others' strengths will make the actors stronger. But here again, the alliances will taken on different forms.

It is also this movement that has put forward the word "partnership". A partner is someone who is not hierarchical positioned to another actor, their relationship is based on negotiations. However, caution is needed when using the term "partnership". In the contracting discourse, the word "partnership" is used to the point of becoming, for some, a synonym of contract. "A relationship between two (or more) parties" is effectively a definition that could apply as well to the concept of "partnership" as to the concept of "contract". However, the definition is insufficient:

- When a consumer buys a salad there is "a relationship between two parties" and a "contract"; but could the situation really de described as "partnership"?
- When two hospitals agree on a joint subsidiary for waste treatment, there is clearly a "relationship between two parties" and the agreement probably would be qualified as a "partnership"; still there is no "contract".

Consequently, it seems that 1) not all contracts are partnerships, and, 2) there are partnerships that are not formalized through contracts

It is thus useful to come back to the definition of the word "partnership". It seems to be one of those words for which it is difficult to find definition that makes consensus. However, we can consider the following definition as a fair starting point:

"A partnership is a formalized agreement between two (or more) parties who have agreed to seek together common objectives"

This definition enables us to bring forward several elements that contribute to the definition of the concept of "partnership":

34

- First there is the idea that a partnership is a relationship that has to be constructed. There is a need to create a bond between the parties. A partnership is therefore built through negotiations, through a process. This relationship will be evolving through time; a partnership is never definitely accomplished, there is a constant need of renewing the relationship. On of the consequences of this is that a partnership is necessarily linked to a long time horizon, a partnership can not be a short, time limited, relationship. The time horizon of a partnership can be more or less formally defined.

- A *partnership* is based on non hierarchical, horizontal, relationships between (legally and concretely) equal partners. The principal-agent theory and the concept of partnership are mutually exclusive.

- The actors will seek to attain shared objectives. This point is maybe the most important of the criteria. Outsourcing for example can not be qualified as partnership. The purchaser (tender holder) will seek to obtain high quality services for a lower cost where as the sub-contractor will search for profit; in this case the actors have thus different objectives and the relationship could hardly be called a "partnership".

- *Partnership* requires the acknowledgment of ones weakness. Choosing to enter in a partnership means that there has been a decision to no longer act alone. There difference of the other needs to be accepted and respected

- *How* will the partnership be implemented? It is a matter of getting together and pooling efforts. There are two distinct strategies possible; often they are portrayed as synonyms.

  i) "Cooperation" signifies that each actors brings their contribution in order to attain the common objective; cooperation results thus in a low degree of institutional interpenetration. The partners will act independently but in a coordinated manner - the coordination mechanisms and modalities have been defined in the agreement.

  ii) "Collaboration" signifies a deeper institutional interpenetration between the partners. Collaborating has a larger aspect of "doing things together"; in other words, establishing alliances for efforts to reach common goals.

Considering all these different elements, it is possible to point out several type of agreements that are often mistakenly qualified as "partnerships":

- In essence, the so called "private-public partnerships (PPP)" in the hospital sector do not actually qualify as partnerships. Some of the criteria are fulfilled:

there are negotiations and there is a long term time perspective. But several other criteria are not met: there is no common objective (for the MoH the objective is to reduce the burden of investment while for the private company it is about profit making), there is no collaboration or cooperation, as defined above; the relationship is vertical: there is a purchaser who sets the rules (and price) and a provider who has to obey to these rules (of course this does not mean that the provider's power could not match or even exceed the purchaser's power).

- *Concretely*, there are contracts that should be considered as partnerships but which are not. Lets take the example of relationships between the MoH and NGOs. These relationships are only rarely based on the "doing together" mentality; they are more often linked to the "have it done (by someone else)" type of logic. The MoH can sign a contract with an NGO either for a defined set of activities (service contract) or for the delegation of management of public health facilities. The partner from the MoH point of view is the agent that will carry out the activities in its name. The contract might not have been preceded by an open call for bids; thus the MoH could have identified the NGOs with which it will establish contractual relations. However, the object of the contractual relationship will be based on the logic of "have it done".

The key issue can be summarized by the following figure:

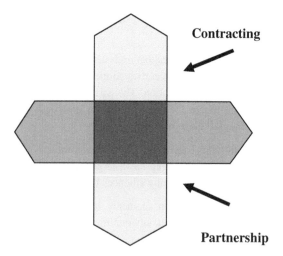

36

From this figure we can see that:

- There are several cases of contracting without a partnership: for example, it is difficult to think of outsourcing as a partnership; this goes also for relationships between health insurances and providers when it comes to setting the price and the package of services covered; finally, the same interpretation applies for most of the performance contracts (for example, when the central level of MoH defines the modalities of awarding bonuses for hospitals that are willing to change their behavior and practices).

- Several cases of partnership do not adopt a contractual approach; the agreement between MoH and the medical board for defining the professional deontology serves as an example.

- However, some contracts can also be considered as partnerships; for example, when two hospitals sign a contract for organizing joint activities or for creating a service network.

In reality things are more complicated. In several cases of contracting, it is difficult to determine if there is a genuine partnership or not. For example, when a Ministry of Health signs a contract with an NGO, some of the aspects of that agreement can be considered as partnerships since the two actors are defining their methods of collaboration, but on the other hand there are aspects that could not be considered as partnership since the contract is destined purely for service purchase.

While the necessity to establish relations is getting increasingly inevitable, the forms taken by these relations are not insignificant. These relations often translate into non enforceable arrangements which do not lead, in a legal sense, to formalize and constrictive mutual commitments between the actors. Here are some of their forms:

- *Recognition of the other* means acknowledging that one's counterpart is a worthy partner. Simple as it may be, in practice this is not always easy: it is hard to overcome a sense of superiority (in the case, for example, of the administration) or of uniqueness (as in the case of a religious NGO). Recognition may even be formalized; a system of accreditation thus becomes a means of coding mechanisms offering recognition. Accreditation constitutes recognition of a counterpart's legitimacy, its skills and activities.

- *Coordination*: through coordination, actors exchange information and opinions both on the fundamental values and the conduct of their activities. The exchange may be very informal (coordination meetings) or lead to the drafting of joint principles of intervention (joint statement, understanding, charter...). There is certainly a moral commitment, but such relations create no obligation in the legal sense.

There are limits to these relations; some actors realize that their relations with others call for more formal commitment. The contractual arrangement is a tool that meets their expectations because it will strengthen their relationship.

Thus, the development of contracting is parallel to the general evolution of health systems, as demonstrated above. Contacting has not come out of nowhere, it is a response to the evolution of health systems.

CONCLUSION

It was important to start this book by an overview on why and how the concept of contracting has come to the fore. Contracting and contracts are undoubtedly as old as the world itself. Since the dawn of ages, individuals and social groups have discussed and negotiated in order to reach agreements that are increasingly formalized. But what has to be acknowledged is that until recently contracting was rarely used in the health sector. In the name of public interest, the State had taken over this sector considering it self as the only provider of health services, even though, for pragmatic reasons, it had to accept the existence of a private sector. At the same time, the State, like private companies, was organized through the logic of hierarchical authority - a model that was supposed to guarantee efficacy.

In the last few years, the evolution of health systems has been characterized by a diversification of actors and a contestation of the organizational principles. This evolution has of course taken different forms in different contexts. In order to implement these changes, a tool was needed. Contracting emerged as one of the tools that enabled these changes to happen. Thus, contracting is not an artificial tool, a tool that would have been entirely created in the minds of more or less knowledgeable technocrats. On the contrary, it is a logical answer to changes that have occurred during the recent years.

Notes

[1] The World Health Report 2000 - Health Systems: Improving Performance. XIV. 2000. Geneva, World Health Organization.

[2] For a detailed description of this integration of health systems functions, see Murray, C. J. L and J Frenck. 2000. A framework for assessing the performance of Health Systems. Bulletin of the World Health Organization 78:717-731.

[3] Muschell, J. Privatization in health. WHO/THE/TBN/95.1. 1995. World Health Organization.

[4] In the context with which we are concerned, the terms "institution" or "organization" are quite close in meaning. According to dictionaries, an institution may equally designate a legally constituted body and the set of rules and customs required for it to function. For its part, an organization is characterized as a group of persons or individuals brought together deliberately to further the group's interests. For some people, the difference between the two terms lies in the fact that an institution imposes its will on individuals while an organization is a reflection of a choice by them. Thus, hospital autonomy or decentralization comes under the category of institutional arrangements whereas provident arrangements (such as mutual health insurance funds) represent organizational arrangements. In the interests of simplicity, we have used the expressions "institutional arrangement" throughout the document.

[5] Cassels, A. 1995. Health sector reform: key issues in less developed countries. Journal of International Development 7, no. 3:329-347.

[6] Van Balen, H and M Van Dormaael. 1999. Health service professionals and users. International SS journal.

[7] The 1991 NHS reform inspired a multitude of articles in both the specialized and mass circulation press. Using the Internet and a search engine (entering simply "NHS"), it is possible to come up with several hundred documents. We shall simply mention a document on the redirection of the health service introduced when the new Labour Government took power: Department of Health, The New NHS (London: HMSO, 1997)

[8] Depending on the legal structure adopted, this management team will be more or less subservient to the regulatory authority (the State) or the board of management.

[9] Affane, S and A Allaoui. 1998. the experience of the Federal Republic of the Comoros. Paper presented at the technical meeting Towards new partnerships for the development of health in the developing countries: the contractual approach as a policy tool, WHO/ICO, Geneva, 4-6 February 1998

[10] As part of new entrepreneurial theories, these considerations are addressed in what is known as the property rights theory. We should mention two seminal articles illustrating this theory:

Alchian, A. A. 1969. Corporate Management, and Property Rights. In Economic Policy and the Regulation of Corporate Securities, edited by Manne, H (Washington: American Economic Institute).

Demetz, H. 1967. Toward a Theory of Property Rights. American Economic Review.

[11] Entering the 21st Century. In Decentralizing: Rethinking Government, World Development Report 1999/2000

[12] Musgrove, P. Public and private roles in health: theory and financing patterns. discussion paper n°339. 1996. The World Bank , Washington. The World Bank discussion papers.

[13] Mills, A., S. Bennett, and S. Russell. 2010. The challenge of health sector reform. What must Government Do?: Palgrave.

[14] Mayntz, R. 1993. Governing Failures and the Problem of Governability: Some Comments on a Theoritical Paradigme. edited by J.Kooiman Modern Governance ed. (London).

[15] Papadopoulos, Y. 1995. Complexité sociale et politiques publiques. Paris. Montchrestien.

[16] Senant, Ph. 2000. Évolution de l'approche contractuelle dans la province de Mahajanga (Madagascar).

[17] Williamson, O. E. 1979. Transaction-Cost Economics: the Governance of Contractual Relations. Journal of Law Economcis XXII, no. 2:233.

[18] Kettl, D. F. 1993. Sharing power : public governance and private markets. Washington: Brookings Institution.

Part I

Chapter 2

Contracting and contract: concepts and new developments

Jean Perrot

INTRODUCTION

The previous chapter pointed out the fact that contracting had emerged progressively as a quasi-natural answer to the evolution of health systems and, more widely, to the evolution of organizations. The discussion at that point was more or less suggesting that contracting and its tool by excellence, the contract were synonyms.

Contract and contracting are indeed often seen as synonyms. However, this chapter's objective is to demonstrate that one should be cautious with these concepts. A couple of examples hereunder will demonstrate why:

- *Some* decades ago, when a French peasant wanted to sell a horse he had to go through an intermediary dealer with whom the deal had to be closed. The horse dealer took out his thick wallet, paid the peasant and rode off with the horse. The understanding between these two actors enabled the transaction. However, no contractual document was signed. The instantaneity of the event made a written document unnecessary. Conversely, when the action has a long term perspective, it becomes important to formalize the agreement with a document - a contract - that will mutually oblige the actors to respect their agreement.

- Two hospitals are willing to work together on waste discharge. They can establish a contract that defines their roles; but they can also create a new structure with a defined legal status: a syndicate, a joint venture, etc. There is no contract in this scenario. The agreement is materialized by the legal entity's statutes that define the roles of the two hospitals.

In these two examples, there are no contracts. Still, there is a genuine agreement between the actors. This calls for a clarification of terminology. The first part of this chapter is focused on the concept of "contract" and the second part on the concept of "contracting".

1. CONTRACT

The generic concept of contract seems to be simple. Our common understanding of a contract is defined by a visualization of a contractual document which has a certain number of clauses and which is signed by the contractual partners. This simplified vision often leads to the misunderstanding that it is easy to come up with a standardized contract, in other words, an all-round document that would be suitable for each situation.

The contract was originally conceived as a mechanism to secure commercial exchanges of goods. It marks an agreement on the exchange which is protected *a priori* by the law which only fixes the limits of possibilities for mutual commitments and *a posteriori* by the justice system that guarantees the fulfilment of contracts and allows to settle disputes.

This conception of a contract is of course still prevailing; however, nowadays, the contract has become increasingly a multiform concept of coordination between actors: it is thus a mechanism through which actors exchange promises of behaviour.

The current literature on the concept of contract is very rich; different disciplines contribute from their specific points of view to this literature - law, economics, sociology. The objective here is not to enter into a sophisticated conceptual debate, but rather to offer some precisions for those who are responsible for action.

1.1   Terminology

The notion of "contract" is principally related to legal considerations. Or, differences will inevitably arise between countries concerning these legal aspects; while medicine, economics, physics, or chemistry are realms of knowledge in which thinking is global, the same cannot be said of law, where there are numerous differences. It is impossible to go through the specifics of each country; but as an example, the French and English legal traditions are contrasted below.

French legal tradition	English legal tradition
All definitions refer to Article 1101 of the French Civil Code: *"A contract is an agreement whereby one or more persons make a commitment, to one or more other persons, to give, do or not to do something."* For example: *Dictionnaire encyclopédique Quillet*: "A pact between two or more people" *Grand dictionnaire encyclopédique Larousse*: "Agreement, or coincidence of wills, to create an obligation on one or more persons towards one or more others."	The Oxford English Dictionary: "A mutual agreement between two or more parties that something shall be done or forborne by one or both"; also "An agreement enforceable by law" Encyclopedia Americana: "A promise or set of promises creating a legal duty of performance" Webster's Third New International Dictionary: "An agreement between two or more persons or parties to do or not to do something" Collier's Encyclopedia clearly defines the

43

Encyclopédie Bordas: "Type of agreement in which one or more persons make a commitment to one or more other persons to give, transfer, do or not to do something. It entails a manifestation of wills involving at least two persons. The will is the source of the obligation that will result from the contract"	elements that should be present within a contract: "A valid contract must be: 1) by mutual consent, 2) founded on an exchange of value, 3) in a specified form, either written or oral, 4) executed by legally responsible persons, and 5) for a legal purpose.
E. Littré Dictionary of the French language: "Agreement between two or more willing parties, which aims to create or cancel an obligation."	

At this point it is worth highlighting the differences that exist between the English word "agreement" and the French word *"agrément"*.

French word *"agrément"*	English word *"agreement"*
English translation: "consent", "approbation", "acceptance"	French translation: "*accord*"; a contract is an "*accord*." It is therefore a synonym of "*contract*"
"Agrément": In French administrative law, the word *"agrément"* represents a unilateral act corresponding to two possible cases. It either refers to an authorization given by public authority to exist or to carry out an activity; e.g. to open a private pharmacy requires an "*agrément*". Alternatively it may concern a recognition by the public authorities of something that already exists but which will enjoy special recognition under the "*agrément*". For example, an authorized (*agréé*) health centre is a private health centre that the public authorities recognize as valid. Under private law it might refer, for example, to a manufacturer that recognized a distributor of its products. The distributor authorized (*agréé*) by the manufacturer has been given the opportunity to distribute that manufacturer's products.	An "agreement" is defined as follows: Oxford English Dictionary: "a contract duly executed and legally binding on the parties making it" Webster's Third New International Dictionary: "a contract duly executed and legally binding on the parties entering into it" But also: Oxford English Dictionary: "a mutual understanding, accordance in action or purpose"

44

Some near synonyms:

- *Accord*: Defined by the *l'Encyclopédie Bordas* as, *"a generic term referring to the coincidence of two wills. An "accord" makes it possible to come to an arrangement, to enter into a convention, treaty, or any other type of contract; and, more generally, to establish a new legal relationship between two or more partners."* This term corresponds to the English word "agreement".

- *Protocole d'accord*: This is a verbal procedure describing the resolutions of an assembly or conference, and reporting the consent of the contracting parties. A *"protocole d'accord"* is therefore an agreement that has not yet been accomplished — an agreement that is still a work in progress.

- *Convention*: According to the *Grand Dictionnaire Encyclopédique Larousse*, this is "an "*accord*" reached between persons, groups or subjects under international law, for the purpose of producing legal effects, and which in principle imposes an obligation on the persons signing it." Essentially, the meaning of term "*convention*" is very close to "*contract*", but the two terms can be distinguished in three ways: (1) The term "*contract*" is less frequently used than "*convention*" in international agreements; (2) A *convention* can be seen as possibly less constraining than a *contract*; (3) A *convention* often engages many more parties than a *contract*. Oxford English Dictionary, "A convention is an agreement creating legal   relations."

- "*Accord-cadre*" (framework agreement): According to the *Grand Dictionnaire Encyclopédique Larousse,* this is an "Agreement in which the terms used are sufficiently general to serve as a framework or model for subsequent more detailed agreements."

- "*Charte* (or *chartre*) (charter): According to the *Grand dictionnaire encyclopédique Larousse*, this is a "formal written document used for the purpose of assigning rights or reconciling interests."

- "*Traité*" (treaty): Official agreement between States.

The differences between all of these terms clearly are often tenuous; and usage and custom will play an important role. For example, in the health insurance domain, one generally talks of an agreement (*convention*) between insurance and a provider, whereas the term "*contract*" is seldom used.

1.2   What is a contract?

Four conditions are therefore essential for a valid contract to exist: acquiescence among the parties, capacity to contract, a defined object, and a lawful cause:

- *Acquiescence among the parties*: No one can be forced to sign a contract. This element is very important: a Health Ministry may encourage health sector actors to develop contractual relations, and it can take all measures to facilitate these relations; but it cannot force anyone into a contract, which means that all parties are independent or a least autonomous.

- *Capacity to contract*: A contract signatory must have legal status; without it, that party has no authority to sign. Nonetheless, this aspect must be clearly distinguished from the person who is actually going to sign the contract. For example, if in the Health Ministry only the Minister has authority to sign contracts, he or she may also delegate such authority to any person of their choice; the holder of signatory power must therefore have proof of such a delegation.

- *A defined object*: This element is important and frequently source of dispute. In a commercial contract, for instance, it is quite easy to specify the object of the contract; e.g. a supplier agrees to deliver so many refrigerators of a given type on such and such a date. In contrast, while it is easy to reach agreement on the fact that an NGO that manages a health centre must supply a minimum package of activities, divergences may arise as to how this minimum package should be provided.

- *A lawful cause:* Despite its importance, this clause fortunately does not pose too many problems.

We propose the following definition of a contractual arrangement:

"A voluntary alliance of independent or autonomous partners who enter a commitment with reciprocal obligations and duties, in which each partner expects to obtain benefits from the relationship."

An important distinction: public contract-private contract. A public contract can be defined by three criteria:

- It necessarily involves a person defined under public law — i.e. the State, or subnational or local entities; this is a necessary but insufficient condition, because such persons can also enter into contracts under private law;
- Its object is in the realm of public interest;

- The contract contains clauses that depart from common law. These are prerogatives of public authorities, which means that the public party can alter the execution of a public contract at any time, provided it is in the general interest.

If, following amicable attempts to settle a dispute, litigation occurs before the higher authority, a full appeal is heard by the administrative tribunal, unlike private contracts where appeals are heard by courts of common law.

Contracts are of different types. There is no lack of typologies; the aim here is not to propose a new one, but instead to find highly operational criteria for distinguishing between contract types.

To gain an idea of these differences, consider the following situations:

- *Situation 1:* A medicine purchasing centre signs a contract with a supplier, which stipulates the type of medicines to be supplied, their prices, the delivery date and the payment conditions. The contract also provides that any disputes will be settled by the competent courts. The contract is signed following an international tender. It is complete and detailed.

- *Situation 2:* The Ministry of Health signs a contract with an NGO, which undertakes to operate a specified public health centre. This NGO uses the health centre's existing infrastructure, and commits to provide the Minimum Package of Activities as defined in the national health policy;

- *Situation 3:* A hospital in a southern country signs a twinning contract with hospital of the north, involving the exchange of medical staff, specifying two exchanges each year in each direction;

- *Situation 4:* The central administration of the Health Ministry signs a contract with a Regional Health Authority to implement medium-term strategic planning.

Two key elements distinguish these situations:

- The first distinctive feature concerns the level of detail and planning contained in the contractual understanding, i.e. the contract's degree of **"completeness"**. In situation 1, and in situation 3 also, the contract is precise: in such cases, the contract is referred to as complete in the sense that all potential situations affecting the contract have been provided for. In contrast, in situations 2 and 4, the contract is imprecise: it is considered "incomplete" because not all possible situations have been provided for. The contract describes the spirit of the contractual relation; the parties involved can adapt their behaviour on the basis of numerous criteria, and it is impossible to say whether such behaviour patterns are opportunistic or the best response to the specifics of the situation. In some cases, certain aspects of the object of the contract are not really verifiable: e.g. a contract that requires the supplier to take all steps to deal with a health problem. If a dispute arises, for example, how can the judge decide whether the surgeon has done everything possible to save his or her patient (where does the reasonable end and extraordinary efforts begin?) In such situations, the judge will rule that the contract is unverifiable and will tend to declare it void;

- The second element is the degree of **enforceability** i.e. the extent to which non-compliance with one or more of the contractual clauses by one of the parties can trigger appeals to the judicial system to enforce commitments or impose a sanction. The contract itself should make provision for the relevant penalties and their mode of application. In situation 1, this enforceability is complete; non-compliance with the contract will immediately give rise to an appeal to the legal system, which in turn will define the penalty. In the extreme case, in situation 4, there is no *de jure* enforceability, since there is only one legal person involved. In situations 2 and 3, although the possibility of enforceability exists; it would be very hard to implement. In situation 2, it would look bad for the Health Minister to take legal action against an NGO that is well established in the country: such action would be legally possible but politically delicate. In situation 3, it would also look bad for a hospital to apply to the courts (and which court anyway?). The penalty would simply entail the renunciation (i.e. the end) of the contractual relation. In these two latter situations, enforceability can be said to be *de facto* impossible;

Taking these two elements into account at the same time produces the following table:

	Completeness	Incompleteness
Enforceability	*Situation 1*	*Situation 2*
Non-enforceability	*Situation 3*	*Situation 4*

These contracts are clearly not alike, so how can they be classified? Situation 1 corresponds to what the literature generally calls the "classic contract" — a form of contract that is recognized in civil law in all countries throughout the world. Situation 4 represents what is increasingly referred to as a "relational contract". Some legal experts are reluctant to classify relations of this type as contractual. Intermediate situations give rise to greater debate. Jurists specializing in frustration of purpose will tend to consider the contract in situation 2 as a relational contract and therefore unverifiable. In contrast, they will consider situation 3 as a real contract despite the fact that its enforceability is hard to put in practice. Contracts can be summarized as follows:

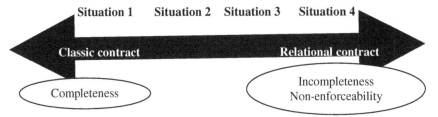

Based on the above, it has to be said that very few contracts in the health sector would be recognized as such by classical jurists. In many situations, the strict requirements are not satisfied; and yet it is clear that these situations really benefit from the use of contracting.

This does not mean that contracting should be ignored. Firstly, it needs to be remembered that the legal world is itself evolving; and the notion of a relational contract is increasingly being recognized following the work of I.R Macneil[1] in particular. Secondly, persons who enter into contractual relations that display a certain lack of foresight or non-enforceability should be aware of the limits of their contracts and accept the consequences.

As shown in the above diagram, the reality often lies between the two extremes of "classic contract" on one hand, and "relational contract" on the other. This continuum needs to be understood, and the following table indicates the elements that tend to occur more frequently on one side or the other.

Classic contract	Relational contract
• Instantaneous or short-term transaction • Completeness of the terms of the contract: no lack of planning • Simple activity - clear mandate • Separation of parties involved: no contacts between them • Suspicion: opportunistic behaviour • Contract enforced by court: penalty • Have something done *(faire-faire)*	• By nature incomplete • Long term objectives • Complex activities - broad mandate • Cooperation -interdependence • Trust • *De jure* or *de facto*, it is impossible to apply to the court to have the contract enforced: self-enforcing • No penalty possible • Ruling or non-renewal • Do something jointly *(faire ensemble)* - cooperation
Agency theory *Market – tender*	*Negotiation* *Partnership*

The classic contract is thus defined on the basis of the following characteristics: the object of the contract is clear; the contract is of limited duration; the parties know exactly what they are expecting from the time the contract is formed; the outcome is predictable and can be described in the contract (completeness of contractual clauses).

But the reality in the health-care sector is different. In many cases, the future outcome cannot be known with certainty, hazards may arise (e.g. an epidemic): these possibilities lead economists to appeal to the bounded rationality hypothesis, which postulates that economic agents are incapable of correctly comprehending all the alternatives offered to them, or all the consequences of their choices. It is impossible to predetermine all actions that will need to be taken; and it becomes impossible and/or too costly to foresee all situations that could arise (i.e. incompleteness of contracts). This is particularly true in the case of complex relations. The willingness to enter into a contractual relation is no less real: one speaks therefore of a relational contract. A relational contract is based on the trust that leads parties to act in pursuit of a common interest, so the contract does not need to be complete and detailed. It will be sufficient to understand the broad objectives of the relation, the working methods, and the resources to be used to undertake the actions in question. The flexibility and cooperation that characterize this type of contract are meant to be guarantors not only of the permanence of the contract but also contractual efficacy and peace.

A relational contract is therefore a negotiated agreement between parties, generally belonging to the public sector, which clarifies each party's role in a common enterprise or action. The strength of these agreements does not depend on the potential imposition of sanctions by a court, but more on the fact that the parties have to work together. Relational contracts give pride of place to the relationship between the contracting parties, thus giving up a degree of precision to rely more heavily on the spirit of the agreement reached. This allows some latitude in the event of contingencies (i.e. the *incompleteness* of the contract). Relational contracts basically rely on trust and flexibility, and they use general formulas to deal with contextual uncertainties (political and financial) and the difficulty of setting precise goals and measuring results. Although the commitment of the parties cannot be legally binding, it is no less real but simply follows other paths and is based on other mechanisms: the value placed on a promise, credibility and reputation, which is based on that party's track record of respect for commitments, but also on social control. For a relational contract to achieve the expected results, it needs to be set in a framework of continuous management of relations, dialogue and negotiation. These are the elements that compel actors to respect their commitments, maintain their cooperation and eschew opportunistic behaviour: the theory of "relational signals" is based on this logic, in that the contracting parties must permanently refer to mutual signs through which each seeks to assure the other of their cooperative intentions. In some cases, an overly detailed contract, in which the details of dispute resolution mechanisms are emphasized, may be a sign that the contracting parties do not trust each other.

The relational contract forces a certain degree of co-operation to emerge between the actors. When considering this dimension, it is useful to evoke the notion of partnership, which normally suggests the idea of collaboration or cooperation. A partner is a person who stands alongside you, with whom you are going to "work together". The notion of partnership represents a common enterprise involving multiple partners. Problems are solved jointly; effort, work and information are shared; and the parties support each other in achieving acceptable results for all. A partnership involves a number of common elements: the parties depend on each other; solutions emerge from each party's constructive criticism; responsibilities are shared and decisions ratified by all. All of these aspects represent what is generally meant by the term "partnership". Nonetheless, in reality, partnerships of this kind are few and far between. The situation is more often one of being face to face. The partner is more likely to be a person facing you, although not considered as an enemy. An example can illustrate this. One often hears of the partnership between the Ministry of Health and NGOs, yet it is very seldom that the contractual relation is based on "working together" it much more frequently involves "having something done". The Ministry of Health enters into service contracts with NGOs, for the latter to undertake certain activities; or the Ministry can establish a contract for delegating the management of its public health care facilities to an NGO. In this case, the partner of the Ministry of Health is the agent that will carry out activities in its name. Clearly, the contract will not necessarily have been established on a competitive basis; the Ministry of Health could have pre-identified the NGOs with which it intends to develop contractual relations. Nonetheless, the object of the contractual relationship will be based on having something done. Partnership in this sense means that dealings with this partner will not take place under competitive conditions but more in the form of negotiation, based on a certain level of trust.

What is it that compels parties to fulfil the contract they have signed?

In the **classic contract**, the answer is simple: a party that fails to fulfil the contract faces the certainty of an adverse court ruling. This sanction is powerful, for not only will the contract have to be executed, but the party will also have to pay penalties. Furthermore, the court's decision cannot be evaded.

In the **relational contract**, as it is impossible (either *de jure* or *de facto*) to apply to the law to enforce the contract one might expect the parties to try to avoid fulfilling the obligations they have entered into. The reality is different however: while a party can evade obligations if it so chooses, it knows that the other party will cancel the contract and/or not renew it. Nonetheless, as a party only signs a contract when it perceives net benefits in the long term, it is not in its interest to fail to fulfil the agreement. On the contrary, it is in that party's interest at all times to demonstrate fulfilment of undertakings, and of being a trustworthy partner that can be depended upon. Renewing of the contract is an important element to take into account. For certain contracts no renewal is foreseen: the contract is related to a task, once this task is accomplished there is no reason for the contractual relationship to continue. In this type of situation the contractor, the one who should accomplish the task, can be tempted by an opportunistic behaviour - only the menace of a sanction can be dissuasive. On the other hand, there are contracts that are renewable, at least if no unusual event occurs. In this case the sanction is situated at the end of the contract period: the contractor knowing that there is a possibility of renewal will have a disincentive for opportunistic behaviour. This depends of course if the contract is being renewed tacitly or through competition.

In short, the concept of contract is more complex than it seems to be. However, the fundamental element to be considered is that a contract is defined as a tool that permits to formalize and agreement between two (or several) parties.

2. CONTRACTING

We shall now turn our attention to the concept of "contracting". We shall consider two approaches:

1. The first one is technical. From this point of view, contracting relates to a process of elaborating and implementing a contract. The contract is at the centre of the process of contracting; it is the tool and everything revolves around it. Simply, contracting is not reduced to the contractual document; it is linked to the upstream process of elaborating the document and to the downstream process of implementing and terminating the contract.

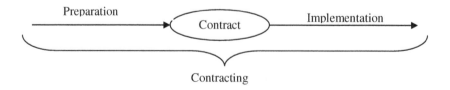

Preparation ⟶ Contract ⟶ Implementation

Contracting

Observing contracting from this point of view will bring us to consider the entire process. In operational terms, this means that the concerned actor has to be involved at each step of the process. It has to invest itself in the preparation of the contract, it has to draft the contractual document and it has to participate in the implementation of the contract until the termination of the contract. All these aspects are further discussed later on in the part II of this book.

2. The second approach is based on a reconsideration of the very foundations of contracting. The element that really matters in a relationship between two or several actors is not the contract but the agreement between the actors. The relationship between actors can be based simply on an exchange of information or points of view; what is important to consider here is that the relationship is based on an understanding, an agreement. There has been a coming together of actors who have reached an agreement[2].

- In some cases the agreement will inevitably make use of the contractual tool. After an understanding is reached, a contract that defines all the elements of the understanding will be signed. The contract is therefore the tool that materializes the agreement. A commercial contract follows this logic: in order to buy goods or services, there is a need to materialize the agreement by a contractual document. There are no other solutions. Moreover, if the agreement is governed by public procurement rules, the Ministry of Health will not have even the possibility of choosing the modalities of establishing the agreement.

- In other cases, an agreement materialized by a contract is one solution among others. For example, if a Ministry of Health wishes to withdraw itself from the management of one of its hospitals, it has several solutions: privatization (selling to a private actor), creation of a autonomous status, transfer to a territorial administration or delegated management. The choice of delegation of management will induce an agreement, but this was not the only option. These considerations bring up the notion of strategy; contracting was chosen among several possible solutions.

- In other cases, an agreement based on negotiations and a contract is a way to establish, between the actors, a relationship that substitutes to hierarchical commandment. For example, a Ministry of Health can no longer use the hierarchical commandment with the public hospitals to which an autonomous legal status has been given. The agreement based on a contract is a strategy that substitutes to a hierarchical command and control method. This logic is based on the fact that rather than imposing, it is preferable to convince the actors to get involved in the actions.

- In some cases the agreement will be materialized by a document which, in some circumstances, will be called a "contract", but in other circumstances will have another name (charter, convention, treaty, quasi-contract, etc.). They are all agreements, in other words, mutual commitments between actors. This is also the case for all types of internal contracting. They are clearly based on an agreement between actors; but as the parties belong to the same legal entity, the agreement is not enforceable. The agreement is genuine and often the actors have put in a lot effort in order to establish it. However, this agreement - this contract - has its specific features that should not be ignored.

- Finally, in some cases, there is an agreement that is not materialized by a contract. Let's take the example of two hospitals who are willing to reach an understanding for joint actions on waste disposal. They can establish a contract which will define their roles; but they can also create a new structure to which they confer a legal status and personality: a syndicate, a subsidiary company, etc. In this case there is no contract even though contracting has happened since there is an agreement of intent between the actors. The agreement is materialized by the legal entity's statutes which will define the roles for both of the hospitals. Depending on the national legislation, several legal statuses can give expression to this type of agreement: a cooperative, a community based health insurance, an association, a group; but also a semi-public company which are increasingly often described as institutional Public-Private Partnerships which differs from contractual Public-Private Partnerships.

Thus, when observing the issues brought forward above, the term "contracting" is often too simplistic. The materialization of the agreement is important; this can take, as demonstrated above, different forms of which the decider has to choose to most appropriate one. Since no better terminology is available, we could refer to a concept of "agreementing" which could include all the aspects discussed earlier. For the remainder of this book the denomination "contracting" is retained; but the lector must always keep in mind that contracting can not be reduced to a classic contract.

Moreover, often one hears that : "contracting is a tool for health services", and that as such it is neutral. It is true that a hammer can be used for building a wall but also for breaking into a house. In these cases, the hammer is a neutral tool. Therefore, contracting and contract should not be confounded. A contract is a tool, and is therefore neutral: anything can be put into it (in the limit of existing laws and regulations). But contracting is not a tool: it is a strategy and as such it is not neutral. Why to use contracting? When faced with a given situation, the actors can use different strategies: they need to make choices. After a detailed analysis of the situation, it might turn out that contracting is the most promising strategy (but there is never certitude on the result). It is only after the analysis that contracting and its implementation modalities are chosen. Thus contracting is neither good nor bad as such: it is a strategy that will be more or less adapted to the context and to the capacities of the actors involved.

"Strategic contracting"

Strategic contracting is a concept that answers two questions:
- is contracting the best of the solutions available for me?
- if yes, what type of materialization should I consider for the agreement?

Sometimes the designation "contractual approach" is used. The rationale is the same as above, namely that contracting is defined as an approach, as a manner to tackle a situation. This approach of a situation has to be balanced against all the other possible options. "Strategic contracting" and "contractual approach" follow thus the same rationale; simply, the emphasis on strategy is most probably stronger than a mere "approach" which is more neutral.

CONCLUSION

For conclusion, the author would like to share an experience that has repeated itself several times. He receives a telephone call during which the person on the other end says "I have heard that you work on contracting. I would also like to put in place an experience. Could you send me a model for a contract?" Once he has answered that things are not as straightforward as that, the person on the other side of the line is generally disappointed. At this point he has to explain that there are no standard contracts since each case of contracting is the result of an analysis of a given situation to which contracting strategy has been deemed the best option.

The use of a contract needs technical capacities that should never be overlooked: this will in fact be discussed in the Part II of this book. But above all, it is important to realize that in the health sector contracting is a strategy that has to be contextualized; its use has to be weight against the advantages, the inconveniences and the risks of all the other possible solutions in a given situation.

Notes

[1] Macneil, I. 1978. *Contracts: adjustments of long-term economic relationships under classical, neoclassical and relational contract law. Northwestern University Law Review*, no. 72:854-905.

[2] We are not of course talking about illicit agreements such as those between companies for **artificially** increasing prices.

Part I

Chapter 3

Typology of contractual relations

Jean Perrot

INTRODUCTION

The scenario comprising a public sector occupied only by the Ministry of Health and a private sector which is either for profit or denominational, where the two either ignore one another or compete to provide health services is increasingly unrepresentative of reality. By increasing the organizational complexity of health systems, the gradual transformation that has affected the roles and status of traditional operators and the emergence of new ones, some of them from outside the sphere of health (health financing entities, decentralized local authorities), have brought about interactions between these different operators as well as encouraging and occasionally necessitating cooperation and collaboration. Consequently, the emergence of these interactions is not a mere trend but the consequence of the reorganization taking place within health systems.

As already discussed (Part I, Chapter 1), although the need to build relations is increasingly obvious to health operators, we nevertheless need to consider their actual form. The forms taken by these relations are not insignificant. One path taken to emerge from isolation is coordination. Operators enter into non-enforceable relations, in other words, relations that do not involve formal and binding obligations in the legal sense. Here are some of the forms these may take:

- *Recognition of the other* is the first phase; it means quite simply acknowledging that one's counterpart is a worthy partner. Simple as it may be, in practice this is not always easy: it is hard to overcome a sense of superiority (in the case, for example, of the administration) or of uniqueness (as in the case of a religious NGO). Recognition may even be formalized; a system of accreditation thus becomes a means of codifying mechanisms that offer recognition. Accreditation constitutes recognition of a counterpart's legitimacy, its skills and activities.

- *Coordination*: through coordination, actors exchange information and opinions both on the fundamental values and the conduct of their activities. The exchange may be very informal (coordination meetings) or lead to the drafting of joint principles of intervention (joint statement, understanding, charter,...). There is certainly a moral commitment, but no legally enforceable one.

There are limits to these relations; some actors realize that their relations with others call for more formal commitment. The contractual arrangement is a tool that meets their expectations because it will strengthen their relationship. Nevertheless, interactions between the actors differ in nature and scope. This diversity of contracting represents the richness of this instrument; however, in order to better understand this diversity, it is important to bring out the differences and to establish a typology that gathers the different types of contracting according to their resemblances. The first part of this chapter will thus propose a typology that will answer this question.

When faced with all the different opportunities for contracting, the decider has to ponder on the choices that lay ahead: why to use contracting instead of another strategy, why to use one form of contracting instead of another? These questions will de addressed in the second part of the chapter.

1. TYPOLOGY

There are numerous typologies for contractual relations: some are based on the nature of the contract (public - private), others on the actors involved, and others on the scope of the contract (hospital contracts, drug supply contract…). We propose to group them into three categories depending on the object of the contract, i.e. depending on the primary purpose of the contractual relationship: a) a delegation of responsibility, b) a purchase of services, and, c) cooperation. Besides, the strategies followed by the actors may respond to two rationales:

- The rationale of *"having it done"*: realizing that it is not efficient enough, a health actor, will come to an agreement with another actor to perform the activity in its stead. This is the rationale of what economists refer to as the agency theory, in other words, the actors are not on the same footing: one of them -the principal- seeks a solution to its problems from an agent who will act on its behalf. In order to secure the best possible service, the principal will take the best bid, and to this end set the providers in competition with one another.

- The rationale of *"working together"*: after having determined where their synergies lie, partners cooperate for a common purpose. The actors in such a relationship consider themselves to be partners who, each in their own way, contribute to solving the problem. Relations between these actors are based on cooperation.

Depending on the nature of the situation, an actor will adopt what it considers to be the most appropriate solution. Whenever (at least) two actors come up with the same analysis, a contractual relationship may come into being. The following examples illustrate the diversity of solutions to which actors resort.

1.1   Contractual relations based on delegation of responsibility

For many years, the State felt responsible for providing populations with the health services they need. Specifically, it endeavoured to provide the best possible coverage of health services throughout its territory. To do so, it provided health services directly through health facilities. Under this welfare-state vision, its mission would be accomplished only when the health infrastructures it had defined for each level of care were present everywhere. At the very most, it would agree to the presence of private actors until it was able itself to acquire the means of achieving the universal coverage it had decided upon.

There is no need to go into details at this point, as the arguments are well known; the State realizes its limitations and the impossibility of providing universal coverage in a timely manner on its own. It also has to admit that the services directly provided by it are not always sufficiently efficacious.

This leads some countries to opt for privatization. However, few countries will opt for "active" privatization, i.e. selling off public-sector health facilities to the private sector. The approach adopted will be more insidious and more or less officially recognized; it will be to allow the private sector to expand.

However, at the same time, countries will take another track - delegation of responsibility. The rationale is as follows: rather than itself managing the health facilities it owns or pursuing on its own the development of health coverage, the State will seek out an actor to do it in its stead. In contrast with passive or active privatization, the State retains control over the development of health services by establishing contractual relations with actors who will agree to the delegation of responsibility.

This principle of delegation of responsibility takes various forms depending on the context in countries:

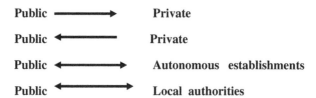

Contracts delegating responsibility to a private actor

Rather than setting up and operating a service itself, the State negotiates with a private actor. However, we need to distinguish between an existing service and one that is to be created:

Contracts for devolution of public service: a private organization (such as a private company, association, foundation, trade union or mutual fund) manages a public service on behalf of the State. In such cases, the State delegates or devolves its prerogatives to a private organization. An operating agreement designates the organization as the operator of the public service which is entrusted to it together with specifications determining how it is to be operated. Examples of this are the contract with a midwives' association to operate the Bardot maternity hospital in Côte d'Ivoire,[1] and contracts for a private company to operate hospitals in South Africa. Mali has committed itself to a more systematic approach, because its national health policy stipulates that the State will no longer operate basic health centres whose management is to be entrusted to community health associations (ASACO).

Community Health Associations (ASACO) in Mali

In 1990, the MoH, having realized the limits of a centralized health system, based on hospitals and free care, was to adopt a new sectoral policy, the main thrust of which was greater responsibility for the populations who would henceforth be responsible for managing the Community Health Centres (CSCOM) through the intermediary of an ASACO. The ASACOs manage CSCOM; both bodies were set up simultaneously in a thirteen-stage process codified by the Ministry of Health and culminating with a mutual assistance agreement signed by the ASACO and the State. This approach is based on shared responsibilities and financial commitments between the population and the State, which are formalized in the standardized mutual assistance agreement providing for the following: definition of the health and managerial missions of the CSCOM, 75% funding for the infrastructure and equipment, including the initial stock of drugs, with the ASACO funding the difference; the CSCOM operates with the revenue from fee paying. Lastly, the agreement sets the terms under which the Ministry of Health is to exercise its supervisory authority, through the district management team and the provisions applicable in case of non-fulfilment or termination of the agreement. Partnership based on the contractual approach has thus been instituted as a principle of national health policy and is applicable to Mali's primary health care system as a whole. This strategy has implied a thorough review of the roles of the State and of the population, with the State abandoning its role of direct provider of basic health care. Nevertheless, there are numerous problems: i) there are zones that are not viable or barely viable; the ASACOs have essentially developed in the financially best off districts, ii) the problem of the mutual assistance agreement which over time has become a standard contract restricting negotiations to a minimum; this has created too many grey areas (such as poorly defined methods of evaluation and control and no details of the qualifications required of the staff hired). If it is to last, this model must evolve, and in particular incorporate the new partner to have emerged from administrative decentralization: the local communities.

There is a similar experiment in Côte d'Ivoire: the community-based health facilities (FSU-Com) whose management association signs an agreement for the "concession of a public service" with the Ministry of Public Health[2].

Delegated management of public health facilities, i.e. of facilities performing a public service mission, may adopt a diversity of forms which are themselves determined by national contexts and legislation. We shall focus on two situations determined by the degree of involvement of the private entity (the assignee) in the infrastructure and equipment:

- The private entity receives from the Ministry of Health the existing resources - the buildings and equipment- as they stand in order to perform the public service mission, but the resources remain the property of the State. As a rule, responsibility for the upkeep, maintenance work, and renewal are shared by the delegator and the assignee in the manner laid down by the contract. Technically speaking, and in legal systems inspired by French practice, this is known as *affermage*; in the English legal system, it is referred to as *lease contract.*;

- The private entity takes responsibility for constructing the buildings and procuring the equipment. These will revert to the State when the agreement (which is generally a long-term one) expires. Under French law, this is known as *concession*; under English law, it is referred to as *Build, Operate, Transfer (B.O.T.)*.

In all cases, the State remains the project manager; it negotiates directly with the contractor. his type of contractual relationship does not necessarily entail the withdrawal of the State, but a change in its level of involvement; the contract will in particular need to ensure that the operator undertakes to fulfil the public service mission characteristic of the care facility. Besides, in most cases, the State remains the owner of the infrastructure (land, building, major equipment) and is thus better able, if necessary, to reconsider the delegation of management.

Contracts for the concession of a geographical area: As with an oil or forestry concession, the State may grant the exploitation of a geographical area it considers to be inadequately served and which it does not wish or is unable to serve itself. For example, contracts to provide primary health care services in certain parts of Bangladesh[3] and contract leasing a whole health district to an NGO in Cambodia,[4][5].

Concession of an entire health district to an NGO in Cambodia

Beginning in 1999, and with the support of a loan from the Asian Development Bank, the Cambodian Ministry of Health started drawing up four-year contracts with NGOs to provide health services for an entire health district. The contract covers health workers' wages, recurrent costs, drugs and consumable medical supplies. As for activities, the

---

contract stipulates that the health services must deliver the minimum package of activities for health centres and the supplementary package of activities for district hospitals.

The local administration, which depends on the Ministry of Health, retains responsibility for data collection and for supervision of the health facilities under contract. It is also required to report on the implementation of the contract and its smooth operation.

From initial analyses, it would appear that the changes in the methods of work are so far-reaching that both the NGOs and the Ministry of Health have difficulty in fully appreciating their new roles. The analyses also show that by adopting this geographical approach the Ministry of Health offers the assignee the possibility of adopting a systemic approach to the district for which it is responsible, thus making it better able to organize the local health system.

This rationale also underlies certain measures designed to help young physicians set up their practice in rural areas where health facilities are lacking. For example, in Mali and Madagascar, the Ministry of Health has helped young physicians to set up practice by signing with them a contract specifying that they are the only health personnel in a specific geographical area, and that in exchange they must provide primary health care as defined by the national health policy.[6] Analysis of these experiments has shown that even if it initially meets with difficulties, the introduction of private medicine under contract is nevertheless possible, even in poor rural areas, and is a potential solution when the conventional approach using health facilities is not possible for financial reasons.

Contract of inclusion with the public service

A private organization, which owns its structures and possesses its own resources, collaborates, is associated with and performs a " public service mission" Under contract with the State, it thus becomes a public service concessionaire. For example, the church hospitals in Tanzania[7] and Ghana[8] are contractually the only referral facilities in a determined geographical area. In Zambia, the Memorandum of Understanding signed in 1996 by the Ministry of Health and the Church Medical Association of Zambia stipulates that the boards of management of the church-owned hospitals have the same powers as those in the public sector.[9] In many countries, these are actually implicit contracts. In Chad, the country's health map is organized around existing health facilities, whether public or private; the responsibility[10] for the health of the population in a given area can thus be assigned to a private health facility, although the responsibility remains implicit. In order to avert numerous problems, it would often be worthwhile formalizing such arrangements through contracting.

Significantly, it is possible that private institutions, which own and manage health facilities, may not perform a public service function. This does not prevent the Ministry of Health, in addition to recognizing their activities through a system of accreditation, from developing contractual arrangements with them in order to determine what collaboration or support they require in exchange for the activities they perform.

Moreover, it has to be underlined that delegated management concerns not only the function of health services provision, but also that of health administration. One of the main functions of devolved health administration is to manage health facilities operating within its area. This is a relatively simple function when the Ministry of Health manages health facilities directly (in which case they are merely administrative services), it becomes more difficult when the health facility has autonomous status. When the management of the public health facility has been delegated, it is rare for habits to have become established. In contrast, the contract associating private health facilities to the public service makes devolved health management easier.

Contracting out health facilities, whether in the form of delegated management or inclusion with public service, means that certain actors, especially the NGOs, will increasingly place their action within the public service framework. The contract signed by them concerning this delegation will determine their role in the provision of health services.

However, these entities may wish to commit themselves still further and to participate in the devolved health administration. The rationale is the following: as they are already managing health facilities in the area, they also wish to become involved in the devolved health administrative function. This role may remain on the level of coordination, although it may also lead to a specific contractual relation:

- This contractual relation may define the modes of collaboration or of participation in the running of the devolved health administration. For example, NGOs already running health facilities will define, in this ad hoc contract, their relations with the district management team, and in particular the role of each entity;

- The same contractual relationship may also adopt the form of delegated management: in this case, the manager of the health facilities in the area is given a contract to assume the devolved administrative function. This may be done in two ways: either by drawing up specific contracts for each function (management of health facilities and devolved health administration) or by drawing up a single contract simultaneously defining both the roles assumed by the manager. It should be emphasized that, as with any principle of delegated management, the manager assumes responsibility for the devolved administrative function. Contractually, the manager takes over the State's regalian functions.

This type of contractual approach is determined by the vision held of the health district. Simultaneous contracting of both functions - the provision of health services and health administration- corresponds to integrated models, i.e. systems in which both functions, while clearly identified, are closely linked or highly dependent on one another. In such systems, it is assumed that it is impossible for the two functions to be taken on by different entities. For example, under the "classical" model of the health district, sole responsibility for the administration and management of health facilities is assumed to lie with the Ministry of Health.

Contracts binding the State to the local authorities

An alternative approach comes under the trend of providing certain public institutions with autonomy. Recognition that one of the weaknesses affecting the organization of public health services lies in the concentration of all functions in the hands of a single entity - the central State - results in a proposal to create distinct entities. Because they have their ears closer to the ground, these entities are directly responsible either for a specific activity (such as procurement and distribution of medicines) or for a health facility (such as an autonomous hospital). For example, in Morocco, the Ministry of Health is currently drawing up contract-plans with the autonomous hospitals. Likewise in Tunisia, plans are afoot to gradually introduce target-based contracts (over several years) between public health establishments (which are autonomous entities) and the department of stewardship in the Ministry of Health.[11]

However, such situations lead to a special kind of arrangement since they involve only public operators. If a public operator is autonomous it does not mean that it is independent: there is always some form of stewardship. In many cases, this approach remains at the experimental stage: many countries are turning towards reforms that grant autonomy to their local hospitals, without at the same time organizing the contractual relations that will inevitably spring from this new institutional set-up. When such contractual relations exists, as for example in Zambia where autonomous hospitals have signed agreements with the Ministry of Health,[12] the State, because of budget constraints, has a tendency to neglect its financial commitments, thus undermining the credibility of contractual relations.

Contracts binding the State and its autonomous institutions

Within the broader framework of State administrative reform, the trend is to bring the administration closer to the population whenever possible (principle of subsidiarity). Thus, in the field of health, numerous countries have transferred or are in the process of transferring responsibilities to the local authorities. The State's health facilities are transferred to the local authority, which becomes responsible for running them. This is currently under way in Madagascar and in Senegal.

The contractual arrangement in Mahajanga district in Madagascar[13]

In Madagascar, a 1995 law and the 1996 decree bringing it into force entrusted management of basic health care centres to the communes. The instructions determining the extent of the responsibilities and resources transferred are however somewhat vague. The GTZ project in Mahajanga province is designed to put into practice this political desire for decentralization. The aim of the project is to develop collaboration between the district management team (technical oversight) and the communes to which the centres are handed over. In addition, the project proposes management models for these health facilities, in the form of two types of agreement: under the first of them, the health centre is managed by a users' association which enters into a lease contract with the Commune and in the second the centre is managed as an autonomous communal administration with a board of management where the population is represented. The contractual framework, which is relatively complex as it involves several tiers of contractual relationship, was thus determined from the outset. It is subsequently operationalized through as many contractual arrangements as are necessary.

Evaluations carried out by the GTZ team responsible for the support have shown that decentralization brings about a far-reaching redefinition of the actors' roles and that the contractual approach is a potential strategy for understanding the new relationships that emerge between these actors.; although it is not always easy to simultaneously control institutional reform (decentralization) and the implementation of a new strategy (the contractual approach).

Because local authorities generally lack the financial resources required for carrying the burden of these new responsibilities, and also because the central State wishes to maintain its capacity to harmonize practice within its territory, the need to set up links between the central State and the local authorities responsible for these basic health care facilities is recognized. While such links may be of a conventional administrative nature, they increasingly take the form of formalized contractual relations designed to serve as tools to assist with the transfer of responsibility to the local communities.

Internal Contracting

Delegation of responsibility may be internal, in other words it may operate within what for legal purposes is a single unit. The adjective "internal" needs to be defined depending on whether:

- There is only a single entity in the legal sense, but contracting operates between distinct parts of the unit. This is the case, for example, when the central echelon wishes to enter in a contractual relationship with the peripheral level (province, region or health district). For example, in Burkina Faso, the central echelon has drawn up performance contracts with the health districts, which have no distinct legal status. Under the contract, the central echelon delegates to the devolved level its responsibility for attaining specific results. In strict legal terms, this is not really a contract, because it is not "enforceable". Nevertheless, it is a contractual relationship because it involves negotiation and agreement between the parties concerned.

- There is only a single entity for legal purposes and the relationship is established between elements of this entity answerable to the same authority. For example, internal contracting inside a hospital; in this case, each of the services is answerable to the same management authority: the contract is established between the management and the different services. In this way, France has developed internal contracting within public establishments on the basis of the 1996 reform. The contract is binding on the head of the establishment and the heads of the medical and non-medical services. Under the internal contract, management authority is delegated by the Director of the hospital to the centres of responsibility, i.e. the services. This contract determines the objectives, the means and the indicators for monitoring the centre of responsibility, the incentive to interest them in the results of their management and the consequences of failure to fulfil the contract.

This type of internal contracting has numerous advantages but also poses its own specific problems: what type of incentives (individual or collective) will persuade the actors effectively to implement the contract? What contract monitoring mechanisms are sufficiently effective?

The first two categories above involve relations between the public and private sectors. The State considers that it is vested with a public service mission but entrusts management thereof to private bodies. The contractual relationship governing this delegation of responsibility follows the rationale of concession and will adopt specific legal forms depending on the national context. In contrast, the

67

latter two categories concern relations between the State and public entities that possess legal status (autonomous structures or territorial communities). Transfer of responsibility is effected by the law. However, responsibility is not transferred in full; there are still links between the State and these entities. It is difficult to regulate these links through a conventional hierarchical relationship: the contractual relationship offers itself as the tool for addressing them and making them operational. However, in all cases the State will ensure that the assignee complies with the public service mission: the contract exists to ensure this.

Programme-budgets in Morocco

The new results-based budgetary management which the Ministry of Health is endeavouring to introduce may be defined as a formalized process designed to determine each year, albeit within the framework of a sliding three-year programme and with annual budgeting, the respective responsibilities of the central administrative departments and of the departments of the Ministry of Health to which responsibility has been devolved and which are coordinated by health regions to which power has been delegated for the attainment of mutually defined objectives. The process thus concerns the relationship between the central echelon and the services to which responsibility has been devolved, i.e. the health regions. In order to encourage the actors to assume their individual responsibilities, it is intended to formalize this relationship through a contract between these two levels of the health administration.

1.2 Contractual relations based on an act of purchase

This category corresponds to situations in which a fundholder prefers to purchase the services rather than producing them itself. In this case, the rationale is based on a simple principle: rather than *"doing"*, in other words providing the service itself, a health actor will entrust a partner with providing it, in exchange for remuneration. The fund holder seeks to make the best possible use of its partners by choosing the one offering the best service (the same service at a lower cost or a better service for the same budget). To do or to buy that is the question. This strategy may take different forms. In particular, we shall need to distinguish between cases in which the actor used to perform the activities itself and has decided to cease doing so (generally known as *outsourcing*)[14] and those in which the activity is new.

This purchasing strategy applies at two levels, depending on the object of the purchase:

68

- it concerns itself with how fundholders (individuals, but also their representatives (the State, health insurance systems)) use their funds to procure health services from health service providers; in this case, the purchase concerns a final product – the health service;

- it also concerns itself with the mode of production chosen by the health service providers; in this case, the purchase concerns production factors.

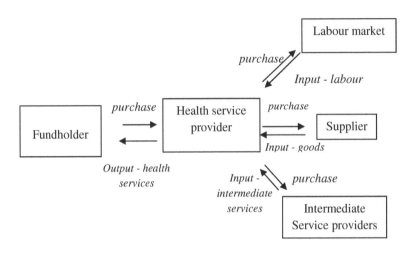

Relations between fundholders and health service providers

Individual fundholders may decide themselves to purchase the health services they require from a health services provider. Generally speaking, this purchase does not give rise to a specific contract; however, in certain cases (such as plastic surgery), the client may insist on drawing up a contract. Individuals may also entrust their funds (voluntarily in the case of non-compulsory insurance systems or involuntarily in the case of mandatory or tax-based systems) to an institution that will decide whether to provide the health services itself or to purchase them from a provider. In the public sector in particular, the functions of fundholder and health service provision have long been integrated and still frequently are. However, recent trends in health systems have revealed a growing separation of these functions. Fundholders will adopt "strategic purchasing" to use the expression used in the World Health Report 2000[15] whereby they will decide that they are best able to supply the service themselves or that there is another provider that is able to deliver services with better value for money . In the latter case, individuals delegate to the fundholder the authority to represent them in all their relations with health service providers. However, these relations between the fundholder and the service provider are determined by the status of the fundholder:

The Ministry of Health: the Ministry of health which, through its budget, holds public funds, may decide that it will no longer undertake certain activities itself but use its budget to purchase services from providers. This approach is common for certain specific and focused activities; for example, tuberculosis, leprosy, malaria and AIDS control,[16] immunization, integrated management of childhood illness or elimination of malnutrition.[17] In Namibia, the Ministry of Health signs contracts with private practitioners to perform surgery in isolated rural areas.[18] Such contracts may be signed with all types of actor. In some cases, the Ministry will purchase services from NGOs. In this way, contracts have been drawn up between the Ministry of Health and NGOs to provide reproductive health or AIDS control services within the framework of the World Bank funded PDIS project in Senegal. In Latin America, several countries (Colombia, Costa Rica, Guatemala, Peru and the Dominican Republic) have implemented contracts with NGOs in order to expand health coverage or improve the quality of care.[19] In other cases, the Ministry of Health will reach agreements with private physicians: for example, the draft agreement between private physicians practising in rural areas of Mali and the Ministry of Health to provide immunization as part of the EPI programme. In the field of reproductive health, Ministry of health contracts private providers to perform certain activities (such as antenatal care).[20]

It is also important to consider who takes the initiative for this contractual relationship. In some cases, it will be the fundholder, i.e. in this case the Ministry of Health; the latter, holding funds, wishes to have certain activities performed and makes proposals, through a call for tenders or via negotiations, to providers wishing to carry them out. In other cases, the providers take the initiative of offering to perform certain activities for the Ministry of Health and the Ministry responds to the proposal.

Administrative decentralization and the ensuing transfer of funds to the local authorities introduces a new dimension into this type of contracting. In particular, whereas providers such as NGOs previously had a single correspondent - the Ministry of Health - they now have to deal with a multitude of deciders, each of whom potentially has its own rationale, and to adapt to each local context.[21]

Government funding agencies: this approach is based on the following principles: i) within the State itself, in this case the Ministry of Health, the separation of the provider and purchaser function, ii) the creation of State-run funding agencies as autonomous entities within the public sector. These agencies receive allocated public funds, of which they have to make the best possible use to purchase services from the best service providers for their population. In developed countries, the English model is without a doubt the best-known example and has given rise to numerous publications.

In England, this trend is part of the new public-sector management and the concept of "managed competition", (Enthoven 1993).[22] The public sector endeavours to introduce market inspired[23] operating mechanisms that are capable of improving the system's efficiency. According to the authors, this involves introducing into the public sector the concepts of "planned" markets, (Saltman and von Otter 1992),[24] "internal" markets, (Enthoven 1985),[25] "quasi markets", (Le Grand et Bartlett 1993),[26] "managed competition"), and "manacled competition", (L.E.Brown, V.E.Amelung).[27][28] More or less controlled competition should lead to greater efficacy and consequently provide the population with better service.

The British National Health Service (NHS)

The national health service reforms introduced by the former Prime Minister Mrs Thatcher are based on a clear distinction between providers and fundholders or purchasers and on the introduction of competition among the actors through "quasi-markets". The purchasers are either district health authorities or groups of general practitioners who purchase hospital services for their community from providers whom they pit against one another. Contracts are then signed by the actors. The general framework and principles of this reform were laid down in a 1990 act. Numerous evaluations have been made of these contracts.[29] Many of them emphasize the difficulty of creating authentic competition and the possible negative effects (collusion between providers, selection of low-risk patients, etc.)

In 1997, Tony Blair's Government established the "new NHS" based on the quest for a third way. The principle of the internal market was abandoned; competition was replaced by cooperation and trust between partners.[30]

However, the most recent reform to date[31] has reintroduced a degree of competition among providers and extended the "concordat" between the public and private sectors (collaboration between the two sectors is encouraged); this reform bears a strong resemblance to the "internal market" introduced by Margaret Thatcher in 1990.[32]

A series of articles published in 2001 by the journal *Social Science and Medicine* highlights the difficulties encountered by countries that have implemented these reforms during the past decade.[33] These reforms have been introduced with the primary aim of reducing health-care expenditure; however, the experience analysed shows that this has not been the case. However, the reforms have transformed the institutional culture, no longer based on an administrative hierarchy but on competition, and have led to a redefinition of the role of the State, especially at the level of health-care providers. Sweden has also begun reforms based on the separation of service providers from purchasers and the introduction of market-inspired mechanisms. After a period of competition (1989-1993) Sweden, without calling into question the contractual approach, is moving towards more cooperative relations between health-care purchasers and providers.[34]

In the developing countries, reforms of this kind are few. In Ghana, the "Ghana Health Service", a Ministry of Health implementing agency, was established in 1996, one of its roles being to procure health care services from providers on behalf of the Ministry of Health. The implementation of this reform is still in its infancy.[35] In Zambia, the results of a similar process are equally ambivalent.[36]

Insurance systems: in developed countries where the health service is not State-funded, health care is financed by insurance systems that are semi-official, autonomous or private. The population is required to contribute to these insurance systems.[37] There are differences in the way health care expenditure is covered by them. There are three main models:[38, 39]

- The reimbursement model: the patient pays the health-service provider and is reimbursed by the insurance system. This model is analogous to the French social security system: there is no link between fundholder and provider;

- The integrated model: the population chooses an organization that is both purchaser and provider: the Health Maintenance Organizations (HMO) in the United States are found under this category;

- The contractual model: the insurance system purchases the health services directly on behalf of the policy-holders: the German model is a prime example.[40]

In developing countries, insurance systems are only at an incipient stage and are characterized by the fact that they are not obligatory and provide cover only for a small part of the population. Nevertheless, these systems are taking shape.[41] Once they have been created, such insurance systems will look into the practical details of how to cover their members' health-care expenditure. One current method is to draw up agreements with public or private health-care facilities as well as private practitioners. Such agreements covers rates, terms of reimbursement, admittance of policy holders, quality of care etc. One example is the agreement signed by the mutual insurance societies belonging to the support fund for remunerative activities by women (Fonds d'Appui aux Activités Rémunératrices des Femmes – FAARF) and public health centres in Burkina Faso.[42] The first evaluations of this experiment highlight the importance of the contractual approach as a strategy for improving the quality of care, since it has forced the health services to take a hard look at themselves and to adapt to the needs of the population. As for mutual health insurance societies, the contractual approach has forced policy-holders to clarify their needs and priorities. In Romania, since 1994 for eight districts, and as of 1998 for the entire country, the health authorities and the health insurance systems have drawn up contracts with independent physicians for the provision of primary health care.[43] Another example is the PRIMA in Guinea, where the mutual health insurance society has established contracts for the provision of services with the prefectural hospital on the one hand and the health centre on the other.[44]

Whether the State itself, official agencies (such as Regional Health Authorities in New Zealand or Health Authorities in Great Britain) funded from the State budget or health insurance funds financed by contributions, all these entities are gradually becoming "pro-active" purchasers. [45] They are no longer content with simply distributing budgetary allotments or reimbursing their members' expenses. Through contractual arrangements, they negotiate conditions with providers (private or public) for access to care either for the population under their responsibility or their members.

Moreover, it is worth taking a closer look at what purchasing actually encompasses. It is extremely simplistic to look at this in purely monetary terms. When institutional purchasers purchase health services from providers, they naturally agree on the price of the transaction, while taking into account the quality of the service provided. However, it is worth keeping in mind that the act of purchasing is a complex one involving many elements. Economic theory, especially concerning marketing, shows that the act of purchase, even for relatively simple goods, brings a number of elements into play; for example, purchasing a car does not only depend on the relatively objective criteria of its transport function, but equally on subjective characteristics such as the image produced by the car (age, social class, and gender of the owner are characteristics that are linked to a car). The same goes for health. For instance, when a health-insurance company agrees on a contract with a health-care facility, it is likely that the negotiation will not relate to the rates for medical procedures (these will have been set already) but to the service « purchased »: conditions of admittance of policy-holders, terms of payment by policy-holders, etc. In this way, purchasing health services is a powerful means of addressing the quality of care. Through contractual arrangements, purchasers can put quality of care first in their dealings with providers.[46] These quality elements may be addressed either in the initial stages of the relationship with the provider (in which case, quality standards can help to choose the provider) or later on in the relationship (in this case, part of the provider's remuneration depends on the results in terms of quality of service).

Moreover, it is worth highlighting that this type of contractual arrangement between a fundholder and a health-service provider is necessary in all health systems that adopt capitation.[47] The contract specifies the obligations accepted by the health-service provider in exchange for the lump sum it will receive in advance for each registered member in any given system. Many developed countries have adopted capitation (USA – HMO and Great Britain); others are considering introducing it, or at least partially (Canada and France for example). ; There has been a considerable increase in the use of this provider payment method in middle-income countries: several Latin-American countries have developed such procedures (Argentina and Nicaragua),[48] and they have also been developing in Thailand.[49] However, in developing countries, capitation is rarely used on account of the weakness of their insurance system.

Lastly, the health-service procurement function should not be viewed simply in quantitative terms, but also from a quality perspective. Clients are not indifferent to the quality of the services they purchase. Viewed in these terms, contracting is a tool that permits providers to offer high-quality services.[50]

Health service-providers' production processes

The health-service provider, and the same applies to the administration, has at its disposal funds received directly from individuals or from fundholders, to carry out its key core functions. The health service provider or operator can act as a conventional producer that assembles items to produce the product it wishes to supply to its clients. These items will be bought either on the labour market, as far as human resources are concerned, or on the goods and services market, for other supplies; to achieve this, conventional contracts will be negotiated. It may also approach specific providers for certain intermediary services. In this case, a contract will be drawn up in which one party undertakes to perform work for a fee which the other undertakes to pay; this is known as **sub-contracting** in the field of business. Examples are: maintenance contracts (a scheme in Papua- New-Guinea), catering (schemes in Bombay, India), laundry services provided for a hospital by a service firm (a scheme in Thailand).[51] The aim of this approach is to improve the use of scarce resources. Assessments of these arrangements, though in need of further evaluation, are yielding valuable lessons.[52] These evaluations show that signing a contract with a reputable business does not necessarily guarantee good service; the entity proposing the contract should also be capable of monitoring each stage.

Contracting of non-medical services in public health facilities in Tunisia [*]

Public Health Establishments *(Etablissements Publics de Santé* - EPS) are university teaching hospitals under the supervision of the Ministry of Public Health. They were set up under an act adopted on 29 July 1991; they have a high degree of managerial autonomy, are governed by commercial legislation and run by a board of directors. Since 1993, EPS have resorted to contracting for certain non-medical activities: catering, cleaning, security and assistance with accounting. In 2001, 16 of the 21 EPSs resorted to contracting.

There are a number of reasons why the EPS decided to subcontract some non-medical services: i) the mediocre quality of catering and cleaning services in hospitals is a source of discontent for patients and of wasted resources, ii) the shortage of skilled staff on account of budget cut-backs, iii) the commitments made as part of support for hospital reform, iv) the bandwagon effect, fashion and mimicry, which have played a significant role, based on biased belief that private service is of a higher standard than public service.

In conjunction with the central Ministry of Health administration, the EPS have set out terms and conditions of contracts as a reference guide to help each establishment draw up specific contracts. These terms and conditions stress the following: i) specific technical considerations for each activity, ii) the requisite resources to be provided by each party, iii) the division of tasks between the contracting parties, and, iv) the control mechanisms to be adopted by those hospitals concerned.

Each EPS is required to monitor work being carried out by external firms and to train its staff properly to take on these new tasks. Technical and administrative services are involved in day-to-day monitoring of the contractual arrangement. An administrative and technical monitoring committee is charged with regularly following-up the progress and evaluation of services, improving the internal administration of subcontracted services and with reviewing the terms and conditions of contracts. We may draw the following conclusions from this experience:
- According to general professional opinion, the quality of services from subcontracted providers, especially catering and cleaning, has improved. The costs, however, are relatively high, leading to successive increases in unit costs;
- The staff freed by contracting have filled other roles, thus resolving problems of labour shortages in other areas;
- While in the majority of EPS, contracting is the subject of close follow-up and regular supervision on the basis of the terms of the contract, negligence still occurs in subcontracted work;
- Relations between subcontracted staff and the institution's staff are often strained, primarily on account of the lack of a clear definition of roles and responsibilities;
- Patients, confused by the differences in staff, may ask for services from the subcontracted staff who are unqualified for certain tasks, thus creating tense relations with the institution;
- The lack of experience of the contractor staff to work in a hospital environment, the lack of supervision and the instability of their situation are the main risk factors that should be addressed by the EPS administrators in their contractual relationships.

To conclude, experience of subcontracting non-medical services in public hospitals in Tunisia reveals certain advantages in terms of improved quality as long as it is accompanied by efficient and rigorous monitoring by those in charge of the hospital. However, costs are still relatively high since the number of potential providers is too small to allow real competition to take place.

[*] *H. Achouri, A. Jeridi, respectively Director and Head of Unit of the Hospitals Administration Service - Ministry of Public Health, Tunisia*

This outsourcing of auxiliary services does not always yield the expected results: for example, in the Czech Republic, hospital catering services were recently subcontracted to SODEXHO, a French multinational company; however, in the light of the high cost of subcontracting, these services have once more been taken over by the public hospitals.

These service contracts can also apply to other areas. For example, in Chad, as part of the health-sector support project (HSSP) funded by the World Bank, the Ministry of Public Health has signed contracts with partners such as international NGOs, United Nations agencies (UNICEF), bilateral cooperation organizations (Germany) to enable them to provide their technical support to prefectural health directorates (at regional levels): supervision, management, drug supply, cost recovery, etc. In Cambodia, as part of a project funded by the Asian Development Bank, a contract gives an international NGO authority over staff from the Ministry of Health, in particular for the award of bonuses (linked to giving up private practice and the improvement of services).[53] As part of decentralization, NGOs such as BEMFAM in Brazil, CEMOPLAF in Ecuador, MEXFAM in Mexico, and CARE in Bolivia, have signed contracts with local councils to train their staff in areas such as reproductive health.[54]

It is worth looking at the way in which these contractual relations are established. The literature on the procurement function has increased considerably in recent years.[55] The debate on the issue may be summarized by two main trends: competition and partnership.[56] Competition is the traditional approach to relations between purchasers and providers: each party keeps its distance and the purchaser encourages competition in order to obtain the best possible service for the lowest price during the transaction and then renews the competition as often as possible during the competition: "Arm's length relationships; frequent tendering which is risky and costly; reliance on price; spot contracts or complex contingent claim contracting; multi-sourcing; lack of trust; reluctance to share information; adversarial attitudes ("win-lose" outcomes)".

Conversely, in the partnership or "co-maker" approach, the purchaser forms relations based on confidence and trust with specific providers: "avoiding unnecessary costs of excessive tendering and frequent competitions; fewer, dedicated suppliers; long-term contracts; coordinated strategies between buyers and suppliers; a sharing of risks and rewards; trusting relationships; single sourcing; resulting mutual benefit ("win - win" outcomes)". The evolution of the British NHS reveals the transition from relations based on competition to those based on trust;[57] instead of "purchasing", we will refer to "commissioning" i.e. the act whereby an authority hands over responsibility and power for a limited period, to an entity who acts on its behalf. "Commissioning" is thus a strategic activity for assessing requirements, resources and existing services and for making the best use of available resources in order to satisfy the needs identified. "Commissioning" involves defining priorities, purchasing the appropriate services and evaluating them.[58]

As a rule, relations based on competition are suited to the first of these categories, purchasing raw input. However, the available evidence on the provision of intermediate services reveals the limitations of relations based solely on competition and that a degree of partnership is proving a prerequisite for satisfactory results. The resulting contractual approach will be related to this distinction: in the first category, we will find mainly enforceable contracts which will fully set out all the conditions of the relationship; in the second, we will adopt "head of agreement" relational contracts.[59]

1.3   Contractual relations based on cooperation

In the previous two types of contractual relations, we have, as far as possible, referred to the "actors involved" rather than the "partners". This latter term can in fact have two distinct meanings. In one sense, a partner is your counterpart. This tells us nothing about the situation of that actor: he may just as easily be an enemy as a friend. The term "partner" simply indicates with whom he has a relationship. This is the meaning that corresponds to the two types of contractual relations above. In the second sense of the word, the partner is the person with whom you are associated. To be a partner means to work together towards a common goal while respecting each partner's identity. The contractual relations to which we will now turn our attention to are based on this second meaning of the word "partner".

At the heart of contractual cooperation lies a desire for organizational interpenetration. This can be interpreted in many ways. Firstly, it is generally characterized by lasting commitments by the actors; relationships take time to form, but equally to develop and produce results. The actors, aware of their past relations, meet to exchange ideas and look ahead to continuing a relationship in the future. Secondly, and most importantly, the degree of cooperation between actors varies. Therefore, after having identified their synergies, the actors work together towards a common goal. However, in some cases, each actor, in its own way, will play an active yet autonomous part, in producing this result, while in other cases, the actors will work together to perform all or some of the tasks needed to reach the objective.[60] Lastly, this contractual cooperation implies that at each stage in the contractual relation, the actors are fully involved in decisions concerning the implementation of the contract and in making the necessary adjustments for unexpected circumstances that may arise during the contract; the complexity of these contracts makes it impossible to completely finalize them and demands a certain degree of flexibility, calling for constant decision-making.

In this way, cooperation can be defined as a "long-term agreement which involves interactions between members of independent organizations that combine or pool their forces".[61] In concrete terms, contractual cooperation can be expressed in different ways: we shall distinguish between the two main categories according to the degree of organizational interpenetration.

A minimalist vision

Since the beginning of the 1990s, in some OECD countries the concept of Public-Private Partnership (PPP) has developed. In comparison with the forms of contract explored above, PPP is distinguished by the fact that the private operator is not remunerated by users or by the public, but by the public entity who drew up the contract. To take the example of a Ministry of Health or a public health establishment that wants to build new infrastructure. Traditionally, they would first of all have to come up with the necessary funds before, as the client, finding a designer to draw up the project then a principal contractor to manage the building work. On completion of the building work, they would then have to find a firm to ensure maintenance of the infrastructure (in all respects: maintenance of the buildings and equipment, but also catering, caretaking, laundry services etc.). There are several drawbacks to this kind of arrangement, not least of which is the search for funding, as public institutions do not necessarily have easy access to financial markets. Moreover, it is no easy matter for small hospitals to take on the responsibilities of client and they have to delegate this responsibility. The hospital finds itself handling numerous separate contracts. The PPP approach makes it possible to simplify this process. The public actor passes through a private partner (or a group (consortium) of private actors) who will assume responsibility for all the separate functions described above. It will finance, design, build and maintain the infrastructure; to use the infrastructure, the public actor will pay a fee to the private company. The hospital is thus freed of any concern with running the hospital and is able to fully assume its main role providing care. Since the PPP approach is relatively recent in the health sector, it will be further discussed in a separate chapter (Part II - chapter 1).

Agreements with weak organizational interpenetration

These agreements correspond to situations when actors reach an understanding on the framework of cooperation (aims, means); however, putting these into practice affords each actor a high degree of autonomy. Their complementarity has to be taken into accounts.[62] Without going into too much detail, we can place the following agreements in this category:

- Franchising:[63] a franchise differs from a classic contractual arrangement between two partners in the following ways: i) the franchiser must be able to offer something to the franchisee (a financial and material contribution, know-how), ii) the concept of the network: at the heart of the system is the idea that a higher authority wishes to harmonize a network of legal entities sharing a common goal. The franchiser is the coordinator of the network and therefore endeavours to ensure consistency. The franchisees know that they all belong to the same network; this identification with a network is important. In this way, the Ministry of Health can resort to franchising to further involve the private sector. Even if the State is not the service or health-care provider, it may wish to maintain its role as a leading actor in the proceedings.

Implementing the DOTS strategy

The "Directly Observed Treatment Short-course" strategy, DOTS is now considered to be one of the most effective and low cost means of controlling tuberculosis. It involves providing TB screening tests and ensuring that patients follow a course of antibiotic treatment. In developing countries, the National Tuberculosis Control Programmes have difficulty coping with the situation and the private sector, when operating alone, is inefficient (misdiagnosis, late or non-existent referrals, inappropriate treatment, etc.) Collaboration has become thus indispensable. Several countries such as India, Bangladesh, Cambodia and China are trying out types of franchising. The National TB Control Programme (NTP) in each country i) defines a standard treatment protocol and ii) signs contracts with private practitioners who monitor the treatment of a certain number of patients following the treatment protocol. The NTP applies its know-how and supervises the system. The franchisees form a network of medical personnel that work contractually under the label of NTP.

The contractual tool has become an efficient instrument that helps the Ministry of Health and private practitioners jointly to analyse the mutual costs and benefits of their relationship.

Franchising has also developed in areas such as reproductive health.[64] Some countries have tested franchise networks for first-level private health facilities: for example the PROSALUD network in Bolivia and the ZamHealth network in Zambia.[65] There are also experiments with family planning activities.[66] In recent years, the concept of social franchising has developed. While this follows the same rules as conventional franchising, its purpose is social, in other words it does not entail payment by the beneficiaries; for example, distribution of family health products and services in the developing countries. An international NGO that has funds from bilateral cooperation may finance private providers to provide the population with high quality reproductive health products and services. Without this support, the services would never have been made available by these providers, or would have been of poor quality.[67]

Collaboration between health-care institutions and voluntary associations: since 4 March 2002, French law has authorized public and private hospitals to sign agreements with non-profit associations to enable them to intervene in hospitals: for example, the activity of non-profit associations in the field of palliative care for patients, or associations that provide extracurricular activities for hospitalized children.[68]

The network approach: if, in the past, continuity of care was almost exclusively assured by the medical profession, today, the involvement of many professional health-care and social categories is sought. Recognition of the multiplicity of factors determining health leads to multidisciplinary approaches. Comprehensive case-management of patients is becoming more and more necessary; the aim is to coordinate the range of care provided to patients by health-care actors either at the same time or successively. The operational response to this is increasingly taking the form of a care network. The ensuing contracting formalizes the role of each actor in a global and coherent system for dealing with patients. France is currently developing this type of contracting.[69] Within this defined framework, each practitioner maintains a high degree of autonomy for his or her activities.

Strategic planning at the local health system level: the organization of health systems at the district level is currently undergoing a profound transformation with entities that do not belong to the world of health coming into play, i.e. local governments. Administrative decentralization is leading to the emergence of an authority with generally very weak expertise in health issues (except in big cities).

Legislation on administrative decentralization more or less defines the role of local authorities at the level of health facilities. However, the links with the health district, and consequently with the health management team that ensures consistency, are rarely addressed. Through administrative decentralization, health will find itself confronted with two rationales:

- The systemic rationale, adopted by traditional health care actors (the Ministry of Health but also the health care service providers) which is based on technical considerations;

- The rationale of politics, where health is but one of the mandates of the non-specialized elected representatives of local governments and where the geographical area rarely corresponds to the health district.

The question is how to reconcile the systemic coherence of the health district's traditional health actors with the political rationale of actors responsible for administrative decentralization. The solution is no longer to be found in the channels of centralized and command and control government coordination, as was often proposed by the administration through health district plans. It is here that the approach developed through the concept of "strategic planning"[70] takes on its full significance. It involves bringing together all the actors in a given area (here a health district) and, through negotiations, drawing up a strategic plan that defines the district's main orientations. On the basis of an analysis of the situation and taking into consideration the needs of the health district, the strategic plan establishes the priorities, determines the strategies that will enable it to attain its objectives and indicates the financial implications. It offers a framework, a guide for future actions that will be put into place. This approach, which separates the strategic vision of the evolution of local health systems from the planning of operations, allows different health actors to reach agreement on basic issues before taking action.

However useful it may be, this approach may nevertheless be nothing more than a gentleman's agreement between the actors. Contracting makes it possible to go further by introducing a binding element of formalization into relations. The "performance contract" tool is part of this rationale. While preserving the strategic planning approach, the contractual agreement or "contractual cooperation"[71] binds the actors that have signed to a legally enforceable commitment and to respect the obligations they have freely and jointly accepted. It also has the virtue of establishing a stable relationship between partners and mutual standards of behaviour; in this sense, a contract is a method of organization.

In the sphere of administrative decentralization, some go even further and question the advisability of adopting a sectoral approach which has the drawback of singling out health problems. They advocate the adoption of an approach that starts from the decentralized geographical area and encompasses all sectors at the same time. The resulting contractual cooperation between actors and the central authority allows priorities to be set and creates better inter-sectoral harmonization.[72] However, it is also clear that the main drawback of this approach lies in its complexity and time-consuming nature.

"Sector-wide approach (SWAp)" mechanisms: in conventional negotiation mechanisms between a Government and its development partners, such as UNDP Round tables, the search for a consensus on national health policies does not lead to any formal commitment. One of the characteristics of SWAPs is precisely to overcome this situation and secure a real commitment from both parties, i.e. the

Ministry of Health and the development partners. In this way, both parties formally undertake to respect the national health policy which they have jointly approved. In particular, and this is one of the characteristics of the SWAp approach, they agree to pool their financial resources and to entrust responsibility for managing them to the Ministry of Health. Consequently, the spirit of SWAps is one of contractual cooperation, since it involves formalizing partnerships through contractual relations. These conventions essentially bind the parties to obligations bearing on means rather than on performance.

Health "SWAp" in Tanzania[73]

Tanzania has recently undergone a fundamental health-sector reform; this has been conducted through a SWAp process. Up till now, this SWAp has been set forth in three contractual documents:
- A *Declaration of intent* in June 1998, signed by the Ministry of Health and the development partners, showing their commitment to a reform programme of the health system based on common implementing mechanisms;
- A *Memorandum of Understanding,* in October 1999: this preliminary agreement defines the procedures for the "common-basket" funding arrangements and the obligations and commitments of partners;
- A *Side agreement,* between the Ministry of Health and those partners who wished to add funds to the basket, in March 2000.

These documents are fully consistent with the contractual approach; they show a commitment to clearly defined responsibilities that goes beyond conventional cooperation mechanisms. However, the first analyses to have become available show that however useful these different documents may be, they merely constitute commitments based on good faith between partners, and not enforceable and binding commitments. Thus, even if good faith is present when the documents are signed, it does not mean that it will actually be there in reality.

Furthermore, actual implementation of SWAp at the health district level is part of the spirit of the contractual approach. The approval of an action plan for a health district by a committee that is responsible for the "basket" of funds both from the State budget and the development partners is one of the prerequisites for receiving the funds needed for the district to operate.

"SWAp" in Bangladesh[74]

In Bangladesh, over the last twenty years, development partners have spun an extensive NGO network in the area of reproductive health, which they have often financed directly, thus by-passing the Ministry of Health. The SWAp that was introduced aims to change this situation. After having jointly decided on a health strategy, the funding from the development partners is pooled and its management entrusted to the Ministry of Health . The latter signs contracts for the implementation of the strategy with the NGOs. It should be pointed out that the results are ambivalent due to a certain inflexibility in the development partner's procedures.

General budget support: the new strategy in the relationship between State and certain development partners is based on general budget support (GBS). By essence, GBS is a form of contracting since the State and its development partners agree on a number of indicators, which are generally linked to the MDG. GBS from development partners is contingent upon attainment of these results. A contract is thus entered into by these development partners and the State. This deeply changes the role of the development partners because they are no longer the providers of specific means; they grant their support on the basis of the results attained. The State, via the Ministry of Finance, has to agree with the specialized sectoral ministries on how to use this funding. It is not always easy to reach this agreement, particularly because the Ministry of Health is not always sufficiently prepared to use these new mechanisms. The agreement, which is again in line with the spirit of contracting, signals a marked evolution in the role of the State, which bears greater responsibility for its actions.

Partnership agreements: admittedly, this often-used term frequently crops up in very different situations and can even include some of the cases described above (for example, SWAps can be considered to be partnership agreements). In general, the following agreements are included in this category:

- Partnership agreements between States: these are generally agreements on cooperation between a developed country and the Ministry of Health of a developing one;

- Partnership agreements between a pubic entity and a private entity: for example, the European Union frequently signs partnership agreements with NGOs; the agreement between the Bill and Melinda Gates Foundation and the United Nations Foundation also fall into this category;

- Partnership agreements between private entities: for example, two laboratories from the Merck KGaA group (Théramex, the leader in treatment for the menopause, and Monot, number one at the chemists: these two laboratories have signed a partnership agreement in the area of women's health for the joint promotion of Evestrel (tablets and cream) among doctors as well as in Chemists and at supermarket drug counters;

- Partnership agreements between health establishments: for example, a hospital in a developed country signs a partnership agreement with a hospital in a developing country to conduct training for its medical staff. These agreements can lead to twinning arrangements, where interpenetration is greater.

Agreements with strong organizational interpenetration

These agreements correspond to situations in which actors reach an understanding on the framework of cooperation (aims, means) and carry out some, if not all activities together, allowing them to fulfil the objectives of the contract. Once again, without going into too much detail, the following agreements can be classified under this heading:

Joint management: joint management, understood as a sharing of authority and responsibility, can be seen on a macro-level: where France is concerned, we can point to joint management of the social security bodies by the employers and unions. However, it can also be seen from a micro-level: for example, managing a health institution. Such is the case of a certain approach to community participation: this vision is along the innovative lines of the Bamako Initiative. At the health-facility level, we find a joint management committee or a board of management that is made up both of members of the health staff (manager) and representatives of institutions representing the community: town councils, associations. There should be a balance between, on the one hand the health administration, which should ensure that health facilities fulfil their public service commitments, and on the other, the population, which, insofar as it significantly contributes towards their financing, should be able to decide and control how its financial contribution is being used. In practice, this joint management is expressed in different ways: (i) in everyday administration (for example, shared management of cost recovery revenue by members of the administrative committee and the manager of the health centre), or (ii) with regard to the main policy trends of a health institution (for example, users' associations sitting on a hospital's board of management). Thus, the contract, in its broadest sense, is made up of joint management procedures which are defined by the actors involved.

Alliances: this lies at the heart of "working together". The agreements deriving from this are based on active participation by partners and rely on complementarity between resources, technology and know-how. These alliances can take two forms:

- The first is what the world of industry refers to as "strategic alliances": these are agreements whereby partners determine the terms of their cooperation, i.e. how they pool their resources on a day-to-day basis to reach the target they have set;

- In the second, two entities decide that to carry out a given activity, they will set up a joint subsidiary. This contractual cooperation is not set out in a contract, but rather in the statutes of their joint subsidiary. For example, i) two hospitals may decide to share some of their services: specific laboratory tests, specific aspects of accounting, etc. ii) health-care providers may decide to share drug supply facilities; to do so, their alliance may take the form of a joint subsidiary, for example, an economic interest group (GIE).[75] The spirit of contractual cooperation is evident in the statutes of a joint subsidiary or entity in which each parent entity defines its involvement.

Thus, contracting proves to be far broader and much more elaborate than the concept of a contract in the legal sense of the term. It defines any agreement between actors, whether in the form of a contract, or through other means, such as those examined above.[76]

Finally, each actor who intervenes in the field of health can be seen as an organization at the hub of a web of contracts linking it to all those counterparts with whom it is likely to enter in a relationship. This array of opportunities lies along two axes:

- A "vertical" axis: to explain this, it is useful to refer to agency theory and the concepts of "principal" and "agent". "Downstream" contracting is when the actor involved is in the position of principal; this includes all service and subcontracting contracts. "Upstream" contracting is when the actor involved is in the position of agent, in other words, on the basis of a contract, the agent pursues the objectives defined by the principal;

- A "horizontal" axis: there is no longer an agency type of relationship: each of those involved is a partner who seeks the means of improving their collaboration. through a contractual relationship.

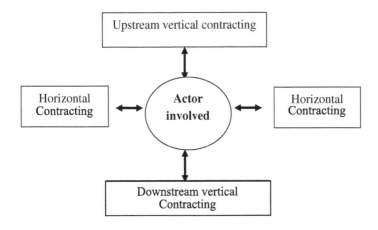

Each actor, and consequently the decision-makers above him, should examine the formal links that they may establish within their environment. In order to use these relationships to their full potential, they should consider all the opportunities available to them, that is to say, study each possible relationship and, depending on their strategies and abilities, develop those which offer them the greatest benefit. To illustrate this point, we refer to the case study of three Colombian hospitals.[77]

Obviously, the contractual relationship will exist only if the potential counterparts aim for similar results. There must be a meeting point between two individual sets of interests and intentions, making it possible to formalize the planned relationship. The approach is pragmatic; it involves the implicit assumption that what is advantageous for each actor is equally advantageous for the system, in other words for the collective interest.

Many countries content themselves with this approach and allow contractual relations to develop on the basis of individual interests. Others, in contrast on the understanding that reconciliation of two individual interests does not necessarily guarantee the collective interest, will try to channel the movement by providing a frame of reference for individual decisions: a contracting policy.

2. STRATEGY

The above typology allows us to describe all the opportunities for contracting that may be used by actors in a country. In respect of all these opportunities, the decision-maker has yet to consider a number of questions.

2.1 Contracting as one of the tools available

When actors in the health system choose contracting, it is always in order to solve a specific problem. This makes it incumbent upon them to consider whether, in each particular case, contracting was the best tool they could have used. For example, the manager of an independent public hospital whose laundry service is not performing satisfactorily needs to ask himself whether sub-contracting is the best solution to the problem and whether it would not be better to review the existing procedure without making any changes in the status, discussing with the manager and staff and examining the service's resources, applying any necessary penalties or introducing a performance bonus system, etc. Perhaps the hospital manager should examine all the possible internal solutions before resorting to sub-contracting for this particular service.

Consequently, sub-contracting is never the only possible solution. Before resorting to it, deciders should examine all the options available to decide whether it is the best solution.

2.2   The absence of a frame of reference

The above typology has illustrated all the opportunities available for contracting, but it has not pointed to any preference. For example, the use of management by delegation for a public health facility has been explained and examples given. This type of contracting is therefore possible. It is now up to countries to determine whether or not they want this type of contracting to develop. There may be many reasons for their decision. Some of them are technical: for example, the absence in the country of any reliable entity capable of taking on the task. Others may be strategic: the country prefers to develop the independence of public health facilities by setting up public establishments. Lastly, there may be political reasons: the country wants the Ministry of Health to be directly responsible for management of the public health service.

As contracting develops in a country, the need for a frame of reference also develops. The country has to clarify its choices. It must indicate those areas in which contracting is to develop, the ways in which it is to be introduced, the role to be played by the Ministry of Health and the positions and roles reserved for other players in the health sector.

This frame of reference is an integral part of national health policy. However, because of the impossibility of adequately setting out this frame of reference in its national health policy document, it will always be in the country's interest to draw up a national policy paper on contracting; we shall examine this aspect in a specific chapter of the second part.

2.3   The absence of a strategy

Let's return to the example of the director of an autonomous public hospital. When he takes office he finds that the laundry service is not performing satisfactorily, and that the same holds for the patients' catering service and caretaking. He also observes that relations with the local mutual health insurance schemes are by and large informal. He would also like to develop twinning arrangements with a number of hospitals in other countries. In such circumstances, the director cannot but admit that it will be impossible to set up all these contractual relations overnight. He will need to draw up a strategic plan for their implementation and to set priorities.

The same is true at the country level. The Minister of Health will need to consider what strategies he or she wishes to introduce. Should the development of contracting be determined by the actors' priorities or should the Minister define them?

One thing that has to be borne in mind is that it will be hard to reverse the choices made. For example, if the Ministry of Health has opted for management by delegation of its public hospitals, it has to remember that it will always be possible to reverse the decision and to revert to direct management. However, any such decision will be difficult to put into place; in the meantime the already limited skills available before the delegation of managerial responsibility will have dwindled *away, and it will take time to rebuild them.*

2.4   The issues at stake in contracting

In the world of business it is clear what is at stake in contracting. Each contracting party strives to benefit from the contract to which it commits itself. Matters are more complex in the health sector. Whether or not it is a party to the contract, the Ministry of Health cannot object to each contracting party endeavouring to seek their own individual benefits. However, as the steward of the public interest, the Ministry of Health must also be concerned with the benefits for society as a whole. It will examine how a contract between two or more actors ultimately helps to improve the health of populations. The following diagram will help to explain this:

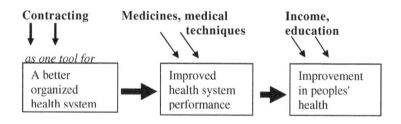

By helping to improve health system performance, contracting, like other determinants, helps to improve peoples' health. Even if this fact is not always easy to demonstrate, health actors considering the use of contracting must always bear it in mind. There is no reason to object to the contracting parties benefiting individually from contracting, provided the community as a whole also benefits. It is in this respect that contracting is a tool of interest to a Ministry of Health.

Provided it continues to improve the health system's performance, contracting will always find a keen advocate in the Ministry of Health; however, if the experiences currently under way in the country fail to help improve health system performance, the Ministry will turn its attention to other tools.

Because contracting changes the organizational and production methods of health services, there are those who wonder what the consequences of those changes will be, and whether what is actually at stake is privatization of the health system and the withdrawal of the State.[79]

The concept of privatization

Privatization is a concept that at first sight appears simple. According to the dictionary definition, privatization involves the transfer of ownership of an entity from the public to the private sector, its opposite being nationalization.

In everyday parlance, this is the sole meaning of privatization, and as such contracting cannot be understood as a form of privatization. This is because privatization involves a transfer of ownership whereas contracting builds on the existing situation, with the stakeholders already present, and seeks to establish relationships among them. Privatization is an institutional arrangement whereas contracting is concerned with relationships.

However, in specialist literature on State reform, privatization is defined more broadly: it is understood as the adoption of a management model that draws on the rules of the market. According to the theories of D. Rondinelli and M. Iacono,[3] this type of privatization can be achieved in several ways:

– By transferring ownership:[4] like a public enterprise whose ownership is transferred to the private sector, the ownership of certain public entities (hospitals, health centres, laboratories, drug distribution services, etc.) is transferred to the private sector. Some authors describe this as State "divestment"[5] since the entity's assets are transferred in whole or in part.

– By ensuring that public entities adopt private-sector managerial practices, while maintaining public-sector ownership: eliminating arbitrary subsidies and public monopolies, according autonomous status, and permitting the outsourcing of certain tasks and the drawing up of employment contracts outside the public administration. The public entity adopts private-sector managerial techniques and becomes an independent enterprise within a larger entity constituting an administration.

– By entrusting the management of public entities to the private sector, while maintaining public-sector ownership, also known as management by delegation.

– By purchasing services from private providers, whether or not they operate from health facilities, while maintaining control over public funding.

– By replacing the public sector with the private sector: in this case ownership is private and will remain so, but the private entity substitutes for the public stakeholder that previously carried out the task.

In each of the five cases above, we can therefore say that the health system would be more privatized in the sense that it would operate more in line with the rules of the market.

However, certain strategies may limit privatization: for example, ensuring that the private sector cooperates with the public sector: in this case ownership is private and will remain so, but the entity agrees to act in accordance with national health policy. This could be described as greater state control.

There are thus three factors to consider in assessing privatization:

– Ownership of the entity: typically, privatization is the transfer of ownership from the public to the private sector.

– Management of the entity: the entity is managed according to the rules of the market and private enterprise. In other words (i) users are treated as clients, (ii) services are determined by client demand, (iii) the production process is designed to respond to demand, and cost control is a major concern. The management must therefore abandon the model of administrative hierarchies to achieve a degree of independence.

– Missions or objectives of the entity: Are service providers entirely free to choose their terms of reference (economic liberalism) or does the State have a say in defining them (through contracting or regulations) and consequently influencing which products are produced and how?

The following table summarizes the above points:

Evaluation criteria Reform	Ownership	Management	Terms of reference
Transfer ownership	**Transition from public to private**	Owing to the transfer of ownership, management becomes private	**-Economic liberalism** *or* **- State intervention through contracting or regulations**
Grant autonomy to public entities	Status quo (public)	**Operates more in line with the rules of the market**	Quasi-status quo (public)
Delegate management of public entities	Status quo (public)	**Transition from public to private**	Quasi-status quo (public)
Substitute private for public	Status quo (private)	**Substitute private stakeholders for public stakeholders**	Quasi-status quo (public)
NB: Areas most affected by privatization indicated in bold.			

As an example, let us examine the case of a public hospital under private management. The effects of this decision, classified according to the three evaluation criteria above, are schematically illustrated as follows:

Degree of privatization

	0%	100%
Ownership		
Management of inputs	███████████████████████████████████	
Mission	█	

In this example, the hospital is publicly owned but management of inputs is delegated entirely (by contract) to a private stakeholder. The hospital's mission, although globally remaining in line with public objectives, may also include private objectives (e.g. accepting that the introduction of cost recovery will entail a loss in equality of access for users).

Contracting is also perceived as a Trojan horse for privatization. Those who hold this view believe that contracting is a strategy whereby it is possible to introduce privatization in two stages. Unwillingness to declare the objective of direct privatization would account for the use, at least initially, of contracting, enabling the private sector to expand its presence within the health sector. On the strength of this position (like the Trojan horse), after some time has passed the private sector would end up occupying the field. From this point of view, contracting is seen as a pernicious means of privatizing, like the Trojan horse, which allows warriors to enter a town without showing themselves. Contracting is thus seen as a form of privatization in disguise, which will come out into the open once it has taken over.

Between those who believe privatization to be the best strategy for improving the efficacy of health systems and those who are convinced that it calls into question the need to develop public health a third trend is emerging, whose rationale is based on the opportunities of developing certain forms of privatization, provided they develop in a defined framework.

The basic assumption of this rationale is that privatization is capable of enhancing the efficacy of the health system provided there is a means of ensuring that the actors work with the interest of the population as their objective. This requires a strong commitment on the part of the State to perform this regulatory function. Nevertheless, there is quite a broad range of tools available with which it may mitigate the potentially harmful effects of privatization, in particular by controlling the use of contracting as a means of introducing reforms that lead to greater privatization:

- When the State adopts contracting policies, it simultaneously takes not of greater privatization of the health sector and develops the means of containing privatization by ensuring that all health service providers act in the general interest, in other words for the good of the populations. Contracting policies ensure that specific contractual arrangements comply with the orientations and strategies of national health policy. These contracting policies may be accompanied by a whole range of regulations to control the practices of operators: for example, when the State resorts to management by delegation or to association with NGOs, it may require them clearly to differentiate their health activities from their other activities;

- Thanks to its overall control , the State has the means to ensure that the increased level of health sector privatization that results from contracting obeys the principles of the national health policy. For example, poorly defined and badly supervised delegated management of a public structure may result in virtual privatization in the strict sense of the word. However, if it is well controlled by the State, management by delegation makes it possible to preserve the health structure's public health objective;

- By building up the technical skills of all the actors. the State may ensure that contracting will be wisely used and that harmful effects are avoided. For example, by facilitating contractual relations based on mutual trust, the State favours contracting that is based on relations other than those of rivalry and competition prevailing in the private sector;

- By conducting evaluations of the reforms that resort to contracting, the State may highlight good practices and draw attention to the kind of experience that ought to be rolled out;

However, contracting may also be understood as a tool for regulation by the State. By making judicious use of the tool, the State is able better to regulate the health system through State interventionism that is flexible, reflective and responsive, and no longer based on authoritarian regulation. The modern State is one that no longer issues orders from above, but agrees to negotiate with its societal environment; contracting is one of the tools that fit this rationale.

Without departing from its role as guarantor of the general interest, the State must define public-service missions, organize the operators who will then be responsible for performing those missions and then monitor and evaluate their practices. In this case, the State need not itself be an operator in order to achieve its ends. However, this calls for a strong State capable of fully performing these roles. It will require appropriate technical skills; to be realistic; it will also need to possess adequate financial resources to tip the scales in favour of its views: if the State lacks the means of its ambitions, it has little chance of success.

Similarly, contracting calls for an honest State. If the State is beset by corruption, contracting will be a means of rewarding private interests (rewards for political parties, interest groups or even individuals) that have proved useful. In this case, it will have been the means of privatizing financial resources and power. As we have seen, contracting is far more than a mere tool: it is a strategy or an approach. Depending on how it is employed, it is capable of bringing about far-reaching changes in the very organization of the health system; and its use yields very diverse results. This is why a ministry of health should always bear in mind the "**strategic contracting**" approach; in other words the need to envisage contracting as a strategy:

> - are there ways of improving a situation without resorting to organizational changes?

> - of the tools available, is contracting the one that is efficacious and easy to implement?

BY WAY OF CONCLUSION, THREE FURTHER CONSIDERATIONS...

1. Throughout the world, including in the developing countries, the way health systems are organized is undergoing far-reaching changes. In this regard however, we need to distinguish between *institutional arrangement* and *contractual arrangement*. The emergence of new actors in the field of health, whether from within the field itself or from outside, results in new forms of organization in the sector and in a redistribution of roles. The multiplication of the number of actors and the diversification of their roles almost inevitably leads to the development of interdependence between the actors, the nature of which needs to be examined. In this respect, contractual arrangements are the outcome of institutional arrangements.

Consequently, while most institutional arrangements carry within them the need to draw up contractual arrangements, strangely enough in actual practice these two elements are by and large independent. In many cases, it would be advantageous to consider the two simultaneously.

The table below sets out the links between both elements, in the areas considered in this document.

Reshuffling within health systems

	Actors concerned	Institutional arrangements →	Contractual arrangements
Internal	Private service providers	Accreditation	Association Concession
	Public health-care establishments	Autonomy	Contract with the Ministry of Health
	District administration	Devolution District Agency	Concession Joint responsibility Contract between the Ministry of Health and the Agency
External	Population	Management committees Associations	
	Institutions responsible for risk sharing	New independent actor (Mutual insurance companies)	Contract with providers
	Local authorities	Transfer of responsibility to decentralized local authorities	Complex contractual arrangement

Lastly, we should stress that as well as reinforcing partnership with the private sector, such reshuffling has also instituted an internal dialogue within the State, in other words, a dialogue between the central State apparatus and its constituent entities.

2. If contractual arrangements are not set within a contractual policy, there is a risk of inefficacy and of misapprehension as to the potential of contracting. It is very important to emphasize that while contracting may prove a highly effective tool for revitalizing the organization of health systems, it is by no means an unfailing universal panacea.

In order to achieve an impact in terms of better health-system performance, the objective towards which we should aim is no doubt the development of contractual policies which follow a systemic approach.

Does this mean then that we should censure any specific contractual arrangements which are not part and parcel of a contractual policy? Is it necessary for any specific contractual arrangement to be preceded by a contractual policy? Recent examples of the use of these concepts and instruments reveal complex situations. In some cases, it is because the actors involved in specific contractual arrangements become aware of the limits of their approach that they suggest a more systemic one. This frequently happens with the "framework agreement" approach; for example, in Burundi as well as in Uganda, the churches felt that specific contractual arrangements were insufficient and instituted a frame of reference for their negotiations. Others prefer to perfect contractual relations through specific contracts, to show the worth of this approach and only then to establish it as the principle through which the health system operates through a contractual policy that is formalized in a national health policy (for example, in Madagascar). Thus, specific contractual arrangements, by which we mean a stage that must be superseded, may prove to be a useful strategy, preferable to the prior development of a purely theoretical contractual policy that will not be followed by any acts. Such a strategy is all the more justified in the context of incipient decentralization, because it makes it possible to preserve the forward dynamic needed by any process of decentralization and thus to foster "negotiated law".

3. Whether it is directly party to a specific contractual arrangement (as in the case of an NGO owning a health facility which signs a contract with the management team of a health district) or not concerned (as in the case of a mutual insurance company which signs an agreement with a private health facility), the State cannot dissociate itself. Its responsibility for the welfare of the population requires it to be capable of exercising control over specific contractual arrangements. Such control must first of all be practiced upstream, and it should not be possible for any specific contractual arrangement to be signed without the "authorization" of the State.[83] However, the same control is also required throughout its implementation via effective supervision and in order to help resolve any conflicts between the contracting parties. In order to perform this monitoring, the State needs to possess specific capacities, and it is often these which are lacking in ministries of health, more accustomed to the workings of conventional bureaucracy[84].

The subsidiarity principle

Subsidiarity means quite simply that a decision must always be taken and responsibility for it assumed as closely as possible to citizens. As low down as possible as and no higher than necessary. The principle of subsidiarity can be addressed in two ways:

- Article 3b (now article 5) of Title II of the Treaty of Maastricht stipulates " In areas which do not fall within its exclusive competence, the Community shall take action, in accordance with the principle of subsidiarity, only if and in so far as the objectives of the proposed action cannot be sufficiently achieved by the Member States ". Thus the European Union must first of all allow its Members States and their national and local institutions to act.
- Subsidiarity may also be defined as the transfer, by the grass-roots level to the level immediately above it, of some of its operations in the interests of greater efficacy. The higher level thus has a mandate from the lower level, contrary to hierarchical relations, in which the opposite is true.
Application of the principle of subsidiarity leads to a fundamental re-examination of interactions between the different actors. For example;
- in respect of decentralization, there is a general tendency to assume that the State has granted to the local authorities those powers it is willing to pass down to them. The rationale of the subsidiarity principle is quite the opposite: because they are closer to citizens, local authorities are able to solve many of their problems. They should delegate to the higher level only those responsibilities they are unable to assume themselves. This is also the spirit of federalism.
- in line with this principal, the role of the State is transformed: it shifts from that of welfare State to that of subsidiary State, i.e. a State that intervenes only when it has determined that civil society, or the local public institutions have failed to provide the populations with a satisfactory response.

Nevertheless, the principle of subsidiarity does not mean either withdrawal or abandonment of responsibility; ultimately, the concept is quite close to those of regulation and advising.
Application of the principle of subsidiarity may adopt several strategies. One of them is laissez-faire; things should be allowed to sort themselves out at the lowest level, i.e. among the components of civil society and intervention should only be a last resort. However, another strategy currently being developed is based on the notion of "coaching". Rather than intervening downstream, it is preferable to prevent upstream. Contracting, of which responsibility for ensuring the public good is an intrinsic part, is in line with this rationale.

However, the role of the State is of even greater importance when these specific contractual arrangements are set within a contractual policy. The development, implementation and evaluation of any such contractual policy is the responsibility of the State and more particularly of the Ministry of Health, who has to be the prime mover of the contractual policy. This role calls up one of the essential functions of the health system: stewardship. This function, whose importance was highlighted in the World Health Organization's (WHO) World Health Report 2000, vests in the State legitimacy to direct national health policy, even though to do so requires the participation of all those involved. Thus the authoritarian State, acting through the general, impersonal and coercive rule of law, is less and less adapted to the context of modern societies which are characterized by their growing complexity. A modern State is one that no longer issues orders from above, but agrees to negotiate with its social environment. Modern law makes greater provision for establishing "game rules" (flexible, reflexive, responsive, etc.), and no longer claims to be all-regulating but simply create (open) frameworks of negotiation in which direct democracy can operate. In practice, this is no easy matter. The State must simultaneously guarantee the consistency of national health policy while allowing room for singularity. In this respect, it is difficult for it to be a real partner, that is to say an actor like any other. Even if it accepts contracting it is almost always a separate partner, beyond and above the parties, reserving for itself the right to intervene if things do not go (as it thinks) they should. Only practical experience, based on mutual respect, will make it possible to strike a balance.

Notes

[1] The Bardot maternity centre (Côte d'Ivoire), an experiment presented by the European Community at the technical meeting *Towards new partnerships for the development of health in the developing countries*, WHO, Geneva, February 1998

[2] Community-based health facilities (FSU-Com), document of the Projet Santé Abidjan (PSA), Côte d'Ivoire

[3] Zakir Hussain, A.M. (1998) "A New Direction Towards Management of Health Care Delivery System", Ministry of Health and Family Welfare, PHC Series – 31

[4] Fronczak, N. (1999) "Description and Assessment of Contracting Health Services Pilot Project", Basic Health Services Project, MOH, Cambodia

[5] Soeters R, F. Griffiths (2000) Can government health workers be motivated? Experimenting with contract management: the case of Cambodia, communication presented at the international symposium on financing health systems in low-income countries in Africa and Asia", France, Clermont-Ferrand 30 November - 1 December 2000

[6] NGO "Santé sud" with the support of French Cooperation and the European Union. Assistance in setting up makes provision for basic medical equipment. The applicant may also request a loan to purchase a motor bike and a cash advance. The rural physician undertakes to comply with a set of «specifications» to satisfy the health needs of his or her area of reference (treatment and

prevention). He is required to make rounds on specific days to the main villages and home visits.

[7] Bura, M. (1998) "Church-related Hospitals contracted as Designated District Hospitals: Tanzanian Experiences", communication presented at the technical meeting *Towards new partnerships for health development in the developing countries, WHO*, Geneva, February 1998

[8] Yeboah, Y. (1999) "Contracting: the case of Ghana from the perspective of the Christian Health Association of Ghana (CHAG)", paper presented to the meeting organized by Medicus Mundi International *Updating heath care development cooperation*, 5-7 November 1999, Dar Es Salam, Tanzania

[9] Hanson, K. L. Atuyambe, J. Kamwanga, B. McPake, O. Mungule, F. Ssengooba (2002) *Towards improving hospital performance in Uganda and Zambia: reflections and opportunities for autonomy, Health Policy*, 61: 73-94

[10] Definition of the notion of public service or what others call, albeit with nuances, the general interest, is not an easy matter and depends on different national contexts. However, what is sure is that the notion of public service is based on the fact that because of their nature, objectives and the interests involved, certain activities in society must be exempt from the rationale of the market and the search for profit, and be managed in accordance with specific criteria ensuring everyone has access to certain goods and services and thus helping to ensure the economic, social and cultural cohesion of society (solidarity and equalization).

[11] Achouri, H. 2001. *Le projet d'appui à la réforme hospitalière: objectifs, implémentation, résultats et enseignements. La Tunisie médicale* 79, no. 5.

[12] McPake B, K. Hanson (2000) "A model of the equity implications of reforms in Zambia", *Paper presented at the international symposium "Financing health systems in low income countries in Africa and Asia, France, Clermont-Ferrand, 30 November - 1 December 2000.*

[13] Bodart, C. B. Schmidt-Ehry (1999) "L'approche contractuelle comme outil de mise en œuvre des Politiques nationales de santé en Afrique" (The contractual approach as a tool for implementing national health policies in Africa), GTZ, Division 43

Ph. Senant, T. Kirsch-Woik (1998) "Aspects juridiques de l'approche contractuelle comme outil de mise en œuvre d'une politique nationale de santé " (Legal aspects of the contractual approach as a tool for implementing a national health policy), paper presented at the meeting *"The contractual approach as a tool for implementing national health policies in African countries"*, Dakar, Senegal, 19-21 October 1998

Senant Ph, Kirsch-Woik Th (2000), "Evolution de l'approche contractuelle dans la province de Mahajanga (Madagascar)" (Evolution of the contractual approach in Mahajanga province, Madagascar), Paper presented at the international symposium on Financing health systems in low-income countries in Africa and Asia, France, Clermont-Ferrand, 30 November - 1 December 2000.

[14] Outsourcing: resorting to an outside operator to perform an activity which an actor has decided to cease performing itself.

[15] World Health report 2000: Health systems: Improving performance, p. 104 et seq.

[16] Several examples of agreements between youth associations and the National AIDS Control Programme of the Ministry of Health of Chad were presented at the Information seminar on the contractual approach in the health sector in Chad, N'Djamena - 4 and 5 November 1998

[17] Marek, T., I. Diallo, B. Ndiaye, and J. Rakotosalama. 1999. *Successful contracting of prevention services: fighting malnutrition in Senegal and Madagascar. Health Policy and Planning* 14, no. 4.

[18] Shaw, P. R. 1999. New trends in Public Sector Management in health - Applications in Developed and Developing Countries. World Bank Institute.

[19] Abramson, W. B. 1999. *Partnerships between the public sector and nongovernmental organizations: contracting for primary health care services.* A study carried out by Abt Associates Inc. as part of LAC Health Sector Reform Initiative.

[20] Lubben, M., S. H. Mayhew, C. Collins, and A Green. 2002. *Reproductive health and health sector reform in developing countries: establishing a framework for dialogue. Bulletin of the World Health Organization* 80, no. 8:667-674.

[21] Kolehmainen-Aitken, R-L. *State of the practice: Public-NGO partnerships in response to decentralization.* 22. 2000. LAC Health Sector Reform Initiative.

[22] Enthoven, A. C. 1993. *The History and Principles of Managed Competition. Health Affairs, Supplement.*

[23] For a detailed presentation see, Sara Bennett, Barbara McPake, Anne Mills (1997), op. Cit.

[24] Saltman, R. B. and C. von Otter. 1992. *Planned Markets and Public Competition: Strategic Reform in Health Care.* Edited by Milton Keynes.: Open University Press.

[25] Enthoven, A. C. *Reflections on the Management of the NHS.* 1985. London, Nuffield Provincial Hospital Thrust

[26] Le Grand, J. and W. Bartlett. 1993. *Quasi-markets and social policy.* London: The Macmillan Press.

[27] Brown, L. E. and V. E. Amelung. 1999. *Manacled Competition: Market reform in German Health Care. Health Affairs* 18, no. 3.

[28] Strictly speaking, these terms are not equivalent. In systems with internal markets (Great Britain, New-Zealand) purchaser and provider are considered t o be completely separate, and it is mandatory for the purchaser to make a contract with the provider; in contrast, in systems in which there is managed competition (Netherlands, United States), vertical integration of the purchaser and provider functions is possible (as is the case of the Health Maintenance Organizations (HMO). On this topic see,

Flood, C. M. 2000. *International Health Care Reform: a legal, economic and political analysis.* Routledge Studies in the Modern World Economy ed.: Routledge, London and New York.

[29] Le Grand, J. 1999. *Competition, Cooperation, Or Control? Health Affairs* 18, no. 3.

[30] The White paper for the new NHS may be consulted on the Internet: web site of the U.K. Department of Health on 2 October 2000: http://www.official-documents/doh/newnhs/wpaper.htm

[31] Department of Health. *Delivering the NHS Plan: Next Steps on Investment, Next Steps on Reform.* Cm 55 03. 2002. Stationery Office, Norwich.

[32] Lewis, R. and S. Gillam. 2003. *Back to the market: yet more reform of the national health service. International Journal of Health Services* 33, no. 1:77-84.

[33] Light, D. W. 2001. *Comparative institutional response to economic policy managed competition and governmentality. Social Science and Medicine,* 52:1151-1166.

Light, D. W. 2001. *Managed competition, governmentality and institutional response in the United Kingdom. Social Science and Medicine* 52:1167-1181.

Lieverdink, H. 2001. *The marginal success of regulated competition policy in the Netherlands. Social Science and Medicine* 52:1183-1194.

Andersen, R., B. Smedby, and D. Vagero. 2001. *Cost containment, solidarity and cautious experimentation: Swedish dilemmas. Social Science and Medicine.* 52:1195-1204.

Cabiedes, L. and A. Guillén. 2001. *Adopting and adapting managed competition: health care reform in Southern Europe. Social Science and Medicine* 52:1205-1217.

Gross, R. and M. Harrison. 2001. *Implement ting managed competition in Israel. Social Science and Medicine* 52:1219-1231.

Fougere, G. 2001. *Transforming health sectors: new logics of organizing in the New Zealand health system. Social Science and Medicine* 52:1233-1242.

Iriart.C, E. E. Merhy, and H. Waitzkin. 2001. *Managed care in Latin America: the new common sense in health policy reform. Social Science and Medicine* 52:1243-1253.

[34] Harrison, M. I. and J. Calltorp. 2000. *The reorientation of market-oriented reforms in Swedish health care. Health Policy* 50:219-240.

[35] Larbi, G. A. 1998. *Institutional constraints and capacity issues in decentralizing management in public services: the case of health in Ghana. Journal of International Development* 10:377-386.

[36] Cassels, A. 1995. *Health sector reform: key issues in less developed countries. Journal of International Development* 7, no. 3:329-347.

[37] In some countries, these systems are a virtual State monopoly, as in France, while in others, there are numerous insurance systems, as in Germany.

[38] Hurst, J. W. 1991. *Reforming health care in seven European nations. Health Affairs*, no. Fall 7.

[39] van de Ven, W. P. M. M., F. T. Schut, and F. F. H. Rutten. 1994. *Forming and reforming the market for third-party purchasing of health care. Social Sciences and Medicine* 39, no. 10:1405-1412.

[40] Von der Schulenburg, J. M. G. 1994. *Forming and reforming the market for third-party purchasing of health care: a German perspective. Social Science and Medicine* 39, no. 10:1473-1481.

[41]For example, the Internet site set up by ILO for Africa is worth consulting: http://www.concertation.org

[42] Thiombiano, A. (2000) "L'approche contractuelle et les services de santé décentralisés: l'expérience des mutuelles de santé du Projet FAARF et les formations sanitaires au Burkina Faso" (the contractual approach and decentralized health services: the experience of the mutual insurance societies participating in the FAARF project and health facilities in Burkina Faso), paper presented at the meeting on "The contractual approach and decentralized health services in Africa, Dakar, 19-22 June 2000"

[43] Vladescu, C. and S. Radulescu. 2001. *Improving primary health care: output-based contracting in Romania.* In *Contracting for public services: output-based aid and its applications* , edited by P.J.Brook and S.M.Smith World Bank and International Finance Corporation.

[44] Criel, B., A. N. Barry, and F. von Roenne. *Le projet PRIMA en Guinée Conakry. Une expérience d'organisation de mutuelles de santé en Afrique rurale.* 2002. Guinea, Conakry, The PRIMA project in : an experiment at organizing mutual health insurance societies in Africa.

[45] C.M. Flood (2000) Op.cit.

[46] In 1988, A. Donabedian suggested approaching quality from three angles: the inputs offered by the provider, the care-production process and the results obtained.

[47]Capitation is a method according to which a health-service provider is paid by a fundholder: the latter pays the provider an amount determined in advance on a per capita basis and paid for a period in the future. Using this amount, the provider undertakes to provide all the care needed by the individuals for whom the sum has been paid.

[48] Telyukov, A. *Guide to prospective capitation with illustrations from Latin America.* 5. 2001. LAC- Health Sector Reform Initiative. http://www.americas.health-sector-reform.org

[49] Bitran, R. *Paying Health Providers through Capitation in Argentina, Nicaragua, and Thailand: Output, Spending, Organizational Impact, and Market Structure.* Technical Paper N°.1. 2001. Partnerships for Health Reform (PHR), Major Applied Research 2.

[50] Waters, H. R., L. L. Morlock, and L. Hatt. 2004. *Quality-based purchasing in health care. International Journal of Health Planning and Management* 19:365-381.

[51] For a review of these services, see, .Mills, A. 1997. *Contractual relationships between government and the commercial private sector in developing countries.* In *Private health providers in developing countries,* edited by Bennett, S., B. McPake, and A. Mills (London: Zed Books).

[52] Bennett, S., B. McPake, and A. Mills. 1997. *Private health providers in developing countries.* chapter 12 ed. London and New Jersey.

[53] Soeters R, Griffiths F (2000) "Can government health workers be motivated? Experimenting with contract management: the case of Cambodia", paper presented at the international symposium "Financing health systems in low-income countries in Africa and Asia", CERDI, Université d'Auvergne, Clemont-Ferrand, France.

Soeters, R and F. Griffiths. 2003. *Improving government health services through contract management: a case from Cambodia. Health Policy* 18, no. 1:74-83.

[54] Kolehmainen-Aitken, R-L. *State of the practice: Public-NGO partnerships in response to decentralization.* 2000. LAC Health Sector Reform Initiative.

[55] In particular, the journal *"European Journal of Purchasing & Supply Management"* has for several years been a source of seminal articles. Although the field concerned is only rarely health, the concepts and tools developed are of I nterest to the health sector.

[56] Parker, D. and K. Hartley. 1997. *The economics of partnership sourcing versus adversarial competition: a critique. European Journal of Purchasing & Supply Management* 3 , no. 2:115-125.

[57] Gilson, L. 2003. *Trust and the development of health care as a social institution. Social science & Medicine* 56:1453-1468.

[58] Peacock, S. *Experiences with the UK National Health Service Reforms: A case of the infernal market?* 1997. Australia, Centre for Health Program Evaluation.

James, C., M. Dixon, and M. Sobanja. *Re-focusing Commissioning for Primary Care Trusts.* 2002. An NHS alliance discussion paper. http://www.nhsalliance.org/docs

[59] Cox, A. 1996. *Relational competence and strategic procurement management: towards an entrepreneurial and contractual theory of the firm. European Journal of Purchasing & Supply Management* 2, no. 1:57-70.

Thompson, I., A. Cox, and L. Andersen. 1998. *Contracting strategies for the project environment. European Journal of Purchasing & Supply Management* 4, no. 1:31-41.

[60] In the sphere of business economics, this issue arises in respect of "subcontracting partnership", where the sub-contractor producing the article on behalf of a principal helps to design the article.

[61] Ingham, M. 1994. *Organizational apprenticeship in cooperation. Revue Française de Gestion* 97:105-121.

[62] Zafar Ullah, A. N., J. N. Newell, J. U. Ahmed, M. K. A. Hyder, and A. Islam. 2006. *Government - NGO collaboration: the case of tuberculosis control in Bangladesh. Health Policy and Planning* 21, no. 2:143-155.

[63] According to the European Code of Ethics for Franchising, franchising is *"a system of marketing goods and/or services and/or technology, which is based on a close and ongoing collaboration between legally and financially separate and independent undertakings, the Franchisor and its individual Franchisees, whereby the Franchisor grants its individual Franchisees the right, and imposes the obligation to conduct a business in accordance with the Franchisor's concept"*

[64] Agha, S., A. M. Karim, A. Bala, and S. Sosler. 2007. *The impact of a reproductive health franchise on client satisfaction in rural Nepal. Health Policy and Planning* 22:320-328.

[65] Makinen, M. and Ch. .Leighton. *Summary of Market Analysis for a Franchise Network of Primary Health Care in Lusaka, Zambia.* Technical Report 15. 1997. Washington, Abt Associates and PHR.

[66] Montagu, D. 2002. *Franchising of health services in low-income countries. Health Policy and Planning* 17, no. 2:121-130.

[67] Ruster, A., C. Yamamoto, and K. Rogo. Franchising in Health. Note Number 263. 2003. The World Bank. Public Policy for the Private Sector.

[68] Jean, Ph. 2002. *Voluntary associations. Revue Hospitalière de France*, no. 487:18-23.

[69] For example, networks in the areas of perinatal care may be consulted on the Internet site of the Rhone-Alps regional hospital agency: http://www.satelnet.fr/arhra

[70] Green, A. 1992. *An introduction to health planning in developing countries.*: Oxford University Press, Reprinted 1995,1996,1997,1998,1999.

[71] Marcou, G., F. .Rangeon, and J. L. Thiébault. 1997. *Contractual cooperation and municipal government.* Paris, France: L'Harmattan.

[72] In accordance with this approach, what matters is avoiding the errors made in the past. For example, the introduction of cost recovery into the health sector without any coordination with the Ministry of Finance or other sectors has led to many problems.

[73] Brown, A. Current Issues in Sector-Wide Approaches for Health Development: Tanzania Case study. WHO/GPE/00.6. 2000. Geneva, Switzerland, World Health Organization.

[74] DFID (2000) "Making the most of the private sector" Report to DFID (Department for International Development), Seminar on 11 and 12 May 2000

[75] An economic interest group (GIE) is a legal entity under French law whose purpose is to employ, for a specific period, all the means necessary to facilitate or develop the activities of one of its members.

[76] Telyukov, A., V. Novak, and C. Bross. *Provider payment alternatives for Latin America: concepts and stakeholder strategies.* 50 LAC-HSR. 2001. Health Sector Reform Initiative. http://www.americas.health-sector-reform.org

[77] Saenz, L. *Managing the transition from public hospital to "social enterprise": a case study of three Colombian hospitals.* 46 LAC-HSR. 2001. Health Sector Reform Initiative.
http://www.americas.health-sector-reform.org

[78] Maarse, H. 2006. *The privatization of health care in Europe: an eight-country analysis. Journal of Health Politics, Policy and Law* 31, no. 5:981-1014.

[79] Rondinelli, M. and M. Iacono. 1996. *Strategic management of privatization: a framework for planning and implementation. Public Administration and Development* 16:247-263.

[80] It is important clearly to distinguish between ownership of a structure and that of an infrastructure. Ownership of an infrastructure concerns built-up property (buildings), unbuilt property (land and major capital investments). Ownership of the structure concerns a legally independent economic unit which is organized to produce goods or services. To take the example of a hospital, the structure may be an NGO that runs the hospital as an enterprise. However, the enterprise may or may not own the hospital buildings (which may, for example. belong to another NGO). What actually matters is who owns the structure and not the infrastructures. This distinction is perfectly clear in the case of shops, in which the goodwill is distinguished from the actual business or of physicians in private practice, who distinguish between their surgery and clientele: in the case of a sale, these two elements are quite distinct.

[81] Savas, E. S. 1990. *A taxonomy of Privatization Strategies. Journal of Policy Studies* 18, no. 2:343-355.

[82] This authorization means that the State accepts the validity of the contract signed by responsible actors

[83] This is valid not only for developing countries; the developed countries are faced with the same problem. This aspect is clearly underscored by the document: "Before you sign the dotted line…ensuring contracts can be managed" (1997), this document may be consulted on the Internet: consultation on the site, Web Competitive Tendering and Contracting Branch (CTC) of the Department of Finance and Administration, Australia, dated 2 October 2000: http://www.ctc.gov.au

Part II

Chapter 1

The different forms of public-private partnership for building and managing health facilities

Jean Perrot

INTRODUCTION

Our starting point has to be the recognition that there are services which, when the requirements of social organization and the expectations of users are taken into account, are such that they cannot be satisfied by the market forces alone. These are activities that the government must to some extent manage and/or organize. In the heyday of the welfare State, it seemed perfectly obvious that it was up to the State to ensure the provision of these economic services of public interest which are still known as "public services ".

Health, and in particular all aspects of public health, are part of this rationale. The State must provide for the population all those services that enable it to enjoy the highest attainable standard of care. In this case, the State will play every role: it will define health policies, promote research, define treatment strategies, ensure the funding of health services and organize and run the provision of health services via health facilities for whose investment, ownership and management it will be responsible. The resulting health system has a top-down hierarchical structure. The State holds all the cards and may issue orders which, originating from the summit, will be passed down to the base of the health pyramid and of its health facilities. This systemic integration is intended to provide for populations the best possible services. The British National Health Service (NHS) was originally founded on these principles.

However, with the passage of time, there has been no lack of criticism. The provision of health services directly organized by the State, i.e. by a decentralized service of the Ministry of Health, is not always efficient. In addition, the budgetary problems faced by all countries, be they developed or developing, make it impossible to ensure the best possible supply of health services.

Hence the need for a response to the criticism; countries' decision makers have several paths to choose from: in many cases, they will resort to contracting.

1. INTERNAL DEVELOPMENTS

The first trend to develop was based on the notion of autonomy. If public health-service providers are to be more efficacious, they must be given greater autonomy:

Devolution: in comparison with direct management by the Ministry of Health or any other local authority, devolution is no doubt the channel whereby the public bodies give up the fewest of their prerogatives. Their aim is to lighten the administrative burden of upstream control and they give health facilities a number of managerial prerogatives that enable them to become more efficient. The forms taken by this kind of devolution vary and depend on national law: they range from mere delegation of authority or signature by the supervisory authority to authentic administrative and financial autonomy (an independent budget) within the public entity[1]. However, the health facility remains under the direct stewardship of the Ministry and of its decentralized services. It has no distinct legal personality. This improves the day-to-day running of the health facility, but the underlying mechanisms remain unchanged. This form of devolution does not radically change the system of incentives. The *régie* (managerial authority) seems to be the oldest form of management of public services. The public service is managed in the form of a *régie* when it is directly operated by the legal person on whom it depends. Although services run in this way may be to some extent individualized depending on their activities, they possess no legal personality. These authorities generally possess financial autonomy in the form of a budget annexed to the State or decentralized local authority's budget;

Autonomy: The public authority may also decide to give greater autonomy to a specific public service provider on account of the nature of its activity. This is the case of a public *statutory body,* an entity with distinct legal personality from that of the State or local authority on which it depends. The *statutory body*, which is specially created to manage a public service, receives its own budget and assets and may exercise full legal capacity (taking legal proceedings, issuing unilateral administrative acts and entering into contracts...). In the same way as a local authority, the statutory body consists of a decision-making body (the board of management) and of an executive authority. However, State stewardship of national public statutory bodies remains a fact, as the most important acts require the prior approval of the Ministries responsible. Despite this, the creation of a statutory body springs from a desire to offer greater flexibility for action by increasing the responsibility of decision makers as well as by fostering staff and user participation in the activity of the statutory body.

Depending on the national legal environment, the legal forms are different. Kenya has opted for the status of "State Corporation";[2] India uses "Medicare Relief Societies,[3]while Zambia has independently managed "national Institutions".[4] In the French-speaking world, after having used the status of "statutory body" (*établissement public*), several countries have now opted for the status of "public health establishment" (établissement public de santé).

Consequently, and depending on the specific features of national law, autonomy is circumscribed by some form of public stewardship; autonomy never rhymes with independence.[5] There are those, particularly in the English-speaking world, who propose a distinction between "autonomization" which corresponds to the notion of statutory body in the French-speaking world and "corporatization", a status under which management authority is more independent from the public purse.[6] Depending on the different national legal systems, this entity will take the form of a private or public limited company whose main shareholder is the State.

The notion of oversight in the context of decentralization and autonomy of providers

In the French speaking tradition the notion of *tutelle* refers to a specific function that gives the higher level public authority a set of control and supervision powers over an autonomous public entity. In the English speaking tradition no strictly equivalent concept exists, we shall thus refer here to the notion of oversight.

The notion of public oversight invokes national law and its specificity. However, at this point we shall recall a number of notions and principles. A public body that possesses a status of autonomy is not fully "independent" since it comes under an oversight authority ; in a manner of speaking it enjoys limited freedom.

1. A distinction is often made between administrative, financial and technical oversight:

- administrative oversight will be exercised by the administration: a representative of the administration will represent the State (the Ministry of Health) on the board of management;

- financial oversight: for example, an accountant will be appointed by the Treasury;

- technical oversight: as a rule, the Inspectorate is charged with technical oversight.

2. How is this (are these different forms of) oversight exercised?

Here too, there are substantial differences depending on the type of statutory body (*public administrative entity, public industrial and commercial entity and public health entity*) and national law. Nevertheless, we shall take a few examples:

- authority to give approval: the most important financial decisions (budget, loans, investments) only take effect after they have been approved by the oversight authority;

- authority to cancel: if the oversight authority considers that a decision is inadvisable, it may decide to cancel it. For example, public bodies operate in specialized fields (a hospital may not commercialize elsewhere its catering capacity): consequently, if a hospital were to open a restaurant, the oversight authority would cancel the decision;

- authority to substitute: the oversight authority may decide to substitute an item of expenditure or a decision with another.

The purpose of these institutional reforms is therefore to make provision for autonomy within the public sector. The two management models referred to above, i.e. devolution and autonomy, refer to unilateral acts by the public bodies that own the health facilities. Relations between the central authority of the Ministry of

Health and autonomous bodies nevertheless continue to be based on foundations that are not very different from the previous ones: for example, staff are often appointed and paid by the central authority, operating budgets are to a great extent determined by the same central authority and decisions on investment remain its prerogative. Nevertheless, there is a growing trend for these relations between public bodies to be governed by resorting to contracting. More and more frequently, health-service providers have to avail themselves of planning tools - operational plans or corporate plans - which form a basis for agreements with the health administration. In some cases, planning is formalized through contractual arrangements.

2. PRIVATE SECTOR INVOLVEMENT

Here, we are dealing with a distinct rationale; rather than seeking to improve things itself, the Ministry of Health will involve the private sector.

Privatization: in this case, for reasons of its own, the Ministry of Health decides that it no longer wishes to be involved in providing health services. It sells off its health facilities to a private for-profit or non-profit entity: this is known as *"divestment"*. The new owner will operate the facility as it wishes, subject of course to the reservation that it complies with the laws and regulations that apply in the country. For example, there may be a legal requirement for the Director of the facility to possess a certain qualification. It will be the responsibility of the Ministry of Health: 1) to ensure that the law is complied with, and 2) to exercise some degree of supervision over these establishments. This of course represents the deepest form of private-sector involvement.

The second possibility open to a Ministry of Health is that based on partnerships between the public and private sectors: this approach is generally described as *"public-private partnership"*. In its broadest sense, the term *"public-private partnership"* encompasses all kinds of association between the public and private sectors for the purpose of providing all or part of a public service. However, the terminology calls for some clarification; part of it poses no problem: the public and private sectors are associated in a common project. However, the word "partnership" is more problematic as well as being ambiguous: it may designate either someone sitting beside you, or someone sitting opposite you, but with whom you have a relationship. In the first case, we are within the rationale of "doing together": two actors reach an understanding to harness their efforts "on a day-to-day basis" to achieve a joint objective; there is an element of complementarity. In the second case, there is no desire to act jointly: the actors are partners simply because they have a relationship; this relationship determines the roles and responsibilities of each of them. We shall see from the situations described below that this is the commonest case. Nevertheless, we shall agree that a partnership exists from the moment that the association of the public and private sectors has made it possible to achieve a result that would have been out of reach without their coming together. However, this does not necessarily mean that they act together on a day-to-day basis to achieve this result. The key factor in the partnership is the explicit and accepted separation of the organizational, regulatory and operational functions of the essential services. By its nature, the organizational function belongs to the public authority. The regulatory function may be performed by the same authority or by an independent entity, depending on cultural or professional factors. The operational function is quite distinct: an operator, whether public or private, has to be chosen on the basis of its professional skills. The best way of choosing is by introducing competition to award the partnership contract, on the basis of criteria of performance. The public entity responsible for organizing or regulating cannot also be the operator without creating conflicts of interest, to the detriment of the service. This Public - Private partnership may take different forms.

Management by delegation

The rationale is as follows: the Ministry of Health wishes to retain ownership but no longer wishes to manage the health facility, either directly (direct management) or indirectly (autonomous entity). The Ministry of Health will seek an entity to manage the health facility in its place and on its behalf:

- In its place: this means that the Ministry of Health no longer takes day-to-day responsibility, if there is no more money to buy medicines, it is not the concern of the Ministry of Health, but of the manager;

- On its behalf: this means that the Ministry of Health is still concerned. Ultimate responsibility lies with the Ministry of Health: for example, if the health facility is not running smoothly, it is up to the Ministry of Health to act: it may, for example, take over management.

We may say that the entity is entrusted with running the facility. How is the assignee to be chosen?

The Ministry of Health has to choose its assignee. It may do so using either of the two main methods: a call for tenders or mutual consent:

- Call for tenders: when it employs this technique, the Ministry of Health relies on competition to produce the best bid. It assumes that there are several potential candidates who will compete with one another and submit tenders and that it will be able to choose the best of them (on the basis of criteria it has determined in advance);

- Mutual consent: The Ministry of Health considers that it knows which institutions are capable of taking on management by delegation, making it more efficient directly to discuss with the entities already identified.

The choice of either technique depends to quite a large extent on the context and consequently on the institutions capable of assuming this function.

It might be important for these methods of selection to have been determined at the national health policy level, or even better, at the level of a national policy on contracting. In this case, the rules are laid down and the Ministry of Health merely has to comply with them. If there are no predetermined rules, the Ministry of Health must each time redefine the methods by which it makes its choice, with drawbacks that are easy to imagine.

In particular, it is important to determine whether absolutely anyone can submit bids, or whether only certain kinds of candidate may do so. For example, it could be specified that only non-profit institutions may be candidates. If this is not specified, it means that for-profit institutions may submit bids: however, it may be difficult to eliminate them if they are capable, at least on paper, of submitting satisfactory bids.

The forms of delegated management: delegated management requires the drafting of a contract in which the Ministry of Health and the assignee agree on how the health facility is to be managed. This may adopt a diversity of forms which are themselves determined by national contexts and legislation. We shall focus on two situations distinguished by the degree of involvement of the private entity (the assignee) in the infrastructure and equipment:

- The private entity receives from the Ministry of Health the existing resources - the buildings and equipment- as they stand in order to perform the public service mission. As a rule, responsibility for the upkeep, maintenance work, and renewal are shared by the assignor and the assignee in the manner determined by the contract. Technically speaking, and in legal systems inspired by French practice, this is known as *affermage*; in the English legal system, it is referred to as *lease contract.* The resources remain the property of the State;

- The private entity takes responsibility for erecting the buildings and procuring the equipment. These will revert to the State when the agreement (which is generally a long-term one) expires. Under French law, this is known as *concession*; under English law, it is referred to as *Build, Operate, Transfer (B.O.T.).* The *concession* is usually reserved for cases in which there is already a public operator and thus the corresponding public service. However, where there is no public operator and the service has to be built up from scratch, we refer to "greenfield" projects;

- The *régie intéressée* (participative managerial authority), another form of contractual delegation of a public service, is distinguished from the other two forms of management by the fact that the assignee (the authority) does not act on his own account but on the account of the public authority. In this respect, he is not paid by the users, but by the public corporation. The level of remuneration depends on the authority's operating performance (improvements in productivity, savings achieved, quality of service provided...), as an incentive to optimizing management of the public service.

In all cases, either the contract will be time limited or the terms for the termination of the contract will have been determined. The Ministry of Health will thus be able to exercise its ultimate responsibility. If performance of the contract is unsatisfactory, the Ministry may take back management of the health facility to run it itself or entrust it to another operator who has been identified. Moreover, as the contract has a term, the operator is aware that it will not be automatically renewed and that the decision will depend on the evaluation made, and thus on the results achieved.

Fulfillment of the public service mission

A public health facility managed by the Ministry of Health fulfils a public service mission.

Definition

Characteristically, a public service is a service whose features, with regard to the needs of social organization and the expectations of users, are such that the mere play of market forces alone is unable to satisfy them. It is therefore an activity for whose organization or management the government must to some extent take responsibility.

The public service does not come into being naturally, it is the result of political will. It is the public authority (whether national or local) that determines the basic mission in response to a general need which it is responsible for identifying.

Constitutions impose on States, and thus on the services they establish, the duties of solidarity, equality and social justice. In most cases, the public service mission develops in sectors which are not covered by competitive market systems. This is because public service missions respond to fundamental social needs requiring long-term investment and hardly compatible with the norms of short-term profitability.

There are three founding principles that must be complied with when performing public service missions:

    a) continuity (the service must be assured round the clock and 365 days per year, it must be available everywhere....)

    b) equality (equality of access and treatment, non discrimination, to each according to his needs...)

    c) adaptability (the ability to adapt to the needs of populations, to the general interest and to technological challenges).

Normally the Ministry of Health wants to ensure that delegated management continues this public service mission. It is important that the rules adopted clearly affirm respect for this mission. This will considerably facilitate negotiations with assignees, as this point will be non-negotiable. Besides, if problems arise over the implementation of the contractual relationship, it will be easy for the Ministry of Health to invoke failure to observe the contractual public service mission clause.

Clearly these two elements - the way in which the assignee is chosen and respect for the public service mission - will make it possible for the Ministry of Health to avoid situations that would be hard to justify before public opinion or social organizations (trade unions, political parties). The task of choosing the assignee will be made far easier if the texts laying down these are clear.

Some actors (trade unions, political parties) see delegated management as a form of privatization and State withdrawal:

- It is clearly not privatization in the strict sense of the word because property rights are not transferred. However, management methods will clearly be more influenced by the private sector: as a rule, the staff will no longer be public servants, the accounts will no longer be kept by the public accounts office and the assignee will not be subject to the public procurement regulations but free to obtain supplies wherever he sees fit, etc.

- State withdrawal. It has to be admitted that in many cases the Ministry decides to introduce delegated management in order to free itself from responsibilities it no longer wishes to, or is unable to assume; in this case, it is fair to talk of withdrawal. However, if the decision has been taken after objective consideration of the strengths and weaknesses of the public and private sectors, it is not really fair to talk of withdrawal. Besides, and above all, there will be no withdrawal if the Ministry of Health fully performs its monitoring and supervisory role over the assignee. Here too, it has to be recognized that in many cases, the Ministry of Health does not actually perform its role but allows situations to get out of hand without acting before realizing, often too late, that the assignee has failed in its duties and obligations. In their defence, it also has to be admitted that the State frequently tends to neglect its commitments under delegated management: often, the State fails to pay to the assignee the promised grant or subsidies.

Finally, there are cases in which the concession concerns not a health facility, but a whole health district. Beginning in 1999, and with the support of a loan from the Asian Development Bank, the Cambodian Ministry of Health started drawing up four-year contracts with NGOs to provide health services for an entire health district. The contract covers health workers' wages, recurrent costs, drugs and consumable medical supplies. As for activities, the contract stipulates that the health services must deliver the minimum package for health centres and the supplementary package for district hospitals. The local administration, which depends on the Ministry of Health, retains responsibility for oversight of the health facilities under contract and for data collection. It is also required to report on the implementation of the contract and its smooth operation. From initial analyses, it would appear that the changes in the methods of work are so far-reaching that the NGOs given the contract by the Ministry of Health have difficulty in fully appreciating their new roles. Analyses have shown that by adopting this geographical approach the Ministry of Health offers the assignee the possibility of adopting a systemic approach to the district for which it is responsible, thus enabling it better to organize the local health system.

The association of a private health facility

From the point of view of the Ministry of Health, this is the opposite of the previous situation. In this case, a private institution owns and manages a health facility located somewhere in the country. The health facility, which has of course been authorized to operate (on the basis of a unilateral decision by the operator) has so far been operating in isolation, in other words it has pursued its activities as it has seen fit. However:

- The private health facility, which is no doubt non-profit (although this is not a sine qua non), wants its activities to be incorporated into national health policy: for example, the facility provides the minimum package of activities, charges the rates determined by the Ministry of Health and has satisfactory contacts with the area's health administration, etc.;

- The Ministry of Health, having considered the situation and observed the private health facility's behaviour, deems that it is not markedly different from any of the health facilities it operates directly. Moreover, the Ministry of Health is aware that in there is no public hospital in this area, that it lacks the means to build one and that even if it had the means, it would be wasteful for two hospitals to cover this area.

On the basis of these findings, the two institutions can collaborate to determine how they may better define their common interests. Rather than leaving the situation as it stands, (and it may well be satisfactory), they decide that it would be preferable to formalize an understanding that defines their positions.

Clearly, the starting point is the notion of "public service mission". The Ministry of health wants the private health facility to continue to perform, or better to perform the public service mission in the geographical area as would a public health facility. On this basis, the Ministry of Health and the private health facility will try to reach an understanding whose aim is to "associate the private health facility with the public service mission". "Associate" means that the private health facility will not be a public health facility: it will preserve its specific mode of operation. However, at the same time, "associate" means that the Ministry of Health recognizes that it performs a public service mission as if it were a public health facility.

Private organization that owns its own structures and has its own resources collaborates, is associated and thus performs a "public service mission " as it is under contract to the State; it thus becomes a contractual public service provider. For example, the church hospitals in Tanzania[7] and Ghana[8] are contractually the only referral facilities in a determined geographical area. In Zambia, the Memorandum of Understanding signed in 1996 by the Ministry of Health and the Church Medical Association of Zambia stipulates that the boards of management of the church-owned hospitals have the same powers as those in the public sector.[9] In many countries, these are actually implicit contracts. Thus, in Chad, the country's health map is organized around existing health facilities, whether public or private; the health map assigns to a private health facility responsibility for the health of the area's population, although the responsibility remains implicit. In order to avert numerous problems, it would often be worthwhile formalizing such recognition in contractual arrangement.

The association thus signifies mutual commitments:

- By awarding recognition, the Ministry of Health commits itself not to set up a public health facility in the area during the next few years. Furthermore, it will commit itself to helping the health facility to perform its public service mission. If this private health facility had not existed, it would have had to do something on behalf of the area's population. The aid may take very diverse forms: assignment of State employees, subsidies for certain activities, provision of certain items of equipment, help with improvements to buildings, purchase and/or supply of medicines, access to training at home or abroad, etc.. Naturally, in exchange, the Ministry of Health will have to agree to this facility's being run along private lines and to accept that certain activities will not be carried out exactly as it would like.

- From the point of view of the private institution, there are many advantages to this association with the State. In addition to the benefits described above, the role of the private institution is reinforced. It may pursue its mission without the risk of being challenged or threatened by the Ministry of Health. It needs no longer fear possible competition in its area. However, in exchange, it must agree to operate as the Ministry of Health wishes and accept a degree of interference, in so far as the Ministry of Health will have requirements which the institution does not necessarily fully agree.

Association is thus a contract which is impossible to fully assess on the basis of financial criteria alone. It is also a form of partnership, in the collaborative sense of the word. It calls for a common vision of the activities and how they are to be carried out. There has to be a common view of future trends; in this respect, it is not a contract that concerns the present.

It should also be borne in mind that private institutions may group themselves into a form of union: for example, AMCES in Benin. This Association brings together several institutions, each of which owns one or more health facilities, including hospitals. It may be in the Association's interest, and in that of the Ministry of Health, not to sign specific contracts on association with each of these facilities, but to sign a framework agreement associating it with the public service mission. This framework agreement may entirely replace specific contracts or simply provide a framework for specific contracts of association to be signed under the framework agreement. The framework agreement thus lays down the main lines of association with the public service mission.

Both the private institutions and the Ministry of Health may achieve economies of scale thanks to this procedure. There is no need to "reinvent the wheel" for each health facility; it will be possible to negotiate many points just once and apply them to several health facilities.

Lastly, we should point out that these private institutions that own and run health facilities may not fulfill a public service mission. This does not prevent the Ministry of Health, in addition to affording recognition for their activity through a system of accreditation, from developing contractual arrangements with them in order to determine such collaboration or support as may be necessary in exchange for the activities they perform.

Partnership contracts

Since the beginning of the 1990s, in some OECD countries the concept of Public-Private Partnership (PPP) has developed. In comparison with the forms of contract explored above, PPP is distinguished by the fact that the private operator is not remunerated by users or by the public, but by the public entity who drew up the contract. To take the example of a Ministry of Health or a public health establishment that wants to build new infrastructure. Traditionally, they would first of all have to come up with the necessary funds before, as the client, finding a designer to draw up the project then a principal contractor to manage the building work. On completion of the building work, they would then have to find a firm to ensure maintenance of the infrastructure (in all respects: maintenance of the buildings and equipment, but also catering, caretaking, laundry services etc.). There are several drawbacks to this kind of arrangement, not the least of which is the search for funding, as public institutions do not necessarily have easy access to financial markets. Moreover, it is no easy matter for small hospitals to take on the responsibilities of client and they have to delegate this responsibility. The hospital finds itself handling numerous separate contracts.[10] The PPP approach makes it possible to simplify this process. The public actor passes through a private partner (or a group (consortium) of private actors) who will assume responsibility for all the separate functions described above. It will finance, design, build and maintain the infrastructure; to use the infrastructure, the public actor will pay a fee to the private company. The hospital is thus freed of any concern with running the hospital and is able to fully assume its main role: providing care. The characteristics of a PPP arrangement are described below:

- The public actor continues to perform the activity carried out in the infrastructure;
- Ownership of the infrastructure, at least for the duration of the contract, is in the hands of the private actor;
- Responsibility for financing the operation lies with the private actor;
- As a rule, the private actor belongs to the for profit sector;
- PPP is not restricted to the health sector: we come across it in sectors as diverse as education, highways, transport, water resources or prisons.

Definition

A Public-Private Partnership contract is a long-term contract whereby a public body associates a private-sector enterprise in the financing, design, construction and operation of a public structure.

Compared to the general public-private partnership concept, the PPP (Public-Private Partnership - the capital Ps are important) has a technical definition laid down above. Some of the literature on "public-private partnerships" is in fact solely focused on the PPPs; where as for some others PPPs are only a marginal element of a global partnership approach including private and public actors. Thus it is important to keep in mind that there exists these two levels of conceptual understanding of what is a public-private partnership.

There are advantages to this technique. It lightens the burden on public finances and thus the public debt. There is no need for the State to come up with the financial resources needed for the investment. At the same time, the State gets over two ideological hurdles: it is able to reduce its influence while avoiding privatization.

The advocates of Public - Private Partnership frequently put forward competition among private actors as one of its benefits. This purportedly enables the public sector to benefit from competition to secure the best service at the lowest cost.

For policy makers, the Public-Private - Partnership is beneficial because it enables short term investment without the need to commit the public purse. This is clearly a short-term advantage; moreover, when the drawbacks appear (the need to reimburse!), the policy maker will most probably no longer be in the same position.

The advocates of Public - Private Partnership stress that the technique makes it possible to shift the risks from the Ministry of Health on to the private partner; the Ministry of Health has nothing to worry about nor need it be concerned about unforeseen events, as these are the responsibility of the private partner.

The Ministry of Health can call on the most competent private actors, who are no doubt more competent than the Ministry itself as they possess specialized know-how while the core concern of the Ministry is with health.

In comparison with a traditional investment, the private actor is concerned by the building of the infrastructure, as well as by its operation. He will be attentive to operating costs and take them better into account when building.

What aspects require particular attention when this type of contracting is used?

The Ministry of Health loses know-how and becomes dependent on the private actors who may in the long run take advantage of this situation.

Supervisory costs: these are rarely included in comparative cost-benefit analyses of the public and private sectors. The difficulty lies in the unpredictable nature of these costs. Moreover, the cost of drawing up contracts and agreements between public and private partners is also frequently not included in cost-benefit models. Even if this cost is taken into account, it is the result of sketchy hypotheses. In addition, those enterprises, which are frequently multinationals, with the capacity to participate in large-scale infrastructure projects, have far greater financial, human and legal resources than the governmental agencies and ministries responsible for negotiating public - private agreements. This is compounded by the experience they have garnered from previous agreements favouring these private firms and detrimental to the public partner. Overall the PPP approach often yields agreements that are poorly put together and restrictive, which do not produce any real savings and which moreover make the public sector dependent on the chosen private partner. This dependence will clearly be of use to the private enterprise during future negotiations. We can thus conclude from the range of experience already available that the actual long-term consequences of Public-Private Partnerships are never taken into account when they are drawn up, giving a positive slant to the purported efficiency of such partnerships.

The short-term benefits may prove to be more than offset by the long-term costs. This makes it imperative to be vigilant and to adopt a long-term view in order to evaluate a Public -Private Partnership.

Illustrative examples

Great-Britain, which introduced the *Private Finance Initiative* (PFI), in 1992, is no doubt the pioneer in this respect. On 1 July 2002, there were a total of 105 PFI contracts in the health sector.

The Barnett Hospital in London and the West Middlesex Hospital in Isleworth signed a PFI contract with the Bouyges Construction group and its English subsidiary Ecovert. The value of the second of these was 110 million euros for the "design-construction" component and 100 million euros for the "facilities management" component. For a period of 35 years, the hospital will pay an annual rent of some 15 million euros (indexed on the cost of living). The maintenance and canteen staff as well as the guards work for a new employer, but not the medical staff. On termination of the contract, the hospital will recover the land and buildings. A major advantage of PFI is that they enable the government to shift onto the private sector any risks deriving from cost overruns and delays. According to the British Treasury, one PFI out of five exceeds its budget, in comparison with seven out of ten when the State was the sole financier. Moreover, almost nine PFI out of ten are "delivered" on time in comparison with three out of ten under the traditional arrangement. Steve Turner, of the West Middlesex University Hospital confirmed "We got exactly what we asked for, on time and without exceeding our budget". There is no doubt that the private sector has every interest in fulfilling its commitments. The consortium receives its first payments only when the work is completed. In addition, it bears the cost of any overruns and the payments may be reduced if the services prove unsatisfactory. Mere failure to replace a light bulb on time gives the public authority grounds for reducing its monthly payment. The formula is a popular one: when it acts as client, the State is compelled to borrow. With a PFI, the loan is taken out by the private partner, the State merely paying "rent". This enables the Government to renew its infrastructure without increasing its debt.

In **Australia**, Public-Private Partnerships have developed considerably in recent years as part of a strategy quite similar to that followed in Great Britain: The State of Victoria pioneered this trend by adopting, in 2000, a detailed PPP policy. We should also mention the experience of the Darent Valley Hospital and of the Berwick Community Hospital. In the case of the latter, the contract with the ad hoc private consortium set up for the operation covers financing, design, construction and maintenance (provision of information services, maintenance of public spaces, security and parking facilities). In exchange, this public hospital will pay a rent for 25 years before ownership of the hospital reverts to the State.

Quebec province has been largely inspired by Great Britain, and is developing the same approach, which it has officialised through Act 61 of 2004, establishing the Quebec Public-Private Partnerships agency. The mission of this agency is to help, with its advice and expertise, to renovate public infrastructure and improve the quality of services provided to citizens as part of the implementation of Public-Private Partnerships. Its role is to provide public agencies with consultancy services of all kinds for evaluating the feasibility of PPP projects, for negotiations and for the conclusion and management of such projects. However, no such projects have so far been signed in the health sphere.

In **France**, the "Hospitals" decree of 4 September 2003 has authorized the use of "long-term *(emphyteutic) hospital leases" (BEH)*, a particular type of partnership contract, and established the National Mission to Support Investment in Hospitals (MAINH). This is a form of contractual arrangement covering the funding, design, construction, maintenance and operation of the building and in some cases the overall provision of services associated with it. However, the BEH strictly excludes care missions, which are the exclusive preserve of the public sector. The hospital establishment thus becomes a very long-term tenant (from 18 to 99 years). At the beginning of 2005, fourteen such projects were being developed.

Except in the case of Great Britain, we do not possess sufficient hindsight to evaluate this strategy. However, we should mention that the strategy has given rise to intense debate or even hostility. Without going into details, the main criticism concerns the level of privatization of the health service as a result of the use of these Public-Private Partnerships. The trade unions, as well as some political parties, see them as an opportunity for the private (for profit) sector to infiltrate public services. Some critics go event further and claim that this strategy is a way of avoiding direct privatization, which is always politically sensitive, while achieving the same result, i.e. de facto privatization. The second criticism concerns the cost of these operations: several analyses have shown that the expected savings are sometimes illusory and that, when all is said and done, these operations are ultimately very costly for the public purse.

Public-Private Investment partnership (PPIP)

Whereas PPPs limit to investments for construction and maintenance, PPIPs go beyond this by adding the element of health service provision. This is thus a case of Design, Build, Operate and Deliver (DBOD), where the word "deliver" is central, since in this arrangement the core activity - health service provision - is operated by the private consortium. Currently, the only existing case in developing countries is in Lesotho where the consortium Tsepong Limited is operating a project involving the national reference hospital and three clinics.

It should be noted that a PPIP is conceptually close to a concession. One of the most important point of distinction lies in the fact that in a PPIP the government takes care of financing, whereas in a concession the users are the direct payers. For example in Lesotho, the government provides the funding which is defined by the number of people covered to whom the hospital must offer a pre-defined set of services. The payment system is defined so that the government will not be paying more than it was paying before the PPIP for the same hospital services.

CONCLUSION

These different forms of public-private partnership for building and running health facilities have blossomed in recent years in the developed countries. However, they are still a rare occurrence in the developing countries, with the exception of arrangements associating private health facilities and the public service mission. There are multiple reasons for this:

- Contractual relations within the framework of public-private partnership are never a simple matter. They call for a high level of technical qualifications from both public and private actors, a requirement that cannot always be satisfied in the developing countries;

- Once this type of operation has begun, it is hard to reverse the process. It is not easy, and it is certainly costly, to terminate a contractual concession or partnership. The difficulty of reversing the process is perhaps one of the reasons why public sector decision-makers hesitate to take the plunge;

- Public-private partnership is to a large extent perceived by public-sector actors as a loss of power. There are also those who would point out that it also represents a loss of the possibility to benefit from the operation of the public service as a source of income and jobs. This potential source of corruption would thus escape the control of public-sector players who will consequently prefer to carry on with operation by the public sector which, although less advantageous for the population, is more beneficial for them;

- Finally, a public-private partnership is still a thorny political choice. Charges of privatization, of withdrawal by the State and of selling off public services are never far from peoples' minds, particularly since there are numerous examples to bolster such charges. For these reasons, policy makers or often reluctant to adopt these new trends which are still perceived as reforms advocated by the adepts of the free market and by the international institutions that seek to promote it.

As we now see in the developed countries, public-private partnership is no longer a tool used at the national level; public-private partnerships are increasingly a global development. Some international firms are developing this type of operation using not only huge resources but highly sophisticated expertise. It is very difficult for the developing countries to handle this. Should they be tempted by the siren songs of these large firms, will they be able to avoid becoming their victims?

Notes

[1] Morocco has adopted this formula by setting up second-level hospitals as autonomously managed services. However, the limits of their performance have given an incentive to assign them autonomy along the same lines as that granted to the university teaching hospitals.

[2] Collins, D., G. Njeru, J. Meme, and W. Newbrander. 1999. *Hospital autonomy: the experience of Kenyatta National Hospital. International Journal of Health Planning and Management* 14:129-153.

[3] Sharma, S. and D. R. Hotchkiss. 2001. *Developing financial autonomy in public hospitals in India: Rajasthan's model. Health Policy* 55:1-18.

[4] McPake, B. 1996. Public autonomous hospitals in sub-Saharan Africa: trends and issues. *Health Policy* 35:155-177.

[5] Bossert, Th, S. Kosen, B. Harsono, and A. Gani. *Hospital autonomy in Indonesia.* 1996. USA, Harvard School of Public Health. 1-30-0010.

This document may be consulted on the Internet: consultation of the web site of the Harvard School of Public Health, USA, dated 30 January 2001:

http://www.hsph.harvard.edu/ihsg/publications/pdf/No-39.PDF.   This study stresses that within the framework of this autonomy, the Ministry of Health continues to supervise the planning procedure and budgeting of revenue from cost recovery.   In this way, the directors of these autonomous hospitals are required to submit an annual plan for the use of their own funds.

[6] Mills, A., S. Bennett, and S. Russell. 2001. *The challenge of health sector reform. What must Government Do?*: Palgrave.

[7] Bura, M. 1998. *Church-related Hospitals contracted as Designated District Hospitals: Tanzanian Experiences.* 1998, at WHO Geneva.

[8] Yeboah, Y. 1999. *Contracting: the case of Ghana from the perspective of the Christian Health Association of Ghana (CHAG).* 5 19990, at Dar Es Salam, Tanzania.

[9] Hanson, K., L. Atuyambe, J. Kamwanga, B. McPake, O. Mungule, and F. Ssengooba. 2002. *Towards improving hospital performance in Uganda and Zambia: reflections and opportunities for*

[10] As a rule, a new corporation is set up for each PPP: an SPV, (*special purpose vehicle*). It comprises a builder, an operator (frequently a subsidiary of the builder) and one or several financiers (usually banks). There are two components to operations: building and operation

Part II

Chapter 2

Hospitals and contracting

Eric de Roodenbeke & Jean Perrot

"The hospital is one of the original creations of Western Christian medieval towns. The etymology of the word hospital is illuminating, not only from a historical perspective, but also as regards the modern concept of hospitals. "Domus hospitalis", or "guest house", became "hospitalis" in the Middle Ages. The word itself comes from "hostis", the stranger, whether friend - "guest", or enemy - a "hostile" being. The hospital does, indeed, have two sides, the two faces of Janus, that simultaneously attract and repel. It embodies all the ambiguities of a place that is primarily intended for the poor and elderly, regardless of infirmity. Afterwards it became a place to treat highly complex diseases, before returning to its original role of admitting vulnerable people, for whom hospitals are very often a last resort"

French Hospital Federation

Hospitals have always occupied a particular place in health-care systems. They are places where great medical experts work, and the population, particularly when in need of their services, generally affords them respect and consideration. Furthermore, hospitals have always taken in indigents afflicted by illness. Today the expertise and complexity of hospitals has increased considerably, but this does not mean that they are an ivory tower for the professionals who work there. Needs evolve and hospitals must adapt and modernize,[1] without necessarily associating modernity with the introduction of advanced technology, particularly in low-income countries.

This need to adapt is realized through ongoing reforms, which affect the most advanced and developing countries in equal measure. While the scope and context of these reforms varies, two questions are always at the heart of the reform process: What place and role should be given to hospitals, and how can the production process be optimized while meeting the needs and expectations of the population?

In recent years, contracting has increasingly been used as a tool to undertake these reforms. It provides hospitals with a formal framework for its relationships with stakeholders. However, this tool presents different facets depending on how it is used and what are its predetermined objectives.

Contracting opens up a range of possibilities for improving hospital performance. However, while the advantages of using contracting are many, the difficulties, misgivings and political issues that underlie contracting need to be emphasized. One should never underestimate the fact that the large-scale use of contracting requires technical expertise that is not always present in modern

126

hospitals and entails costs for formalizing and developing contractual relationships, especially for implementing and monitoring them.

1. STATUS OF HOSPITALS

Considering hospitals in regard to their form of ownership, there are two main categories, namely public hospitals and private hospitals.

> - *Public hospitals are public corporations: in many countries the national government owns public hospitals. But public hospitals can also be owned by regional and local authorities. They can also be autonomous entities under public law*

> - *Private hospitals are privately owned. They are not-for-profit if owned by NGOs, associations, foundations or religious communities. They are profit-making if owned by private individuals, private companies or businesses.*

Table 1: Wide variation in the status of public and private entities:

Public hospitals	National hospitals	Specialized hospitals	Municipal hospitals	Autonomous hospitals	Military hospitals
Not-for-profit private hospitals	Institutions run by not-for-profit associations	Institutions run by foundations	Institutions run by religious communities	Cooperative-based institutions	
Commercial hospitals	Group-owned networks	Clinics in individual ownership	Clinics in public limited company ownership	Clinics in civil real estate company ownership	Clinics attached to companies

Considering mission rather than status, hospitals can also be divided into those that operate according to a public-service mandate, and those that provide private services. As we will show later, distinguishing between types of mission is more useful for distinguishing between types of contract, rather than describing all the elements of the contractual approach. The distinction between different types of ownership status will be a recurring theme when describing contracting arrangements in the hospital sector.

127

1.1 The public sector

For a long time public hospitals were devolved from the Ministry of Health, and in many countries this is still the case. Depending on their size and status, they are administered directly by the Ministry of Health or by the administrative subdivision representing the Ministry; the hospital director and staff are appointed centrally by the Ministry of Health and public finance rules apply. This model gives the central authorities the power to control the hospital's activities and the allocation of public funds. But obviously this system generates a lot of red tape and inefficiency. As a reaction to this situation, various developments are currently taking place.

Privatization of the public sector is the most radical solution. The State, aware of its own inefficiency, lets the for-profit or not for-profit private sector, expand into the provision of health services. It might even go as far as to transfer ownership of its hospitals to the private sector. The degree of formality or competitiveness of the sale may vary. Thus privatized, the hospital leaves the public domain and enters the private sector. The new owner manages it directly. In reality, relatively few countries have actually taken this approach: we will see for example that some socialist bloc countries such as Romania, opted for this radical solution after the fall of communism.

To offset the poor performance of public hospitals without resorting to privatization, the government (not the Ministry of Health) may, in the context of general administrative decentralization, decide to transfer responsibility for hospitals to local authorities. Although there exist many permutations depending on the type of decentralization envisaged, generally speaking, first-tier hospitals are transferred to municipalities, second-tier hospitals to regional authorities, while in most cases national referral hospitals remain under central control.

However, as stated in the previous chapter, local authorities will face the same issue as the Ministry of Health, i.e. how should they manage the hospitals under their control? Assuming that they refrain from direct administration, the Ministry of Health or the local authorities, as hospital owners, can use the following management models:

Devolution: compared with direct management, devolution is without a doubt the method through which the public bodies give up least of their prerogatives. The administrative burden associated with control is lightened by transferring certain management prerogatives to the hospital, thereby enabling it to boost its efficacy. This type of devolution takes various forms depending on national law; it can range from a simple delegation of powers or signature from the administrative controller for a set of actions to full-fledged administrative and financial autonomy (a separate

128

budget) within the public body.[2] At the same time, the hospital remains under the direct control of the Ministry and its decentralized services. It has no separate legal personality. The day-to-day management of the hospital is improved, but the underlying operational mechanisms remain the same. This type of devolution does not radically change the incentive regime. The overall strategic stewardship remains the responsibility of the State or the local authority;

Autonomy: This concept takes various forms, but the idea behind it can be readily defined.[3] Dissatisfied with direct management, the government prompts the hospital to show greater enterprise while ultimately remaining under its control. Autonomy goes much further than devolution, while keeping the hospital in the public sector and under public control. The main features of autonomy are:

- The autonomous hospital stays in the public sector, even though its assets are owned by the legal entity that has been established;

- It has a specific legal personality governed by public [administrative] law;

- There is a separation of the roles of the board of directors, which defines the institution's policies and sets its strategic direction, and the hospital management, which ensures day-to-day management and implements the board's decisions,[4, 5]

- The hospital's budget is drafted and administered separately;

- However, human resources issues are dealt with in a multitude of ways: some autonomous hospitals are almost entirely responsible for their own recruitment and human resources management, whereas at other hospitals only certain posts[6] are left to the hospital's discretion;

- Legal forms vary in accordance with the national legal order. Kenya has "State corporations".[7] India has "Medicare Relief Societies".[8] Zambia has independently managed "national institutions".[9] In the French-speaking world, a number of countries have switched from "Public Administrative Institutions (PAEs)" to "Public Health-care Establishment (PHEs)". This is the case in France and a number of French-speaking countries in Africa, for example in Senegal.

Public health-care establishments. Case study: France

Public health-care establishments (PHEs) are legal entities under public law, responsible for managing a public service defined by law. The management autonomy granted to PHEs does not free them from the oversight of the public authorities, which supervise core operational issues such as finances. PHEs have a legal personality and financial autonomy, but are accountable to the representative of the public authority who ensures that they are fulfilling their public service obligations properly.

The creation of a public establishment reduces administrative burdens, increases managerial flexibility and promotes greater responsibility and involvement of staff.

The governing bodies include:

- A deliberative body, the board of directors, comprising local authority representatives, staff representatives (physicians, nurses, etc.), qualified experts, user representatives, and financial bodies. The board of directors defines the institution's general policies and approves its budget. The deliberative body has limited authority and little room for manoeuvre, owing to the national statutes and rules applicable to the institution and owing to the fact that .the executive body, which has the technical expertise, can play a major role in setting the general strategic directions of the institution.

- An executive body headed by a manager a professional hospital administrator who is appointed by the Minister of Health on the recommendation of the chairman of the board of directors.

Its operations are based on three core principles: autonomy, specialization and administrative attachment:

- Autonomy allows the institution to have governing bodies and to manage its own assets and legal, material and financial resources. Financial autonomy is essential to enable the institution to draw on the resources it needs without being permanently dependent on its supervising authority.

- The specialization of a public institution is outlined in its statutes, which confer upon it a specific mandate and define the nature of its activities. It cannot operate in other areas (there are a few historical exceptions to this, managed autonomously).

- Administrative attachment enables the authority that set up the institution to exercise supervision over it, specifically by approving the budget and the important decisions of the deliberative and executive bodies. This linkage may be more or less constricting depending on the institution's statutes. Public health-care establishments are supervised by the public authorities, namely:

     o   Public health-care establishment accountants work for the Treasury, thus following the well-established principle in French administrative structures that the executive (in this case the hospital director) should be kept separate from the accounting arm;

     o   The budget must be submitted to the regional hospital agency, which has the power to request any changes it deems necessary (for example certain expenses connected with national commitments);

     o   Public health-care establishments must follow regulations on public procurement;

     o   Decisions of the board of directors must be approved by the supervisory authority.

Consequently, and depending on the specificities of national law, autonomy operates within a public oversight framework; it is never synonymous with independence.[10] Some, particularly in the English-speaking world, propose a distinction between "autonomization" (corresponding to the concept of a public establishment in French-speaking countries) and "corporatization", in which management has more independence from the treasury.[11] Depending on national law, this entity will take the form of a limited company at private or public law in which the State is the principal shareholder.

The two management models outlined above, namely devolution and autonomy, concern unilateral actions by the public bodies that own the hospital. In the third model proposed below, namely delegated management, contractual arrangements play a significant role in the relationship between the public authorities, the funding body, and the service provider.

Delegated management: The public body delegates to an external body the responsibility for managing, on its behalf, an activity of public interest and the related infrastructures. Although the initiative to delegate management originates with the public authorities that own the hospital, they cannot impose it, as in the two models outlined above; they must negotiate with an operator and establish a contractual relationship to formalize the nature and scope of the delegated management. Through the contractual relationship, the operator (the party that has agreed to manage the hospital) assumes responsibility for the management of the service entrusted to him; accordingly, the operator will be responsible for his actions and will be answerable to service users. Notwithstanding this, the public authorities do not withdraw completely from the process; ultimate responsibility still lies with them. So if the operator falls short, the public authorities have the opportunity and in some cases the obligation to intervene and regain control of the activity delegated to the operator.

Two models can be distinguished, according to the extent of involvement of the private body (to which the management has been delegated to) in the infrastructure and equipment:

- The private body is entrusted with existing assets (buildings and equipment) by the Ministry of Health, in their current state of repair, in order to perform its public-service mandate. Repair, maintenance and renovation work is normally shared between the parties, in accordance with the terms of the contract. The technical term of this arrangement in the French legal tradition is *affermage* and in Anglophone legal tradition it is referred to as *lease contract*. The assets remain the property of the State.

- The private body is responsible for constructing the necessary buildings and acquiring equipment. These then revert to the State when the contract (usually a long-term one) expires. This is referred to as a Build-Operate-Transfer (BOT) contract in the Anglophone legal tradition and *concession* in the French legal tradition.

A number of criteria can be applied to gauge the degree of independence enjoyed by a public hospital. D.Collins et al. (1999)[12] suggests three:

- Governance: who owns the hospital and sets its policies;

- Management: how are the different management functions (human resources management, supplies, logistics, maintenance, etc.) carried out; -
- Funding: what are the hospital's sources of funding, in particular budget allocations versus patient fees.

A combination of these three criteria is very useful for determining the extent of a hospital's independence. As D. Collins et al. point out, there are cases in which there is no autonomy with respect to governance (the hospital continues to operate under the direct authority of the Ministry of Health), whereas day-to-day management is to a great extent delegated and funding comes mainly from patients, either directly or through insurance.

The diagram below, which summarizes the concepts explained above in respect of public hospitals, can also be used to help better identify the status of hospitals and the degree of their independence:

Diagram 1: Arrangements for organizational reform of public hospitals

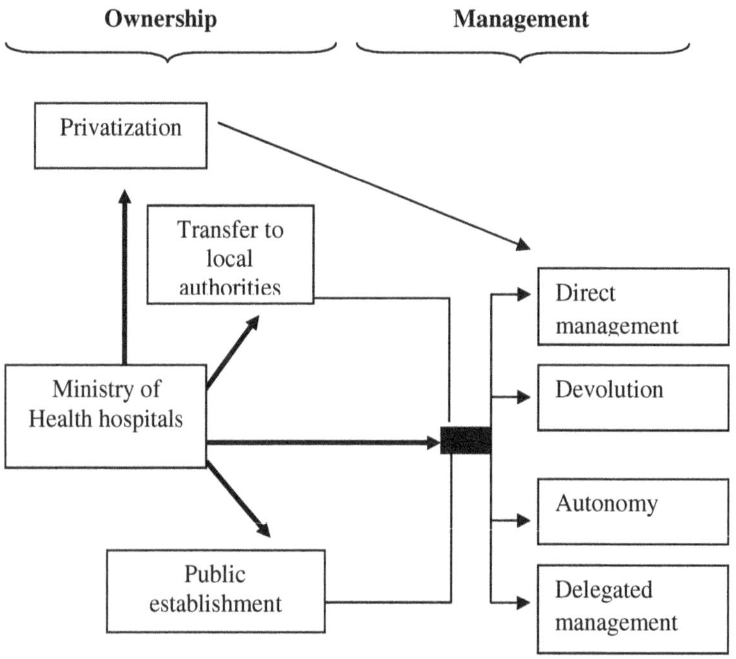

Ownership   Management

Privatization

Transfer to local authorities

Direct management

Ministry of Health hospitals

Devolution

Autonomy

Public establishment

Delegated management

1.2   The private sector

Private hospital facilities exist in most countries. They are often the result of history and market opportunities. Their private owners built them, acquired them from other private owners, or may have acquired them during the privatization of public hospitals.

Private owners manage their hospitals directly. However, the legal status of the hospital determines the operational details of this direct management. A hospital owned by one person will be managed by its owner (which is relatively rare), a commercial hospital will be managed by its board of owner-directors, which will establish an executive body, and a hospital belonging to a NGO, association, foundation or religious community will follow the rules of these organizations (a distinction is generally made between deliberative and executive bodies). The Faith Based actors often establish "subsidiary" associations which are responsible for the management of these hospitals.

A hospital, however, is not a business like any other. Since it deals with public health, it cannot function independently of all social monitoring. Its activities may be framed in the following contexts:[13]

- *Laws and regulations*: any business must respect the laws and regulations of the country in which it is based. In the health sector, however, laws and regulations are generally greater in number and more restrictive than in the rest of the economy. The scope of these legal obligations will depend on the oversight capabilities of the public authorities.

- *Licensing*: owing to the specific nature of the health sector, prior authorization is often required for operating health activities. Licensing enables an organization to conduct its activities lawfully. Licences are normally issued by the Ministry of Health. The criteria for issuing licences are usually defined by regulations and concern mandatory requirements regarding qualifications, types of facilities and premises, operating procedures, etc. Licensing tells the population that the hospital fulfils minimum safety requirements and that the professional staff working there have the necessary qualifications.

- *Accreditation*: is an external evaluation process, conducted by an independent organization separate from the hospital and its supervisory bodies, and covering all its operations and practices. Accreditation aims to ensure the safety and quality of care provided, and also to promote an ongoing policy of quality development within the health-care institution. Accreditation is a unilateral act: it is granted or refused by the organization mandated to do so. The hospital cannot negotiate the terms or rules of the accreditation process. Accreditation may be required to obtain funding, either in exchange for services or to develop new activities. It can also form part of national health-care priorities, to promote hospitals that contribute to these priorities. In theory, accreditation procedures should be identical in the public and private sectors.

- *Association*: when a private hospital and the Ministry of Health wish to strengthen their cooperation, they can formalize this relationship in the form of an association. When the modalities of this association are specifically set out in a legal framework, the association will result in a standard-form contract. If the possibility of association is broached without any major legal constraints, a contractual relationship that results from freely entered-into negotiations will formalize the terms of the agreement between the public authorities and the private hospital. The association between them may be:

    - Full and entire. In this case, the hospital commits to operating in a public service context; on the other hand, the Ministry of Health recognizes that the private institution is carrying out a public service mandate on an equal footing with public hospitals. The contract will set forth the commitments of each party to fulfil this public service mandate. In practical terms, this is quite similar to the delegated management model discussed above. The main difference, however, is that the hospital remains in private hands. The public authority (central government or local authority) that signed the contract may terminate it, but the ownership will always stay with the private sector operator (unless nationalization occurs);

    - Limited. In this case, the private hospital does not commit to performing all its activities in a public service context. However, since the Ministry of Health recognizes the health facility's contribution to public health, and because the private hospital wishes to integrate more of its activities into the framework of national health policy, both parties are able to conclude a contract that sets out the scope and details of their collaboration.

Association leads to greater recognition of the private hospital's contribution and might help it to acquire the resources to make this contribution. For its part, the Ministry of Health is able to persuade the private hospital to make a bigger contribution to implementing national health policy.

1.3   The "public/private" distinction according to status, mandate and funding

Legal form of ownership enables a precise distinction to be drawn between the private and public sectors. When considering types of mandate, the division is not so obvious. Funding arrangements must also be taken into account, since they guide hospital practices and can blur the line between public and private.

With respect to the legal environment, some of the rules governing the hospital sector apply to the private and public sectors in equal measure. In certain cases, however, public status implies an obligation to serve the public interest. This can negate the need of formulating legal constraints that should apply when a hospital's activities are profit-driven (for example limiting the risk of multiplying unnecessary but lucrative procedures).

The most restrictive rules in the public sector apply to production factors and management methods (staff status, public accounting, government contracts, etc.). In the private sector, constraints primarily affect production conditions (licensing, safety standards, etc.). This distinction should be borne in mind before concluding a contract, since it will determine the areas in which the contract can have the greatest impact.

Mandates play a major role in examining the scope of contracting. Indeed, the contractual approach goes beyond the economic rationale of governing production activities through contracts under common law. It also deals specifically with the strategies that organizations use to increase their performance. This approach is particularly interesting because it touches on areas that mainly lie outside market mechanisms. Thus, contracts can be fully applied in a range of legal contexts, but the same theme reappears time after time: the optimization of hospitals' performance to serve their public interest mandate. For example, in order to ensure a certain equality of access to services, it might prove useful to give prominence to the public interest. An accident and emergency service can be used to illustrate this situation. Billing users of the service at cost recovery basis would make it unaffordable for many; impeding access   in this way would go against the very reason for the service's existence. The emergency service can be regarded as a public good, since its existence also benefits those who do not use it (i.e. it provides a sense of security). The distinction between public good and private service is important to bear in mind when drawing up contracts with hospitals, irrespective of their status. The emergency service example demonstrates that, it is the supply of service rather than the activity itself that needs to be funded. The table below

135

summarizes the permutations of status and mandate and their impact on the contractual context.

Table 2: Impact of status and mandate on the contractual context

Status Mandate	Public hospital	Not-for-profit private hospital	Commercial private hospital
Public interest activity	Public hospital service	Full association	Limited association
Private activity	Subject to special provisions	General legal structure	General legal structure

The issue of funding, which has not been explicitly mentioned, underpins the contractual relations that have been developed in the hospital sector. Depending on the funding mechanism in question, contractual agreements will be more or less effective, particularly as regards the relative weight of public money, payments by individuals or insurance (social, private commercial or cooperative) that are used to fund the hospital's activities.

Without detailing the impact of various funding mechanisms, it is important to recall that contractual arrangements are based on the mobilization of resources in exchange for the provision of services. Contractual arrangements are only credible when they result from voluntary actions by the parties involved, each of whom must have the means to uphold their commitments.

Where a paying third party is present, the formation of a contract is more complex than in bilateral situations. However, as we shall see subsequently, it is precisely in this situation, where market mechanisms are less effective, that contracting offers the most possibilities. It prompts the service provider to seek performance, while the oversight authority has no direct control over the funding of activities. France is a good illustration of this, in that contracting enables the public authorities to promote developments without making direct use of constraints or developing a client-provider relationship in respect of purchasing hospital services.

The hospital contracting context is rooted in status, mandates and funding arrangements, whereas the legal context underpins the way that contracting arrangements function. Together, these different aspects generate so many permutations that it is not possible to propose a globally applicable contracting policy. It is therefore preferable to list the different types of contractual relationship and their implications, so as to enable interested parties to identify the solution best suited to their priority objectives in the light of possible developments in their respective legal frameworks.

2. USE OF CONTRACTING BY A HOSPITAL

In the previous section, we sketched the institutional context in which hospitals operate, from the perspectives of ownership, management and mandate. We shall now consider the hospital as a health service provider. A hospital can thus be seen as the centre of a node of contracts connecting it to all the partners with whom it could potentially establish a relationship. Here we shall expand on all of these possibilities. In reality, a hospital will not necessarily use all of them. The hospital's institutional policy, based on detailed analysis of its situation, will enable it to determine which contracting scenarios to pursue in the short and long term. This contracting potential is even more important when the hospital is independently responsible for the use of production factors as well as its mode of production. Contracting means that a client/supplier relationship is central to exchanges within the institution, as well as those between the institution and external parties.

Diagram 2 : Contracting possibilities

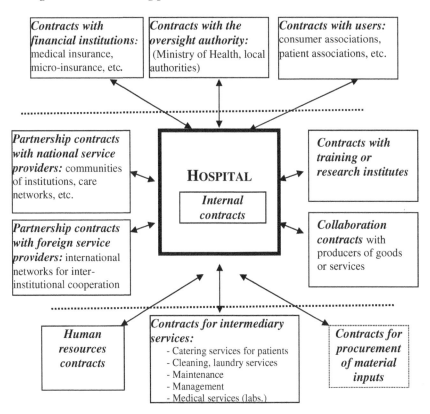

2.1 "External" contracting

External contracting refers to all contractual relations that a hospital develops with external partners.

"Vertical" external contracting

It is useful to refer to the theory of agency and the concepts of "*principal*" and "*agent*". Vertical external contracting places the hospital either in the position of a *principal* ("downstream") or that of an *agent* ("upstream").

Downstream vertical contracting

Downstream vertical contracting refers to the relationships that the hospital develops with the partners who provide the hospital with the resources it needs to function. It involves basic inputs, both physical and human, and also the provision of intermediary services, which can include logistical and administrative activities as well as health-care activities.

The table below summarizes the different possibilities depending on the object of the contract and the hospital's status.

Table 3: Downstream vertical contracting options

Ownership	PUBLIC (State, local authorities)				PRIVATE	
Management	*Direct*	*Devolved*	*Autonomous*	*Delegated management*	*Direct*	*Direct with association*
Material resources	Procurement contracts under the government contracts code				Procurement contracts under the private commercial code	
Human resources	Public service		Public service and labour market		Labour market: Private labour contracts	
Intermediary services	Not always authorized. Contracts managed by admin.	Depends on delegation of powers	Service contracts that can be broad in scope		No restrictions: service contracts	

Downstream contracting is the scenario in which an autonomous hospital operates in the role of the *principal*. The health service provider seeks to mobilize production factors as efficiently as possible. In order to guarantee service production, the hospital requires various inputs:

- *Material inputs*

In perform its work, the hospital requires a wide range of material resources: medical and surgical supplies, miscellaneous consumables (water, electricity, telephone, maintenance products), etc. It purchases them on the goods and services market in accordance with regulations that normally differ depending on whether the hospital is privately managed (classic market) or publicly managed (public procurement contracts). When the purchase is not immediate, it is the object of a *supply contract*.

Purchasing and the contractual relationship

An act of purchase can be defined as a voluntary exchange between two parties. When this exchange is immediate, the terms of exchange have been negotiated and implemented immediately and therefore do not need to be formalized. Although a contractual relationship is established, its immediate nature means that the relationship does not need to be formalized. On the other hand, when there is a time lapse between the negotiation of the purchase and its coming into effect, the relationship must be formalized through a document (a contract) which is intended to reduce uncertainty regarding the behaviour of either party, but also covers the consequences of events that could affect the performance of either party to the exchange. As a result, any purchase necessarily results in a contractual relationship, but the question is whether this relationship should be formalized or not[1]. Furthermore, the contractual relationship works in two ways: when a first party purchases a service from a second party, this means that, simultaneously, the second party has sold this service to the first. The analyst must decide from which angle to approach the transaction; here, we will choose to look at health-care services purchased by individuals or their representatives, but we could just as easily consider the sale of health-care services by their providers.

[1] Conversely, not all contractual relationships necessarily involve an act of purchase.

- *Human resources*

In many countries, particularly developing ones, the Ministry of Health and the Ministry for the Civil Service share among themselves the role of recruiting, assigning and managing human resources. The Ministry for the Civil Service normally regulates the pattern of employment and sets the legal framework. The Ministry of Health states its needs in respect of employment categories and assigns posts within its services and institutions. Career management and remuneration are more or less centralized and are to a greater or lesser extent the responsibility of the Ministry of Health. In this system, public hospitals have little room for manoeuvre with regard to posts and individual appointments. However, depending on the extent of their autonomy, public hospitals can have a say on several factors influencing the productivity of human resources. Although some of these actions belong to management strategy within the existing legal and procedural framework, others can be situated in a more contractual context.

Employment management policy is clearly within the legal framework, but anything related to internal incentive schemes can fall within a local contractual context. While this comes within internal contracting, such measures have a considerable effect on productivity. It is important to distinguish between measures that fall within the scope of an overall policy, which are decided by the authorities after possible negotiation with the social partners, and one-off actions left to the discretion of the administration. Within the context of overall measures, some types of incentive are implemented on a collective basis, whereas others are directly linked to individual results. The latter arrangement is often applied to medical practitioners to give them the incentive to develop their activities within a hospital framework rather than resorting to outside practice, which may or may not fall within the law.

We should also mention the arrangement adopted by some institutions that are unable to make ad hoc incentive payments to attract health-care professionals in short supply. A form of external contracting enables them to get round this limitation by offering various fringe benefits such as housing and childcare, which are added to the statutory rights of agents. These fringe benefits are written into a contract that specifies the conditions for receiving them (e.g. length of service). These few examples show how public hospitals can better mobilize their human resources when they are given the discretion to explore different ways of establishing contractual relationships with their employees.

In the context of external contracting, it is important to emphasize two components that are important for ensuring good human resources management. Firstly, the contracting of services described in the paragraph below should be viewed in conjunction with human resources policy. The subcontracting of logistical services involves the optimum redeployment of the agents that perform this work. Second, the civil service cannot always provide the staff required to perform certain activities. Recently, developments in information technology (IT) have prompted institutions to seek qualified personnel on the private market. In this situation, as for any recourse to the labour market, contracts stipulate terms of employment as well as the responsibilities entrusted to the employee. The nature and complexity of the responsibilities will influence the decision whether to establish a labour contract between an individual and a hospital, or to contract with a business, to provide services.

In many private hospitals, medical practitioners practise on the basis of ad hoc arrangements. Charging practices and income-sharing arrangements will vary depending on the type of contract. The nature of the sharing is generally determined by the level of competition. Practitioners benefit the most when they are few in number and demand is high.

In charitable institutions, as well as contracts in line with applicable national employment legislation, staff members are also often bound by a moral contract that goes beyond their legal obligations. This contract, which is never formulated in writing, can be implicitly omnipresent, to the extent that those who do not abide by it may actually be excluded. This personal commitment to the hospital's objectives goes some way to explaining the very positive image that some of these institutions enjoy. It goes beyond what businesses try to achieve through commitment to a set of values supported by strong internal communication and sometimes the signing of an agreement to respect a charter of company values.

- *Intermediary services*

For certain intermediary services, the hospital will be able to use specific providers. This is the case for non-medical services: for example, a hospital might contract with a specific company to provide hospital catering or to clean patients' rooms. It can also be the case for medical services: a hospital might recruit a specialist surgeon who is not on its staff or subcontract testing to a private laboratory. In certain cases, hospitals may go as far as contracting out a portion of the medical services that they need (e.g. laboratory testing, medical imagery). This is justified if the activity involves heavy investment or rare qualifications which the institution is not in a position to use to its full capacity.

These types of externalization are generally used more in respect of logistical functions, which do not come within the service provider's primary mandate. This category is different from those referred to above in that it concerns an "organized" intermediary service which itself combines different inputs. The concept of agency is particularly relevant in this context; the health-care service provider acts as the principal, and the ad hoc providers are the agents.

The resulting contractual relationships concern the provision of miscellaneous hospital services:

    - non-medical services: the hospital can enter into a contract with one or a number of external service providers for the maintenance of hospital buildings or facilities (medical or non-medical), or hospital catering. Service contracts of this type are very common nowadays.

Contracting out hospital catering, Bombay, India[14]

This study shows how several public hospitals in Bombay have contracted out their hospital catering services. The results have been mixed. For example, although service costs appear lower, quality has also declined. Above all, the study shows that hospital administrators did not have the capacity to oversee this contracting arrangement and were not sufficiently involved at each stage, for example during the execution of the contract.

Contracting out cleaning services in hospitals in Papua New Guinea[15]

Public hospitals in Papua New Guinea have contracted out premises maintenance to private firms. Although contracting enables the hospital to be rid of a tiresome and ultimately quite costly task, the results have been mixed. For example, when the State did not pay the sum stipulated in the contract on time, the company immediately ceased operations, creating serious hygiene problems. The trial also shows that it is difficult for a private company to observe the hygiene standards that are required to prevent the spread of disease.

Again, these studies demonstrate that contracting does not mean that the hospital can transfer full responsibility to the contracted company, and steps should be taken to adhere to the contract at all times.

Contracting out non-medical services in Tunisian public health-care institutions *

Public Health-care Establishments (PHEs) are public university hospitals under the authority of the Ministry of Public Health, established under an Act of 29 July 1991; they enjoy considerable management autonomy, are regulated by commercial legislation and administrated by boards of directors. Since 1993, PHEs have used contracting for some non-medical activities: hospital catering, cleaning, security, and also accounting assistance. In 2001, 16 of the 21 PHEs used contracting.

A range of factors have prompted PHEs to subcontract certain non-medical activities: (i) the mediocre quality of catering and cleaning services in hospitals, which are a source of dissatisfaction for patients and a waste of resources, (ii) a shortage of qualified staff owing to budgetary restrictions, (iii) the commitments decided upon in the draft project for support of hospital reform, (iv) the important ripple effect of the stereotype that private services deliver better quality than public services.

PHEs, in coordination with the central administration of the Ministry of Public Health, have developed model contracts that provide a starting point for each institution to draft specific contracts. These model contracts place special emphasis on: (i) specific technical considerations for each activity, (ii) the resources required of each party; (iii) the distribution of tasks between the contracting parties; and (iv) the oversight arrangements that the hospital should put in place.

Each PHE must monitor the performance of the tasks entrusted to external businesses and develop its staff resources to accomplish these new tasks properly. Technical and management services are involved in the day-to-day monitoring of the implementation of the contract. An administrative and technical monitoring commission is responsible for periodic monitoring and evaluation of activities, improving procedures for in-house management of subcontracted activities, and review of contract specifications. These experiences have revealed the following:

- According to the general opinion of professionals, the quality of subcontracted services has improved, particularly in respect of catering, cleaning and hygiene. The costs are relatively high, however;

- Staff whose time has been freed up by contracting have been assigned to other duties, thus solving staffing shortages in certain other areas;

- While in the majority of PHEs contracting is subject to effective monitoring and there is regular supervision of activities under the contract, some duties entrusted to subcontractors have been neglected;

- Some tensions have surfaced in the relationship between subcontracted and in-house staff, particularly owing to shortcomings in the precise specification of tasks and responsibilities;

- Patients confuse different categories of staff and sometimes ask subcontractors to do certain things they are not qualified to do, which also creates tensions with in-house staff;

- Personnel from contracting firms lack experience of hospital work. Inadequate supervision and instability are the main risk factors that PHEs must address in their contractual relations.

In conclusion, the experience of contracting out non-medical services in public hospitals in Tunisia shows clear advantages as regards quality improvement, subject to the proviso that contracts are effectively and rigorously monitored by hospital managers. The costs, however, remain relatively high, since the number of potential providers is not yet sufficient to allow for genuine competition.

[*] H. Achouri, A. Jeridi, Director and chief executive officer of the Office for Hospital Oversight, Ministry of Public Health, Tunisia.

- Provision of medical services: rather than providing all medical services using in-house resources, the hospital may choose to subcontract for some of these services. Laboratory tests or radiology examinations are a case in point. A hospital that lacks particular specialists can contact other institutions that have them; the required specialist can either visit the requesting hospital or the patient can be transferred to the hospital where the specialist is based.

- Hospital management: Through a contract, a hospital can use an external provider to perform management tasks. For example, following the practice of small businesses, a hospital might ask a management centre to do its accounting. Likewise, a hospital might ask a private firm (for profit or otherwise) to help manage its human resources. In some cases it can entrust activities such as debt recovery to the private sector (this has been done by Douala general hospital in Cameroon, with some success).

While there are many theoretical arguments in favour of subcontracting and outsourcing, all available assessments err on the side of caution. In practice, experience shows that the main causes of failure are not financial, but rather stem from lack of consultation or failure to respect arrangements that have been agreed upon. Furthermore, all these experiences show that even in the case of seemingly quite simple contracts, the hospital must guarantee regular supervision. This is because even straightforward activities such as the maintenance of hospital premises or catering require a specific approach in a hospital environment, which commercial enterprises are not necessarily accustomed to. Furthermore, even when the company signing the contract has a good reputation, this is no guarantee of success. The hospital must constantly monitor the implementation of the contract to get the most out of it. This entails a mode of organization adapted to the involvement of a third party which is helping to achieve the institution's objectives.

Upstream vertical contracting

In this situation, the hospital is an agent vis-à-vis a number of principals: the oversight authorities, financial institutions and users. Each of these institutions will negotiate their relationships with the agent (hospital) that provides health-care services for them. These services should be defined.

The use of this type of contracting will depend, however, on the type of ownership and structure of the hospital, as well as its management methods.

Table 4: Upstream vertical contracting options

OWNERSHIP	PUBLIC (State, local authorities)				PRIVATE	
MANAGEMENT	*Direct*	*Devolved*	*Autonomous*	*Delegated management*	*Direct*	*Direct with association*
Oversight authorities	Not applicable, or internal performance contracts		Recommended	Provided for in the contract for delegated management	Not applicable	Provided for in the association contract
Risk-sharing financial organizations	Contract managed by the Ministry of Health The framework agreement approach is facilitated		Case-by-case contractual relations The framework agreement approach is more difficult			Case-by-case contractual relations Framework agreement approach may be facilitated
Hospital users	The administration prefers prescribed relations (charter)		Ad hoc contractual relationships with associations catering to a particular clientele.			

- **Contracting with oversight authorities**

This type of contracting will depend greatly on the hospital's form of ownership and its management arrangements.

a. Public hospitals with direct or devolved management

By definition, public hospitals with direct or devolved management are directly under the authority of the public authorities responsible for health-care (State or local authorities). The issue of an oversight authority therefore does not arise.

Nevertheless, the growth of internal contracting between administrative services has been a recent development under the New Public Management rationale. This arrangement generally seeks to optimize the allocation of budgetary resources and the use of human resources in the public sector. Such contracts are generally known as *"performance contracts"*.

In recent years, performance contracts have become quite modish in line with the prevailing trend towards optimization of resources. The complex nature of the hospital product, however, makes it difficult to measure performance. This is why a whole chapter has been devoted to this issue. Readers should refer to this chapter for useful information about this process.

b. Private hospitals without association

Private hospitals do not have an oversight authority, but they maintain links in the audit field, in line with their legal obligations. Since they are not involved in activities negotiated with the public authorities, there is no contractual link between them. The public authority exercises its authority through sanctions in the case of activities that are deemed harmful, or through incentives to develop activities of public interest.

C. Public hospitals under delegated management and private hospitals in association with the State

Delegated management for public hospitals and association for private hospitals are arrangements established via a contract with the public authorities (State or local authorities).

In the case of delegated management, the contract normally details the different forms of relationship with the oversight authorities. In the event that the management delegation contract deals solely with the terms and conditions of the delegation, it will state that the hospital subscribes to the regulations and obligations of public institutions that provide a public service. The information on autonomous public hospitals further on in this chapter is also relevant for institutions under delegated management.

In the case of private hospitals, the contract of association with the public authorities responsible for health care confers on private hospitals the rights and obligations applicable to relationships between oversight authorities and public hospitals. As a result, the mechanisms described below for autonomous public hospitals are generally applicable.

In both cases, it should be noted that the contractual relationship as a whole will be more complex than for public institutions. It will include an additional tier. Relationships between the hospital and its oversight authority regarding the provision of services are supplemented by relationships regarding the context of cooperation between the public authorities and the managing body/manager or the owner of the institution and its activity.

D. Autonomous public hospitals

By granting autonomy to a hospital, the State enables it to boost its independence and decision-making responsibility. These autonomous structures, however, are not independent; they must necessarily maintain a relationship with the authority that granted them autonomy (the Ministry of Health or decentralized authorities):

- For legal reasons; the concept of oversight by public authorities varies according to country and context, but generally covers at least the following three points:
    - Power of approval: the most important decisions regarding the hospital's general policy and budget are enforceable only after approval by the oversight authority;
    - Financial monitoring: the public authorities generally establish a financial monitoring mechanism within the autonomous hospital;
    - Power of supervision and inspection: the oversight authority has the opportunity to supervise and carry out inspections. Some countries have adopted a procedure for periodically evaluating autonomous hospitals (results monitoring).

- For practical reasons; particularly in developing countries, autonomous hospitals lack the resources to be entirely independent of the entity to which they are linked, both financially and in terms of human resources. The hospital staff, who are generally paid out of the national budget, are appointed by the Ministry of Health following selection through competitive examination. On the other hand, financial contributions from patients are insufficient to cover all the hospital's running costs. So the Ministry of Health defrays a large part of hospital's operating costs through subsidies. Generally speaking, investment comes entirely from the State or from donors.

- For political reasons; the Ministry of Health, in its capacity as guarantor of the interests of entire population, intends to keep the option of implementing the hospital policy that it has set at national level in the context of the national health-care policy, and to ensure harmonization between hospitals nationwide.

Legislation and regulation do not always specify the form of the relationship between the State and autonomous hospitals, nor the arrangements for implementing it. It is conceivable that conventional administration methods might

147

be adopted, i.e. each issue or problem is studied on a case -by-case basis within the framework of the oversight authority.

However, hospital autonomy also enables this issue to be addressed through contracts that promote a clearer reading of the relationship between the parties. Of course, these contractual relationships fall under public [administrative] law, since they involve two legal entities at public law under the context of a general interest ; they must therefore respect the administrative procedures in force. This type of contracting remains less flexible and open-ended than "private law" contracting. The characteristics of these types of contractual relationships are:

- The need for an institutional policy: to enter into a contract, the higher authority necessarily requires that the autonomous hospital should have a *institutional or strategic plan*, i.e. that it clearly defines its objectives and its current and future position within the health-care system and promotes consistency in its activities and the use of its capacity;[17] Some countries are pressing ahead with this approach. Morocco, for example, has developed "contract plans" between the Ministry of Health and autonomous hospitals. Likewise, since 1998, Tunisia has introduced objective based contracts between its public health-care institutions (autonomous institutions) and the oversight department of the Ministry of Health. These aim to develop a contractual relationship based on the institutions' performance.[18] This contractual relationship should ultimately become the essential tool for negotiating the mobilization of resources.

The French system

Since the mid-1990s, France has adopted the following system:
- Regional health organization plans (*Schéma Régional d'Organisation Sanitaire* - SROS) set the region's priority objectives for public and private hospital services and specify the apportionment of installations, major facilities and equipment, and health services activities that will ensure that the needs of the population are met as comprehensively as possible.
- Institutional plans, developed by each hospital, set the institution's objectives, outline its current and future position within the health-care system, and aim to promote consistency in its activities and the use of its capacity.
Interface between the SROS and the institutional plan is ensured through an "objective and means" contract established between the regional hospital agency, representing the higher authority, and the hospital. When this is well coordinated, the hospital institutional plan should be seen as a technical resource underpinning the contractual relationship for the operationalization of regional health-care policy.

- The opportunity to establish a longer-term commitment (over several years): this obviates the need for annual budgeting (involving annual expenditure bills or programme contracts). Depending on its revenue and economic priorities, however, the State may find itself unable to honour the financial commitments it has undertaken in a multi-year contract. In such cases the State can invoke an "act of State", which permits it to change a clause in a contract on the basis of the public interest.

- The impossibility of action with regard to contractual responsibility; the failure of one party, particularly the State, to uphold part of the contract is difficult to sanction: it is very hard to imagine recourse to law enforcement to compel one of the parties to fulfil their obligations. The parties' obligations towards each other are therefore not full and complete. This is more of a moral commitment than a contractual commitment in the legal sense.

- Equality between the parties: in law, a contract requires the legal equality of the parties. In this case, this equality is far from guaranteed. In fact, as we have seen, the public authority that grants autonomy maintains some control over the autonomous body. The balance of power is therefore distorted, since the autonomous body will have difficulty arguing against the central authority. It is sometimes difficult to draw the line between a negotiated contract (which is a pleonasm) and an imposed contract (which is a paradox). Autonomy indisputably limits the power of the oversight authority; the authority can, however, view contracting as a means of reclaiming by other means the power it ceded by granting autonomy.

These are very real limits to conventional types of contracting, but these should not be used to call into question the concept itself. Vertical contracting enables both actors – the autonomous hospital and the public authorities – to approach their core relations in an ordered and coherent manner. By entering into a contract, they are compelled to define their relationship and the means they require to implement it. The failure of a contract will affect both parties: the hospital will not accomplish the activities planned, and the oversight authority will no longer be able to guarantee the implementation of its health-care policy. The contracting process should not be viewed from a legal standpoint based on contract law. It is a managerial process that prompts the parties to develop a priority-driven solution based on their capacities. This type of procedure, which creates buy-in, makes a considerable difference when using it for implementing priority measures.

- **Contracting with risk-sharing financial organizations**

It is now generally acknowledged that free medical care does not promote hospital efficiency. The failure of the old Soviet system demonstrated this. As soon as hospitals charge users for their services, insurance is required to guarantee accessibility and risk-sharing. The institutions that arrange this risk sharing vary in nature from private commercial insurance, through national insurance schemes, to mutual benefit insurance companies. Various permutations of the latter are currently developing in low-income countries. We will use the term "insurer" to refer to them when it is not necessary to specify the type of insurance mechanism.

Insurers have significant power owing to the volume of finance that they control. They negotiate with health-care service providers to obtain the best advantages on behalf of their clients. They can approach private providers directly. This is harder to do with providers who are directly linked to the Ministry of Health, since in this case they must negotiate with the Ministry. When dealing with autonomous hospitals or public hospitals with delegated management, however, they are dealing with a partner that has the legal capacity to sign an agreement without needing to refer it to the Ministry of Health. These hospitals are thus able directly to negotiate with financial institutions and to draft ad hoc agreements that can be advantageous to both parties.

When there is no mandatory national insurance scheme, these ad hoc agreements have the disadvantage of resulting in possible balkanization and considerable disparities. The Ministry of Health should therefore play a regulatory role and, through national policy, lay down contracting guidelines to prevent such disparities. In particular, the public authorities must ensure respect for equality of access to public services. While a contract might specify disparities in the standard of hospital accommodation, for example, it must not guarantee better medical care. In general, each contract between a financial body and an autonomous hospital should specify certain minimum predefined criteria.

Similarly insurers, particularly through their federations, have the opportunity to draft and sign framework agreements. There are two possibilities:

- Insurers and providers can establish a framework agreement specifying the principal areas of cooperation and the ground rules for their relationship. The framework agreement will define the terms under which ad hoc contracts can be negotiated. This framework agreement will be followed up by ad hoc contracts specifying the relationship between the two entities. This approach has the dual advantage of harmonizing contractual practices and facilitating negotiations. This type of regulated freedom allows considerable leeway for adapting to local peculiarities;

- Insurers and providers can establish a framework agreement setting out contractual details that the parties can either accept or reject. The framework agreement is therefore the same as a standard-form contract, for mutual benefit insurance companies and providers alike. There is no longer any need to draw up a specific contract; it is sufficient to acknowledge the framework agreement as binding for both entities. This type of framework agreement must be as explicit as possible in order to provide for all eventualities.

The choice between these two alternatives is based on the idea of *subsidiarity*: what authority do mutual benefit insurance companies wish to transfer to a union or a federation? Do they wish to grant broad authority, at the risk of forgoing a considerable proportion of their powers of negotiation regarding health care, or do they merely wish to cede a coordinating and guiding function while maintaining their own negotiating power?

The proliferation of ad hoc contractual arrangements also causes problems for health-care providers. Let us suppose that a district or regional hospital has dealings with several mutual benefit insurance companies in its catchment area, and that, over time, it has signed ad hoc contacts with as many mutual benefit insurance companies, the same hospital will find itself in the position of managing a number of contracts, each with its own special provisions: this is time-consuming and occasions high transaction costs and problems for health-care staff and patients alike. Harmonized contracting practices will minimize these problems.

- **Contracting with users**

Aside from technical considerations, an institution providing public health care can only justify its existence if its users are satisfied. According to WHO, this "responsiveness" is one of the three goals of any health-care system [19]

If we wish to build a system of reciprocal responsibility that benefits patients and the hospital simultaneously, this can be formalized through contractual agreements. The establishment of contractual relations promotes a "client/provider" relationship with the aim of adapting services to user requirements. This approach justifies classifying relationships with patients in a context of upstream vertical contracting. The concept of a client, rather than just a service user, gives the patient a status that is often obscured by regulations and, moreover, one that is necessary to protect the patient.

Although curing illness is the priority, the way in which people are treated is also important. This justifies the existence of regulations that compel institutions to give patients due respect. Such regulations set out the institution's obligations, and especially those of health professionals, vis-à-vis users: it includes an important section on ethics and patient confidentiality. The importance of this protection should not be overlooked, since hospitals are places of refuge that can develop practices justified by the delivery of treatment or the need to rationalize resources, albeit contrary to personal autonomy. The Patients' Charter adopted in France illustrates one regulatory approach.

The French Inpatient Charter

In France, the Ministry of Health has spearheaded the development of a Patients Charter which is applicable in all public institutions (all of which have autonomous status). This Charter was debated at the national level.

The core principles of this Charter, dated 6 May 1995, are:

1. Public hospital services are open to all, in particular the poorest members of society.
2. Health-care institutions shall guarantee high-quality care and treatment. They shall put effort into relieving pain.
3. Information provided to patients must be comprehensible and honest. Patients must be involved in selecting their treatment.
4. Medical procedures may be performed only with the free and informed consent of the patient.
5. Specific consent must be obtained, particularly from patients participating in biomedical research, the donation and use of human body parts and products, and screening.
6. Inpatients may discharge themselves at any time, except where the law stipulates otherwise, having been informed of the risks they could face.
7. Inpatients shall be treated with consideration. Their religious beliefs shall be respected. Their privacy and peace of mind will be maintained.
8. Respect for the private lives of all patients, and the confidentiality of any personal, medical or social information about them, shall be guaranteed.
9. Patients may consult the information in their files, including medical information, through a practitioner of their choice.
10. Inpatients may express their opinions on their care and treatment, and have the right to request compensation for any injury they feel has been done to them.

The Charter has been adapted to certain specific areas: hospitalized children, people with disabilities, people living with HIV/AIDS, etc.

This Charter is an example of a two-tier approach. First of all, it is a negotiation between the public authorities and representatives of users that can be turned into a contract that is binding upon hospitals. However, in order to strengthen this commitment, the State wished to enact it in statutory form. Hospitals are therefore bound by the Charter and patients may seek reparation if the Charter is not respected.[20]

Autonomous status provides an opportunity to involve patients, not, as previously, through parallel structures such as management committees, but directly, as members of the autonomous hospital's board of directors. An example of this is the project in Kasongo (DRC),[21] where a contractual agreement has been established between the hospital and the public.

152

In this context, even though patients are protected, their legal status remains unchanged and the hospital is unable to meet their expectations.

Discharge of responsibility in the United States of America

Any patient entering a health facility, including accident and emergency departments, is required to sign a consent form authorizing the treatment that he or she will undergo. This giving of consent is in fact a way of protecting hospitals against possible litigation in a system where lawsuits are very common owing to the dominant position of commercial medicine.

In so far as the patient signs a document, this is a contract. The fact of signing, and the fact that the terms of the contract are non-negotiable, mean that this contract is intended to protect the interests of the hospital rather than help to protect the patient. This type of contract is similar to the commercial practice of many goods and services providers, who require signature of agreement to general terms and conditions of sale.

In this asymmetrical relationship where the service provider dominates the situation by imposing its rules, consumers have no choice but to sign, otherwise they must forgo the good or service. This is not conscionable in the case of health care. Accordingly, the law imposes obligations on the seller, which must be respected whatever the terms of the contract signed by the consumer. This concept of illegality of contractual clauses is particularly important to protect individuals against abuse of power by providers in a dominant position.

It is interesting to note that free and informed consent that protects the patient (evidence of which can be gathered in any form) in a public-service hospital system is expressed by way of discharge of responsibilities in a commercially dominated system. This shows the extent to which contracting is sensitive to legal and economic circumstances.

From being a tool for promoting relationships based on exchange, contracting can become a means of protecting the provider. Thus, paradoxically, increased recourse to contracting leads to an equally significant increase in legal and regulatory activity to avoid abuses by the dominant party. Rather than one replacing the other, contracts and laws feed off each other in a system which becomes increasingly complex for the patient, who must call on a third party (a lawyer, with whom the patient will have to conclude a contract!) to protect his or her interests...

Making specific arrangements that take account of user expectations enables the debate to move beyond a preoccupation with respect for the individual in the context of organizing and providing care. This is a key element in assessing the quality of the care provided. Two mechanisms are possible: a satisfaction survey or instituting a dialogue with user representatives.

In the first case, the hospital is concerned with user satisfaction as an element of quality of care, but does not enter into a dialogue with its users. To promote the integration of the hospital into the community and emphasize its social dimension, it seems important to establish a relationship with users.

However, it is not easy to establish contractual arrangements with users. People in good health are not very concerned about the potential use of hospitals. In fact, there seems to be a natural tendency not to want to acknowledge this undesirable possibility. In this context it is understandable that it can be hard to define the scope of hospital users: anyone could potentially belong to this group. This is why some consider elected officials to represent users by virtue of their mandate. This justifies their involvement in hospital decision-making bodies. However, it is not unknown in an election-based system for the politicization of health-care issues to result in actions that are purely token or media-driven rather than actually solve problems that might be less "visible" but just as important to users.

Defining users as individuals who frequent hospitals poses other problems. These people are often weak and find themselves in a situation that precludes an equal relationship with those who hold their health in their hands. At best, this definition can be applied to institutions for the long-term care of individuals of sound mind. But this covers just a small part of hospital activity.

In some countries, the voluntary sector acts as a mouthpiece for the concerns of civil society. It is not unheard of for health care to be among the issues raised by these associations, but it is rare to find associations that bring together only "health-care users". As the following brief overview shows, this movement is not homogeneous. The form of contractual relationships will depend on the specific nature of the associations.

Generally speaking, health care is covered by the part of the voluntary sector that deals with consumer or family issues. Associations of this type will doubtless have an interest in contracting with hospitals to improve public health care. They generally adopt an activist stance vis-à-vis issues of general interest that goes beyond protection of the actual members of the association. This aspect of their activity confers upon them a degree of representativeness that surpasses the importance given to them by their members.

Of particular interest are associations involved in health service management. These represent primary health-care services that can contract with hospitals. For the hospital, these associations are "patient suppliers" and "service users". This represents contracting between health-care organizations, and as such is closer to the model of horizontal contracting outlined below.

Mutual benefit associations, whether subject to specific regulation or not, enjoy special status. One chapter is therefore devoted to them because they are health care funders too. They enjoy a very specific relationship with the hospital because their financial leverage gives them a particular strength that users' associations do not possess. Contracting is based around a paying third party.

Finally, there are an increasing number of associations for people suffering from chronic diseases. These associations are very active, since for chronic patients relationships with hospitals are not merely an eventuality but part of their everyday life. This ongoing relationship gives another dimension to how they perceive the institution. These associations can make very specific demands depending on the frequency of contact and the type of treatment provided to their members.

In light of the above, it seems sensible to approach contracting with users by concentrating on two targets with special focus, namely consumer associations and patient associations. This approach should not replace satisfaction surveys. These surveys, which are sometimes quite sophisticated, can be carried out irrespective of how rich or poor a country is and provide impartial information with a view to developing dialogue with user organizations.

- *Contracting with consumer associations*: firstly, these associations must be sufficiently well-established in the population to be credibly representative. It is vital that they should be committed to raising the concerns of their members, and that they should be democratic. Associations such as these have some influence over a hospital's activity, but not as directly as associations managed by paying third parties or health services. Their importance resides more in the social and moral pressure that they can bring to bear in the community. So it is on this basis that the contracts are developed. We might envisage the hospital's commitments involving different aspects of reception, access to treatment, and quality of care in general. For its part, the association can play a role by informing its members how to use the hospital, or by circulating messages regarding prevention.

- *Contracting with patient associations*: these associations must be representative of patients. Where a number of associations dealing with the same illness exist in the catchment area of one hospital, it is important to contract with each of them if there is no federative body. In countries where AIDS has spread significantly, AIDS patient associations have an important role to play in promoting dialogue with hospitals to arrange for care. Contracts will be directly linked to the arrangements for treating a particular illness. They will focus on the patient-centric element of treatment at the institution. This is the major concern of chronic patients, particularly when they have to attend different services within the same institution.

Horizontal external contracting

Contracts between hospitals and other health-care bodies, whether at the national or international level, can be distinguished from contracts signed between hospitals and non-health-care bodies. While the focus tends to be on delivery of treatment, it should not be forgotten that hospitals are also involved in training and research activities. They can also be involved in the production of goods and services. While this trend is increasing in developed countries, it remains rare in developing countries.

Table 5: Horizontal contracting options

OWNERSHIP	PUBLIC (State, local authorities)				PRIVATE	
MANAGEMENT	*Direct*	*Devolved*	*Autonomous*	*Delegated management*	*Direct*	*Direct with association*
Contracting with national health-care bodies	Legal rather than contractual framework	Depends on the degree of devolution	Increasingly developed			
Contracting with foreign health-care bodies	Organized by the Ministry of Health, rarely with foreign hospitals directly		Permitted, but sometimes requires authorization from Ministry of Health			
Contracting with training and research bodies	Legal rather than contractual framework	Depends on the degree of devolution	Contracting based on a legal framework, but with some room for manoeuvre.		Rare, unless there is joint activity or remuneration	Depends on legal obligations and possibility for remuneration
Contracting with non-health-care bodies	Organized by the Ministry of Health directly with the bodies involved		Permitted, but under a specific arrangement for operation and revenue		Open-ended in the context of the institution's activities	

Contracting with health-care bodies

• **Partnership contracts at national level**

Hospitals, whether public or private, have long had a tradition of self-sufficiency. Nowadays, self-sufficiency is less and less possible. Firstly, health issues are increasingly interrelated: referral/counter-referral is becoming institutionalized. Furthermore, for reasons of efficacy, a hospital cannot and does not know how to do everything. As a result, hospitals are increasingly forced to establish relationships with institutions that are not in their linked community, i.e. institutions with which they do not have a hierarchical relationship. The purpose of this relationship varies:

- Organization of inputs: two hospitals may agree to place consolidated orders for certain inputs (e.g. consolidated orders for medicines to obtain a better price), or to establish a joint radiology and clinical examination service, etc.

- Specialization-based: two hospitals may contract to share a geographical area (unless precluded by a regulatory geographical distribution of health facilities)) where they can specialize in certain services (sharing specialist surgeons).

- Synergies: two hospitals may join together to launch an awareness-raising campaign.

Public hospitals under direct management, or devolution, owing to their longstanding tradition of self-sufficient operation, have more difficulty establishing these types of relationship. Autonomous hospitals (public hospitals with autonomous status or delegated management, or private hospitals) on the other hand, can establish contractual relationships with other institutions more easily. These forms of partnership are increasing in developed countries, and are also emerging in developing countries.

With other autonomous institutions with the same orientation: it is possible to establish contractual relationships based on complementarity (one hospital focuses its specialization on a particular service while a neighbouring hospital focuses on another) or on cross-over services (a specialist affiliated to one hospital provides services for another and vice versa). This type of inter-institutional contracting can be a first step towards rationalizing health-care provision in a given area. In Douala (Cameroon), for example, the central hospital and the general hospital have established a range of services that allows both hospitals to broaden their scope of service provision and share certain activities. The public authorities will eventually have to decide whether to strengthen that complementarity through contractual arrangements, or to merge the two institutions. In all large cities this issue of complementarity is central to indispensable efforts to rationalize health care.

With partners at different level: this involves the well-known scenario of the health-care pyramid, in which the basic health-care network refers patients to the hospital system. The absence of contractual relationships might explain why the referral system or referral centre fails to deliver. If agreements do not specify the rights and obligations of each party and there are no provisions to promote such exchanges, it is hardly surprising that each organization functions independently. But other functions apart from patient referral could also benefit from being formalized through contracts. Supervision is a function that should be implicitly guaranteed, yet it lacks sufficient recognition to compete with care provided directly at the hospital level. Likewise prevention activities, which would benefit from the technical and logistical support of hospitals. Accordingly, hospitals should not only be seen as components of a health-care pyramid, but also stakeholders in a health-care network.

Contracting to improve the operational capacity of the health district

The district model, which is extensively described and implemented in many developing countries, is based on a dichotomy between a steering body that monitors the activity of the district as a whole (the district management team) , first-line health-care providers (dispensaries) and secondary-line providers (first level referral hospitals). Depending on the country, there are different levels of first-line health-care structures and the technical capacity of hospitals varies significantly. The administration of this structure is directed by the district chief physician. Hospitals are structured as complex organizations employing various physicians, including specialists. Institutions of this type are administered completely independently from the district administration. Furthermore, following on from the Bamako Initiative and the trend towards decentralization, dispensaries have become increasingly independent of the district administration. In addition, private health-care should also be taken into account, since this can account for most of the health care in the area covered by the district . Private health care can be provided by a facility in competition with the district hospital. Sometimes it replaces the district hospital, without being integrated into a national policy of association with the public service. Finally, the referral/ counter-referral system, which has been elevated to the status of dogma, in fact barely functions. There are numerous reasons for this, for example inconsistency between the principle and the funding mechanism, implied competition between levels, the seriousness of many of the cases treated, and lack of will to physically transfer patients.

The health district can therefore no longer be seen as a homogeneous unit operating in accordance with national regulations under the administration of a unitary authority. It is a complex unit in which the prerogatives of the various partners must be clarified to enable it to operate. Under the previous model, conflicts often used to arise in connection with the hospital, which was often managed directly or was under the control of the district chief physician. As hospitals were granted relative autonomy, tensions inevitably surfaced around who had responsibility for decisions on use of resources.

Contracting seems to be an approach that can both preserve the spirit of the health district and ensure that it functions more effectively. Hierarchical dependency regulations (i.e. carrying out the instructions of the district chief physician) and the application of national procedures (in respect of implementing programmes and reporting) are being replaced by contracts between the parties involved. The fundamental advantage of this approach is that it smoothes out conflicts that revolve around power relations: each party is responsible for certain actions to achieve the objectives set forth in the contract. Furthermore, this approach promotes the search for local solutions in line with priorities identified by the contracting parties. National regulations can still be applied, but they are written into the contract as an element of the legal context.

Contracting falls squarely into the principle of renewing the health district, which recognizes the need to organize the supply of health care from a geographical and demographical perspective, while taking into consideration the multiplicity of stakeholders and their increased autonomy in day-to-day management. Contracting facilitates a move away from mere observance of regulations and instructions to seeking negotiated results.

The success of this type of contracting rests on the existence of a moderator whose role is to monitor implementation of the commitments undertaken in the public interest. This is a new role for the district chief physician. Such a development will entail calling into question previous practices, and probably the need to commit stakeholders to a new role in a new environment. From the hospitals' point of view, this involves genuine governance of the organization and increased management skills.

Horizontal contracting differs from upstream vertical contracting in that it involves a partnership in which each party makes a contribution either to the establishment of a joint activity or the implementation of an activity that is equally beneficial to both partners. Whereas in vertical contracting the hospital does not discuss its offer of service with the contactor, since it is purchasing inputs, horizontal contracting involves dialogue between the partners, who jointly define the service and the role that each will play in it. This system has been widely developed in OECD Member States, with the establishment of care networks. It still remains little used in developing countries, although it has considerable potential to reinvigorate certain sectors of the health-care system.

- **Partnership contracting at the international level**

The benefit of hospital partnerships[22]

Markets have become globalized, which promotes optimization of the most complex techniques, and hospitals in developing countries cannot afford to be left behind. These hospitals are often isolated from the international hospital community for want of resources. It is therefore important to improve resource mobilization to enable them to participate in the exchanges that are crucial for the development of techniques.

Although hospital priorities differ between developing and developed countries, the latter have a pool of expertise that can be of considerable assistance to the former. The world of hospitals is particularly open to knowledge sharing, since this enables medicine to progress. The mobilization of this expertise can therefore take place in a context of formal collaboration on shared goals, while specifying the means of achieving them.

A partnership agreement facilitates the establishment of an ongoing collaboration framework that can satisfy the need for expertise in a broad range of areas where it is important to know the context for intervening. The involvement of individuals will depend greatly on the nature of the relationship. A formalized exchange is a more sustainable and intensive way of mobilizing specialists who must respond to numerous invitations.

Setting up a hospital partnership[23]

More often than not, personal relationships between hospital staff in the developing and the developed world provide the impetus for informal collaboration, an arrangement which quickly shows its limitations in terms of both institutions' needs. An effective solution is to use this relationship to formalize collaboration between the institutions on the basis of an agreement. It might also be possible to expand to hospitals the cooperation arrangements that formerly existed between administrative units (town to town or region to region). Isolated hospitals can also seek a partnership arrangement by applying to hospital federations within a given country or internationally. Access to these contact points is now much easier through their web sites.[24]

To set up a hospital partnership, it is important to formalize a project that is of mutual benefit. These benefits are not necessarily of the same nature. They can be mainly technical or economic for hospitals in developing countries and managerial for hospitals in developed countries.

While personal relationships promote the mobilization of parties, institutionalization is a guarantee of sustainability. It also means that the transaction cannot be hijacked by a limited number of people for their own personal interests, however praiseworthy these may be. Institutionalization can begin with a partnership committee comprising representatives of the main units at the hospital. Institutionalization can also be achieved by submitting a cooperation agreement to the various advisory or decision-making bodies that oversee the institution's operations.

Partnerships are possible between organizations with differing legal forms and/or status on two conditions:

- The organizations must be competent to contract by virtue of their autonomous status, or through delegation of decision-making authority;
- the partnership must be part of a non-profit-making collaborative venture (not the purchase of a service, but a genuine exchange between the institutions).

It is important to formalize the partnership through an agreement that lays down the general framework and implementation arrangements: responsibility, a commitment by each party, and funding arrangements. This agreement should be supplemented using a programme of work specifying various operations that over a predetermined time frame.

If a donor is involved, the donor will provide guidelines for partnership contracts and regulations for mobilizing the funds it will make available. The implementation arrangements for this partnership may involve a three-way contract or a set of contracts between the donor and either or both institutions, and between the two institutions themselves. While contracts must specify the implementation arrangements for the partnership, it is also essential to ensure that the relationship does not become overly bureaucratic. Simple and precise should be the watchwords of those drafting the contract.

Hospital partnerships between France and developing countries

Hospital partnerships have been widely promoted by the French authorities, which have given statutory form to international hospital operations and promoted this trend through technical assistance and funding opportunities.

An analysis of over 50 partnership operations funded through French cooperation in around 30 countries shows that these partnerships actually mean something:

The nature of operations falls into one of the following categories: training, know-how (audit, monitoring or evaluation), medical equipment, equipment and consumables (expendables, spare parts and consumables), dispatch of equipment and "miscellaneous" (documentation, subscriptions to scientific reviews, teaching materials).

The recipient: medical, staff, general maintenance, biomedical maintenance, logistics (catering, linen, laundry), management (administrative sector).

The areas of intervention, enabling several aspects of hospital operations to be addressed: techniques, organization, strategy, training and hygiene.

The experience gained over the past five years highlights the following key ingredients for such an arrangement to be successful:

- The commitment of the institutions must be formalized through an agreement.
- The support of national health authorities is required (many institutions are not truly autonomous).
- It is helpful to set up a formal structure responsible for the partnership within each institution (e.g. a twinning committee).
- It is crucial to undertake activities in several sectors in order to mobilize the different professions in the hospital, thereby ensuring that the exercise does not become the preserve of a select few.
- The programme should extend over three to five years.
- A number of hospitals in one country must not be associated with a single foreign hospital, since the sustainability of the partnership depends on a critical mass of exchanges between institutions.
- Ideally, hospital partnership should be combined with partnership between the corresponding local authorities

Source : E de Roodenbeke, Guidance for the technical cooperation department of the Ministry of Foreign Affairs, 2000

With other partners

- **Contracting with training and research bodies**

University hospitals have a clear-cut training mandate, but their actual role in training is much more complicated than it appears on the surface. Most hospitals are involved in the training of health-care professionals, but depending on their status and level, arrangements differ considerably from country to country. Regulations on vocational training are often vague in developing countries, so there are plenty of opportunities for contracting to formalize the relationships between stakeholders. Research is often a part of the hospital's mandate, but the context is frequently left vague, particularly in low-income countries. Contracting can raise the profile of research, thereby ensuring that more research gets done and that the results of research are used more effectively.

For the initial training of health-care professionals (regardless of category: physicians, nurses, ancillary and technical staff), the hospital plays a vital role in transmitting practical know-how. For the purposes of qualifying, this is almost as important as theoretical knowledge. While in English-speaking countries university-controlled hospitals often provide a training ground for professionals, this rarely happens in French-speaking countries. Furthermore, there is another divide in respect of the status of universities and hospitals. While in the English-speaking world it is common for both to be in the private sector, French-speaking countries promote a system in which both universities and hospitals are more likely to be in the public sector with varying degrees of autonomy. In the case of research bodies, a similar divide may exist, with the difference that the former do not control hospitals, even though some specialized-care institutions may be more involved in research programmes dealing with the pathologies that they treat.

In both cases the relationship between the training and care mandates needs to be formalized; this process engages the responsibility of the Ministry of Health and the Ministry of Education. In a predominantly public-sector system, these relationships are often governed by regulations. A hospital/university agreement outlines the institutional relationship between the faculty of medicine and hospitals. While a framework agreement is particularly well suited to promoting a nexus of relationships that extend beyond the university hospital, it can often be nothing more than an empty shell. The framework agreement may include certification criteria and specify supervisory arrangements in order to avoid reducing the quality of the units hosting interns.

Hospitals are obliged to receive students and offer practical training. The nature and length of internships are specified by regulations. However, the regulatory framework deals only with general principles, often leaving hospitals and universities considerable discretion in determining their arrangements for organizing internships. Thus, when the oversight authority is not really involved in the details of organizing these relationships, contracting should focus on two main issues: the hosting of professional trainees and the role of the hospital and the participation of its staff in training arrangements.

Regarding the arrival of professional trainees, an individual contract is established for each intern. These contracts follow a standard format which can be negotiated at both the institutional level (hospital/university) and the individual level (intern/training supervisor). They set out the content and objectives of the training, and the role and responsibility of the training supervisor. They also stipulate arrangements regarding the respective responsibilities of the different parties and remuneration details. It is quite common for interns whose training is almost complete to undertake certain tasks, thus contributing to the hospital's workforce. Rather than letting this activity develop informally or on the basis of direct relationships between hospital staff and training bodies, it is preferable for the hospital to include this activity in its procedures and codify this practice. This approach enables its contribution to training efforts to be quantified while giving in-house recognition to the role of individuals and services.

Professionals are involved in both initial and ongoing training. In developing countries with significant training needs, this contribution can sometimes take up more of a professional's time than their public health-care activities. This is why it is particularly important for contracts to be established with training bodies. The fact that training is an important source of extra income for some professionals should not be neglected or hidden. Contracting is not intended to channel individual resources back into the employing organization, but rather to promote greater transparency in individual activities and a recognition of the hospital's contribution to training (opportunity cost connected with time spent on the exercise). It is not unreasonable to think that hospitals should offer their services for training purposes on the basis of their human potential. An internal incentive system could supplement the contracting arrangements between a hospital and a donor interested in training activities.

Similar considerations apply to hospitals involved in research under the direction of a research body. However, operational research conducted by practitioners to further their reputation, or by the institution to obtain information for decision-making purposes, does not fall within the same framework. This can be dealt with under an internal contracting policy (see below). On the other hand, it is important to emphasize the special case of clinical research based on the patients who frequent the hospital. In developed countries, legal obligations mean that individual contracts must be concluded between researchers and participants. Lack of regulation should not exempt teams working in developing countries from signing similar contracts to inform their patients and obtain their informed consent. In this area there is another significant difference between countries with French-inspired traditions and countries influenced by the American system. In French-speaking countries, participation in research does not involve remuneration, only costs are covered, whereas in countries influenced by the American system remuneration for participation is common practice. The nature and scope of the contract are different if remuneration is involved, because in the latter case the contract falls more squarely under the scope of civil law.

- **Contracting with non-medical bodies**

This element of contracting, which is being developed in industrialized countries, is still uncommon in low-income countries. It concerns the production activity of public hospitals outside their statutory mandate. In the case of private hospitals, provided this activity does not interfere with activities for which the hospital receives public money, it can, like any other enterprise, sell its goods and services. The resulting contracts are commercial in nature.

Some Western hospitals have sometimes inherited property, the exploitation of which implies contractual relationships - nowadays purely anecdotal (apart from the famous case of the Hospices de Beaune which makes wine in the Burgundy region). It should be noted that contracts resulting from agricultural activity are specific and often require specific competences.

Today, research work and hospital technical facilities lend themselves to contracting with biotechnology companies. In this case, the hospital is involved in the production of goods and services which do not come within its health-care mandate, so it cannot exploit this potential directly. For this reason it must join forces with companies working in the commercial sector. These companies will capitalize on these products, which have a market outside the confined scope of health care.

Aside from these examples linked to a hospital's health-care activities, mention should also be made of contracts involving the use of hospital capacities to perform logistical services. In this regard, hospital catering services may sell meals to municipal services, laundry can be done for social organizations, and administrative services can be performed for third parties (payroll operations, for example). These few examples illustrate the scope for potential activity. In contradistinction to upstream vertical contracting, the hospital sells or makes available goods and services that it produces, for intermediary consumption, in the course of its own production process. In developing countries it is perfectly possible for hospitals to contract in order to sell these products and services. This whole area overlaps with subcontracting. Thus, concerning these activities involving the issue of making something oneself or having somebody else make it, the whole issue of making and selling needs to be taken into account. This may be justified in situations where the market is tight for subcontractors, and hospital production might interest other partners. Thus, a hospital incinerator could be of interest to certain private operators, who do not have sufficient waste output to justify an individual investment.

There are no hand-and-fast rules for choosing between hospital production and subcontracting. It all depends on the market and production capacity. On occasion it might be preferable to optimize hospital production, whereas at other times it might be more economical to subcontract part of the intermediary production. However, in order to optimize the functioning of hospitals, they must be competent to sign contracts to sell their services to partners who do not necessarily belong to the health-care sector. The question of subcontracting will be further analysed in this book.

2.2   Internal contracting

The use of this type of contracting, which is being developing at the present time, depends on both the form of ownership of the hospital and its management structure.

Table 6: Contracting options

OWNERSHIP	PUBLIC (State, local authorities)				PRIVATE	
MANAGEMENT	Direct	Devolved	Autonomous	Delegated management	Direct	Direct with association
Internal contracting	Possible but rare, since this is not part of direct management culture	Possible Even desirable, overseen by Ministry of Health			Possible, but depends on the culture of the enterprise	

The context

The hospital brings together a number of heterogeneous units. While it is vital to put in place regulations that ensure good relations and consistency among these units, a

165

hospital cannot simply be administered on the basis of the same procedures applied indiscriminately to every unit.

Although hospital organization varies from country to country, this institution's core element is the service unit: they are a place of treatment and diagnosis which cover an integrated area of activity. It is therefore particularly worthwhile to organize relationships between units and vis-à-vis management. A unit's internal organization depends to a great extent on the nature of its work and how much medical responsibility it has: hospitals can improve the efficiency of their component parts by ensuring that they are responsible for managing their own work. Contracting is a tool ideally suited to this process: it enables each unit to set objectives in line with the institution's priorities and available resources, while leaving it to the stakeholders' discretion to decide how best to organize themselves. Internal contracting formalizes the relations between hospital stakeholders and their respective responsibilities.

We should mention that some countries tend to favour internal contracting at a level that regroups several service units : the departmental or cluster level. It is especially helpful to select as a base unit one that has sufficient resources and the ability to put these resources to best use. The most appropriate level for this type of contracting will depend on the extent of the responsibility subject to contract and the degree of institutionalization of the responsibility devolved to the chosen entity and its management. If contracting goes as far as to establish budgets and confer a degree of authority over the management of production factors (including human resources), then one should opt for the department over the service unit. A service unit lacks the critical mass of resources to deal with the vagaries of activity and resource management.

Implementation

Internal contracting is conceivable in institutions that possess a basic information system for managing their activities, revenue and use of resources. With a view to promoting dialogue, unbiased information is required to avoid conflicting interpretations of the data that will determine whether or not the contract is being respected. However, this does not justify a comprehensive information system or sophisticated accounting analysis requiring considerable IT resources and highly qualified staff. The scope and level of detail of the contract will nevertheless be in direct proportion to the quality of the information system.

It is also important to ensure that roles are clearly distributed among the different parties, preferably through a legal provision that legitimizes their different roles as follows:

166

- The management, under the responsibility of a higher authority (a board of directors or representative of the public authority), runs the entire institution. It sets guidelines and objectives and is responsible for the allocation and use of resources;

- Service units are headed by a manager. They have the power to determine how they will meet their objectives and how to make the best use of the resources they have at their disposal. They are responsible for their own activities.

Contracts are conceivable when the parties share a common objective. The search for consensus must not block decisions when conflicts of interest arise. Management is responsible for running the institution, and must take decisions and impose them when the parties cannot reach consensus. It is therefore vital to proceed with caution when choosing prospective areas for contracting. There is nothing worse than compelling units to participate and subsequently imposing a final decision contrary to their wishes.

Contracts must be clearly drafted without requiring long negotiations to clarify each aspect in fine detail. While negotiation is an important element of the contractual process, negotiating efforts should not be exhausted in excessive legal detail, particularly since the contract will not be the subject of litigation before the courts. The contract is a moral commitment based on ground rules accepted by both parties. Failure by either party to respect the contract in the absence of just cause accepted by the other would create an atmosphere of mistrust harmful to the effective functioning of the institution.

Examples of spheres of application

In some cases, contracting may be used to manage a crisis, especially when dealing with resource cutbacks.[25] While the principle of expanding activities through additional resources attracts support, it is much more difficult to develop activities by cutting back resources. Yet the latter scenario is increasingly common. To address it, the way in which activities are organized needs to be reviewed. By approaching this issue from a top-down, authoritarian perspective, the risk of error is compounded. Change will not come naturally from the periphery, since it is not easy to call one's own practices into question or to adhere to the principle of resource cutbacks. Management and service units must therefore agree on an approach that benefits both parties. Contracting is therefore based on sharing the benefits of productivity, while accepting that the service unit has a certain degree of autonomy over the use of these benefits. The formation of the contract will have instructive value because it will demonstrate to the service unit the reason for the cutback in resources and the need to change.

167

Contracting may also be envisaged in a system which seeks to boost hospital resources without proportionally increasing operating costs. This occurs frequently in developing countries, where the principle of out-of-pocket financial contribution is becoming the rule. The parties commit to a target and the income and expenditure that go with it. The profit margin realized through additional activity may be spent on the service unit concerned (the profit-sharing principle). More often than not, the decision is made to use this extra profit to invest in the service unit or to distribute all or some of it among the staff in the form of a bonus (see the example of Soavinandriana hospital).

Contracting can be a tool for promoting inter-unit collaboration. An increasing number of pathologies require the intervention of various specialisms, or resources can be shared between a number of specialisms from different service units. In both scenarios, a contract would enable terms and conditions to be established for the use of staff, premises and equipment. A contract could also deal with patient care and the resulting arrangements. Management should participate in contract negotiation in order to ensure that the hospital's mandate is respected.

These few examples show that the sphere of application for contracting is very broad, but in all cases there must be a monitoring mechanism such as a committee of representatives appointed by the parties to the contract.

"Means and objectives" contract at Soavinandriana Hospital in Madagascar.[26]

Contracts were signed between the management and various service units. The contracts are built around an incentive scheme based on a list of specified responsibilities and tasks. There are two objectives:

- To institute a management system that strikes a balance between activities and resources;
- to involve the service unit in management by establishing an incentive team.

The adoption of this contract involved isolating the service unit's expenditure and ensuring that its activity was monitored according to the terms of the contract. Specific emphasis was placed on recovering outstanding payments, and changes were made to the operation of the unit responsible for collections. Operating charts were drawn up in order to monitor monthly activity, revenue and expenditure.

The contract was signed for a renewable one-year term, with a three-month trial period.

All available data for the previous year that could be potentially useful in meeting the objectives established by the contract were annexed.

Establishing this type of contract enabled the service unit to lock in its procurements, thereby ensuring better service delivery to users. It also resulted in increased staff premiums, thereby boosting motivation and hence quality of service.

---

3.   STAGES OF THE CONTRACTING PROCESS

The question on most managers' lips when they hear of all the opportunities afforded by contracting is where to start. Clearly, it is not possible to do everything at once. It is therefore worthwhile identifying which contracting opportunities offer the best potential.

Instituting a contracting process means seeing beyond the instrument, i.e. the contract, and focusing on the whole issue of managing a hospital through contracting. This is a comprehensive hospital-wide approach, as opposed to one that requires individual managers to improve the quality of contracts in their particular sector. It aims for coherence and consistency within the institution, as reflected by a certain standardization in the drafting and use of contracts. It also involves a willingness to improve contract literacy for all those involved in drafting and implementing them. Then there is a strategic stage based on a situation report, which is used to make priority-based choices.

Assessment, opportunities and risks

Though managers do not always fully realize it, hospitals are a hub for contracting. Before developing new interventions it is helpful to start with an evaluation of the contracting situation at the hospital. The above-mentioned models for upstream and downstream vertical contracting and horizontal contracting are a good starting point for carrying out this type of assessment. Above all, this approach is time-consuming and managers will tailor their ambitions according to the time they can devote to them. Not too much preparation time is required - the equivalent of a few man-days are sufficient to identify a few activities that might benefit from contracting.

Review of the existing situation

It is not necessary to allocate significant resources to assessing the existing situation using consultants. A meeting of the hospital's decision-making team is sufficient to review current contractual relations at all levels. This meeting can be usefully supplemented by systematically questioning middle managers, so that the scope of the contracts can be better identified with them. This approach also helps to mobilize all the stakeholders and encourages in-house communication about the importance of this issue. The assessment should not simply determine whether or not a contractual relation exists, but should also take into account how long the contract has been in place, whether it has been renewed, how formal it is, and the issues at stake, particularly economic, but also managerial and social.

When carrying out this investigation, attention should be given to the methods of monitoring contracts, i.e : where they are kept (if written), who monitors implementation, is there a mechanism for periodically reviewing contract performance? etc.

The assessment will not only provide an overview of the situation but will also implicitly provide information about current capacity for contractual management, in addition to identifying the weaknesses of the individuals associated with these contracts and the procedures adopted by the hospital.

Aside from classification by type of contract, it would be beneficial to draw a distinction between formal and tacit contracts. Identifying tacit contracts is certainly the most complex, since it requires an analysis of the relationships between all the parties both inside and outside the hospital.

While there is no need to be exhaustive, the main contracts should nevertheless not be omitted. This approach is consistent with the reasoning presented throughout this book: the contract embodies an exchange, not simply a legal act. In the case of tacit contracts, we should identify those that represent an important commitment on the part of the hospital l, whether internally between units or externally between the hospital and third parties.

Opportunities

The aim of the contractual approach is not limited to putting existing contracts in order, rather it involves exploring areas in which it would be useful for the hospital to formalize existing or potential relationships by means of a contract. However, developing contracting does not just mean adopting a consistent policy of routinely formalizing all exchange relationships through contracts. Opportunities for contracting can be identified through a dual-track approach: strategic and economic.

The strategic approach will mirror that used for hospital development. The existence of a formal strategic plan will make it easier to identify contracting opportunities. Failing this, the hospital's development priorities can be identified quite simply by considering its mandate and role in the local, regional or national health-care system. A district hospital, for example, is intended to provide a point of reference and guidance for primary level health-care. Would it be appropriate to formalize the exchange flows between the hospital and the health-care services responsible for dispensaries, or between all kinds of dispensaries? What are the local priorities for improving a coordinated response, with an impact on public health? Do funding arrangements allow the costs of these support and coordination activities to be covered? Etc.

The economic approach will focus more on analyzing the hospital as a business that mobilizes its production factors in order to deliver services. How can production of these services be rationalized by mobilizing production factors as efficiently as possible. Outsourcing is often the first stage in a contractual arrangement of this type. Under this approach, an economic calculation is a prerequisite for any decision. In this calculation it is essential to take into account all elements involved in costs. This is the stage at which transaction costs should be considered.

Furthermore, this economic approach should include activities that result in improvements in the quality of service offered (including quality of care). This is because improving quality for a similar cost increases the value of the service. Measuring an increase in value is a delicate issue if the improvement in quality leads to an increase in costs.

A review of contracting opportunities is based on evidence and an assessment of the objective advantages of contracting, but it must also rely on the knowledge and common sense of hospital managers, which should be guided by the general interest and the interests of the organization for which they are responsible.

These opportunities should be analysed using the same methods that were used to analyse the existing situation, i.e. through mobilization of the institution's in-house capacity.

Risks

Risks will not be minimized simply by wishing contracts into existence and thinking that doing so will give a more modern image to the organization, or that success will be a sure bet.

The first risk concerns the reliability and continued existence of the other party to the contract. A contract, by definition, is established with another party, and it is therefore essential to ensure that the other party is reliable. This does not mean making a value judgement, but rather objectively assessing their capacity to do what is expected of them. This consideration is equally true for both the strategic and economic approaches. It may be desirable to use contracting as a means of innovation, but if this is the case the results must be monitored all the more closely and the contract should specify arrangements for the swift adoption of backup solutions.

The second risk is connected with the weakness of institutional governance. The development of contracting may encourage corruption and reduce managerial liability. The risks are heightened if there are no mechanisms in place to ensure minimal transparency in contracts, and if decisions are not shared or based on objective elements.

The third risk is that people will not buy into the contract. This risk is particularly high in hospitals where there are numerous occupational groups, often enjoying considerable professional independence. It is also accentuated in organizations with strong unions in which poorly explained contracting is considered as a way to circumvent social dialogue and especially to downgrade employees' working conditions.

The fourth risk has to do with the capacity for managing contracts. Whatever the object of the contract, hospital managers must bear responsibility for the results achieved. It is not right that they should develop contracts as a means of shielding themselves from responsibility for the institution's work. It is therefore crucial to ensure the monitorability of contract outcomes. This presupposes an ability to draw up sound contracts and monitor their implementation.

Implementation

There are several ways to initiate a contracting process. The adoption of contracting might signal a desire to renew the management of an institution and may therefore be central to the institution's managerial vision. In this case, there will be a launch phase and communication will be adapted to this change of direction in the way the hospital is managed.

Generally speaking, contracting is just one strand in managerial policy. It forms part of the existing managerial vision and the degree of attention it receives will depend on the importance and nature of the activities undertaken.

Information and participation

In order to launch an institution on the path towards contracting, or to ensure this process goes more smoothly, it is preferable to opt for a minimal degree of formality, using internal communication through the hospital authorities. This information and consultation phase will be prepared using a case statement. As for any activity, the benefit for the hospital must be justified, either from a strategic or economic point of view.

Before presenting this to the authorities, the management must therefore do preparatory work, following the stages indicated in the preceding paragraph.

Efforts to improve an existing contractual arrangement do not require input from the authorities, since these constitute a straightforward management operation.

They can be included in an appraisal of activities and presented in that context. They can thus be used to evaluate the competence of management, which is trying to improve hospital performance in those areas of activity for which it is already responsible. On the other hand, if the contractual process is going to change the hospital's functions, whether internal or external, this should go through the authorities in order to minimize the risks outlined above.

Choice of priorities

Choosing priorities is certainly not a linear process. Firstly, although throughout this chapter we have focused on the logic of giving the hospital the initiative to contract, the actual situation may differ. The systematic establishment of contracts that link resources with results (performance contracts, or objectives and means contracts) are not initiated by hospitals, but rather by fund holders (public authorities, insurers or foreign donors). While under no obligation to accept this solution, the hospital must rapidly decide whether or not it finds this acceptable. If the hospital commits to this arrangement, the provisions stipulated in these contracts will be broadly imposed on the hospital.

Drafting and monitoring

Here we are not referring to situations where a hospital comes under a national policy that defines all these elements and has actually been imposed on institutions. We are more interested in arrangements that give hospitals control over the process, which implies that they must take all necessary steps to implement a structured contracting policy.

Contract management requires a minimum level of competence and is not merely a legal construct. In fact, it is often necessary to mobilize several skills. Technical skills are essential for the contract objectives and implementation arrangements to bear fruit. In the case of human resources contracting it would be useful to have a grasp of labour law and/or the statutory provisions governing public workers, as well as human resources management. In the case of horizontal contracting with a university, competence in teaching and knowledge of training curricula objectives are essential. Generally speaking, these competences are automatically available when contracts are negotiated with stakeholders who have a genuine commitment to the implementation of the contract.

In addition to these technical skills, it is also desirable to have specific competence in contracting. This will guarantee consistency of approach to individual contracts, and specifically the incorporation of each contract into the institution's overall policy. This type of competence should include economic analysis skills and strong institutional knowledge. In order to acquire this competence, contract-specific training is required. Just as in qualitative processes where the need to identify a focal point, the quality control officer, soon becomes apparent, contracting too requires a contracting focal point.

The size of the institution and the number of contractual arrangements do not routinely justify a position, let alone a unit, wholly devoted to contracting. But this competence, with a degree of involvement and expertise that will depend on the volume and complexity of the contractual arrangements, will need to be identified quickly. The establishment of a focal point also helps to evaluate the results obtained and determine the conditions in which the contract provisions can be best implemented.

We cannot overemphasize the importance of monitoring and evaluation. Since a whole chapter is devoted to this subject, there is no need to elaborate on it here. Monitoring and evaluation are not specific to hospitals, except to say that a very large number of stakeholders must be taken into account.

CONCLUSION

Modern hospitals are increasingly moving away from the concept of administration and service governed by hierarchical relationships and coming to resemble firms. However, this should not be viewed in the neo-classical economic sense, where the firm is simply an agent that attempts to efficiently transform input into output, and where the effectiveness of this transformation is analyzed on the basis of cost and production functions. On the contrary, like a firm, the hospital is defined as an organization, i.e. an economic unit for coordination, seeking to meet an objective, or a set of objectives shared by the participating members. In this regard, the hospital is defined by a "node of contracts"[27] that govern all of the organization's internal and external relationships.

More specifically, the hospital must ask itself two questions:

- Which of the functions that it currently carries out itself could be performed by another party? For a long time it was thought that these were limited to non-medical activities, for example laundry, security and catering. Since then, we have seen the development of contractual relationships in respect of intermediary diagnostic services, for example laboratory examinations and radiology. Finally, contracting has developed in purely medical relationships, for example the intervention of specialist physicians in cases of certain pathologies. There are therefore no theoretical limits to outsourcing; there are no activities that cannot be performed by external parties: and thus the idea of core functions is brought into question. Following this argument through to its logical conclusion, we could arrive at a situation in which the hospital itself produces nothing, and all its activities are conducted through subcontracting arrangements. However, when the question arises of whether to make something or have it made by someone else, transaction costs and the margin realized by the contractor must be taken into consideration. The past and future market situation must also be borne in mind. So the answer must be framed in terms of an analysis of the total costs of the operation when there exists a real choice between making something or having it made.

- Since it is an independent or autonomous party, its relationships with the parties around it involve connections and transactions. To what degree should these be formalized through contracts? Users have requirements that cannot be reduced to the mere notion of price; these requirements must be negotiated. Financial partners, as user representatives, wish to negotiate the terms and conditions of their funding. The oversight authority (in the case of autonomy) wishes to reach agreement on its relations with the hospital. Other stakeholders (municipalities, businesses, NGOs, development partners) with a vested interest in the hospital also want to formalize their relationships with it.

When combined, both these approaches reveal a hospital to be an organization that manages a set of contracts. Specifically, the hospital, as an organization, can limit itself to a few administrators in a few offices, who manage all the contracts necessary for hospital production. These administrators should not be confused with those who perform services for the hospital and have signed contracts to enable them to do so.

A wealth of new possibilities is open to a hospital with autonomous status; contracting allows this type of hospital to better control its environment and its relationships with various partners. However, this control mechanism is complex and it is likely that many regional or district hospitals in developing countries currently lack the technical capacity to take full advantage of the possibilities afforded by contracting. Most probably, hospitals will need time to familiarize themselves with this tool and maximize its benefits by drawing on the experience and training of their staff. The final form of contract transactions will depend on the specific context in each country.

Finally, we should not forget that contracting is not limited to outsourcing; above all it is a powerful tool for improving organizational performance, regardless of whether the organization is in the public or private sector. However, contracting will yield the most benefit only if a country has a hospital policy that dovetails the mission and role of hospitals with the social and public health priorities determined by the population. Contracting will be even more effective if the State fulfils its "stewardship" responsibilities by creating a context that promotes initiative and respect for common objectives. It should therefore not be forgotten that contracting is a tool in the service of policy; it cannot compensate for defective policies.

Notes

[1] Some people talk of "reinventing the hospital"; for example, "The reinvented hospital", Montaigne Institute, January 2004.

[2] Morocco has opted for this approach by establishing second-tier hospitals as independently managed services. However, the performance limitations of these institutions is encouraging a trend towards granting them the same level of independence as university hospitals already enjoy.

[3] The broad range of approaches can even result in a situation where independence is not granted to one specific hospital, but rather to an independent institution that manages several hospitals. This model has been used by the Government of Andhra Pradesh in India.

Chawla, M. and A. George. *Hospital Autonomy in India.* 1996. Harvard School of Public Health USA

This document can be viewed online: Harvard School of Public Health USA website, consulted on 30 January 2001: http://www.harvard.edu/Organizations

[4] Govindaraj, R., A. A. D. Obuobi, N. K. A. Enyimayew, P. Antwi, and S. Ofosu-Amaah. *Hospital autonomy in Ghana: the experience of Korle Bu and Komfo Anokye Teaching hospitals.* 1996. Harvard School of Public Health USA.

This document can be viewed online: Harvard School of Public Health USA website, consulted on 30 January 2001: http://www.harvard.edu/Organizations.ddm. This study shows how important and necessary it is to establish a board of directors, but this is not enough to guarantee true autonomy. In this instance, therefore, boards of directors have not been able to capitalize on the opportunity; but it also appears that the Ministry of Health did not really want them to take it.

[5] Larbi, G. A. 1998. *Institutional constraints and capacity issues in decentralizing management in public services: the case of health in Ghana. Journal of International Development* 10:377-386.

[6] Generally speaking, this refers to contractual positions for grades that do not exist or are very rare in workforces managed by the Ministry of Health.

[7] Collins, D., G. Njeru, J. Meme, and W. Newbrander. 1999. *Hospital autonomy: the experience of Kenyatta National Hospital. International Journal of Health Planning and Management* 14:129-153.

[8] Sharma, S. and D. R. Hotchkiss. 2001. *Developing financial autonomy in public hospitals in India:Rajasthan's model. Health Policy* 55:1-18.

[9] McPake, B. 1996. *Public autonomous hospitals in sub-Saharan Africa: trends and issues. Health Policy* 35:155-177.

[10] Bossert, Th, S. Kosen, B. Harsono, and A. Gani. *Hospital autonomy in Indonesia.* 1996. USA, Harvard School of Public Health.

This document can be viewed online: Harvard School of Public Health USA website, consulted on 30 January 2001: http://www.harvard.edu/Organizations. This study shows that, in the context of this autonomy, the Ministry of Health continues to control the procedures for planning and budgeting income from cost recovery. Thus the directors of these autonomous hospitals must submit an annual plan for the use of their own revenue.

[11] Mills, A., S. Bennett, and S. Russell. 2001. *The challenge of health sector reform. What must Government Do?*: Palgrave.

[12] Collins, D., G. Njeru, J. Meme, and W. Newbrander. 1999. *Hospital autonomy: the experience of Kenyatta National Hospital. International Journal of Health Planning and Management* 14:129-153.

These criteria were set by W. Newbrander in 1993 and 1995 for Management Sciences for Health (Boston, USA: and are cited in D.Collins, G.Njeru, J.Meme et W.Newbrander (1999)

[13] It is important to make clear that legal provisions applicable to the private sector apply to the public sector too. The tenor of the legal provisions will be the same or specifically targeted, depending on the field in question.

[14] Bhatia, M. and A. Mills. 1997. *Contracting out of dietary services by public hospitals in Bombay.* In *Private Health providers*, edited by Bennett, S., B. McPake, and A. Mills (London and New Jersey: Zed Books).

[15] Dagam, K. L. *Papua New Guinea experience in contracting for non-health related services in health centers and / or hospitals with private enterprises.* 1998. Geneva, WHO/HQ/ICO. Towards new partnerships for health development in developing countries: the contractual approach as a policy tool. Communication presented in the technical meeting "Towards new partnerships for health development in developing countries: the contractual approach as a policy tool", WHO/HQ/ICO, Geneva, 4-6 February 1998

[16] Collins, D., G. Njeru, J. Meme, and W. Newbrander. 1999. *Hospital autonomy: the experience of Kenyatta National Hospital. International Journal of Health Planning and Management* 14:129-153.

[17] de Roodenbeke, E. *La dynamique du projet d'établissement. Guide en organisation hospitalière dans les pays en développement.* 2001. Paris.

177

[18] Achouri, H. 2001. *Le projet d'appui à la réforme hospitalière: objectifs, implémentation, résultats et enseignements. La Tunisie médicale* 79, no. 5.

[19] WHO. *World Health Report 2000 - Health Systems: Improving Performance.* 2000. Clermont-Ferrand, France, Paper presented at the international symposium on Financing health systems in low-income countries in Africa and Asia

[20] Delaunay, B. *Chartes usagers et engagements de qualité dans le secteur public en France.* 1999. L'Harmattan, Logiques juridiques, France.

[21] These are not autonomous hospitals, rather private not-for-profit hospitals, and the project is managed by the Antwerp Institute for Tropical Medicine (Belgium).

[22] de Roodenbeke, E. 1994. *Une voie d'avenir pour la coopération, le partenariat hospitalier. cahiers santé* 4 ; 105-9.

[23] Guide de la coopération hospitalière pour l'aide au développement - Editions de l'ENSP- 1997

See also www.fhf.fr under "coopération internationale" : protocole de mission exploratoire pour un partenariat hospitalier.

[24] The International Hospital Federation (www.ihf-fih.org) can provide specific assistance in seeking partners through its many affiliated national federations. It can also give advice based on the experiences of its members.

[25] Hubert, J. and R. Dubois. 2000. *Culture de gestion plus que redressement budgétaire: deux ans de contractualisation au CHU de Rennes. Gestion hospitalière*:671-676.

[26] Wetta, C. 1997. *les contrats d'objectifs et de moyens. Coopération française.*

[27] Jensen, M. and W. Meckling. 1976. *Theory of the firm: managerial behaviour, agency cost, and ownership structure. Journal of financial economics 3*, no. 4.

Part II

Chapter 3

Contracting with private sector networks:

franchising reproductive health care

Dale Huntington

INTRODUCTION

The important role that the private sector has in providing health care in low-resource countries is widely recognized.[1] A recent International Finance Corporation report states that of the total health expenditures in Africa of $16.7 billion in 2005, roughly 60 percent–predominately out-of-pocket payments by individuals–was financed by private parties and about 50 percent was captured by private providers.[2] Private sector provision of health care includes sexual and reproductive health services, for which a considerable number of women turn to the private sector. In many Asian and Latin American countries the private sector – through clinics, hospitals, pharmacies or nongovernmental organizations – provides more than 50% of all contraceptives.[3] Recent evidence from sub-Saharan Africa indicates that approximately one third of all family planning methods are obtained through the private sector.[4] Even the poorest households in seek care from the private sector. Data drawn from Demographic and Health Survey (DHS) in 38 countries worldwide show that for children in the lowest income quintile, 34% - 96% of children who sought care for diarrhoea received treatment in the private sector.[5]

One contributing factor to this growth of the private reproductive health sector is a widening gap between insufficient donor and public funding for health care in general, and the rapidly increasing demand for family planning in particular. In many settings the public sector is simply under-resourced to meet demand for SRH services. For example, by 2015 the number of contraceptive users in poor countries may grow by more than 200 million – driven by increasing numbers of couples entering their reproductive years.[6] Yet during the past twelve years, the annual amount of OECD/DAC government funding for family planning as a percentage of total population and AIDS activities has declined from 22% in 1996 to 3.5% in 2008.[7]

The funding shortfall for family planning varies from region to region, but it is particularly acute in Africa. Whereas US$270 million was required for family planning in Africa in 2006, donor funding and domestic resources combined totalled only US$200 million, resulting in a shortfall of US$70 million for that region alone.[8] In part to make up for declining external assistance and in part due to growing economies, national funding for Sexual and Reproductive Health services has increased in many countries, yet consumers contribute disproportionally through out-of-pocket spending for health services -- over 60% of total domestic expenditures for population and AIDS care recorded in 2007 came from consumer payments.[9]

Although many governments, for a variety of reasons, have been slow to react to the expansion of the private health sector there is now widespread recognition of the need to engage the private sector in healthcare delivery. Implementing properly designed and financed public health policies are operationally much easier when private providers are organized into formal associations or networks, yet in many settings the private sector is disorganized or loosely grouped through professional associations. Governments need to carefully examine different policy options that facilitate the formation of private sector networks and work to ensure that any actions taken to engage with the private sector strengthen and expand the development of private provider networks that bring added value to their members, complement the public sector's efforts, address health consumer needs and further national health goals, including ensuring equitable access.

Private Sector Networks

Networks can take many forms but, in general, they can be considered as an affiliation of providers grouped together under a parent organization. One way to categorize private health networks, based on stated objectives and ownership of service delivery points, results in three types of networks: social franchises, not-for-profit networks and for-profit commercial businesses.[10] There are different benefits to each of these different types of networks but all aim to provide a degree of uniformity in the range and quality of health services provided, in addition to passing on savings or other benefits to its members in areas such as training, procurement of equipment and supplies, and advertising. With respect to providing sexual and reproductive health services, social franchises and not-for-profit networks have been the most prevalent. While both types have a social orientation, a key difference lays in the ownership of individual service delivery outlets: in a social franchise outlets are owned by independent health practitioners, in a not-for-profit network outlets are owned by a non-profit organization or NGO.

Reproductive Health Franchises

Social franchising is a variant of the commercial franchise model, which is defined as "a contractual relationship between a franchisee (usually a small business) and a franchisor (usually a larger business) in which the franchisee agrees to produce or market a product or service in accordance with an overall blueprint devised by the franchisor."[11] In a commercial franchise, the range and quality of services are standardized and identified with a branded name (or logo); the overall arrangement is governed by a contractual relationship between the franchising organization and the providers.[12] In commercial franchises the franchisee will commonly pay an upfront fee to 'buy into' the franchise and pay periodic fees (e.g. royalties, membership) in return for receiving a tried and tested operating manual from the franchisor. The franchisee assumes a financial risk, which is mitigated by a proven track record in the franchisor's commercial viability and business plan.

In a social franchise the franchisor is typically a non-profit organization that bears most of the financial risk involved in establishing franchised outlets. Operational support is provided by the franchisor, and typically involves access to commodities, supplies and equipment at reduced cost, in addition to training in clinical and business skills and advertising. In return, the franchisees are often required to pay franchise fees, maintain certain levels of quality standards, and record and report on sales and service statistics. A key distinction of a social franchise lies in the objectives of the franchise, which are based on social, rather than business, motives. In this sense, social franchises are akin to social marketing programmes, although the focus is on health *services* rather than on health *products*.

Historically, social franchises have taken on the responsibility for assuring the availability and quality of services, and also assuring awareness and use of those services.[13] More recently, increased attention has been paid to ensuring the financial sustainability of social franchises, particularly in the light of reduced donor funding for reproductive health and the trend towards upstream funding mechanisms (such as sector wide approaches that include pooled funding, or direct budget support). In addition, social franchises are now challenged to move beyond the pilot stage and achieve economies of scale for making greater health impact. It is this shift towards sustainability and scale which opens the door to the potential for partnership with governments of developing countries.

Franchising Reproductive Health - Lessons from Contemporary Networks

Social marketing programmes for contraceptives are the best example of long-standing social franchises of substantial scale, even though they do represent a variation on the franchise model and have several important distinctions that make their operations somewhat exceptional among networks of private sector providers. In general, however, international experience with social franchises in low- and middle-income countries for sexual and reproductive health programmes is a fairly recent development and most franchised networks are operating at a relatively small scale. Currently, there are approximately two dozen social franchise programmes worldwide that provide reproductive health services, and most of them have been in operation only for less than a decade. Each of these programmes have been developed in response to specific conditions of the national healthcare market and each have a different configuration of services and varying business plans. As such, each social franchise programme is unique and highly contextualized, making generalizations somewhat problematic. Never-the-less, four broad approaches can be used to describe how healthcare franchises and networks have adapted to the healthcare market and achieved greater scale, successfully segmenting their clientele from other private and public sector providers.

- Franchised networks are providing sexual and reproductive health services that government is not able to offer due to socio-political restrictions on public sector operations. For example, the Sun Quality Health Network (Myanmar), RedPlan Salud (Peru) and FriendlyCare (Philippines) networks are providing family planning services in settings where the public sector has limited the range or availability of contraceptives.

- Social franchises are extending the reach of the public sector health system, reducing the backlog of accrediting providers for specific procedures. For example, the Janani franchise programme, in India trains providers in medical termination of pregnancy and works to expand the number of accredited abortion sites in rural and under-served areas.

- In many settings, private sector networks, including franchises, have been developed in response to the need to improve quality and ensure equity through social insurance programmes. In the Philippines the national health insurance programme PhilHealth is partnering with the FriendlyCare network to provide family planning and other services to the poor, for which FriendlyCare clinics will be reimbursed by the national health insurer. Total Health Trust, in Nigeria, is working as a type of 'preferred provider organization' (PPO) to facilitate the reach of the Nigerian National Health Insurance Scheme in order to expand access to priority health services, including reproductive health (as well as to create financial space for the PPO that is favourable to its long-term sustainability).

- Franchises have begun to develop partnerships with the commercial sector to expand people's access to care and ensure sustainability. RedPlan Salud negotiated a partnership with pharmaceutical companies and distributors, whereby the franchisor (INPPARES) purchases bulk quantities of brand-name oral contraceptives at a discounted rate. These are then sold to midwife franchisees at a marked-up price. As a result of its strategic partnerships, RedPlan Salud is able to meet its health objectives and has achieved financial sustainability.

Underlying these lessons is the recognition that trade-offs exist between serving the poor, providing a full range of sexual and reproductive health services and financial sustainability of the franchise. The inherent tension between these goals underscores the importance of public sector support for private sector provision of public health goods, a clear understanding of franchise objectives by senior managements of both public and private sectors, monitoring of the partnership over time, and adapting policy and operations in response to changing market forces and public policy goals.

There are several government policy mechanisms that can guide the development and expansion of franchises providing sexual and reproductive healthcare. Although a ranking of these policies in order of priority is problematic, financing policies are the most critical. Financial transfers of some type are essential if the private sector is to serve the health needs of the poor, as otherwise the poor will either be at risk of catastrophic expenses or simply not utilize needed health services. Additionally, without financial support for reproductive health services, the private sector will not be able to afford to provide unprofitable services and may not include many reproductive health services in its clinical practices. There are a number of mechanisms through which the public sector can provide financial support to the private sector, including :

- **Social health insurance.** The expansion of social health insurance schemes in developing countries reflects important changes in government financial policy towards reducing out-of-pocket expenses in favour of pre-paid, pooled financing schemes.

- **Contracting private health providers.** Another mechanism for working with the private sector involves making direct payments to health providers through various types of contracting mechanisms. Evidence on contracting services by government to the private sector suggests that direct contracting can be effective in reaching underserved populations with reproductive healthcare in many settings. [14,15]

- **Input subsidies and tax incentives.** Governments have a long and successful history of providing subsidies for public health programmes delivered through the private sector, including NGO/not-for-profit networks. Most common are government-supported subsidies for commodities such as contraceptive methods, childhood immunizations, treatment for tuberculosis and, more recently, HIV/AIDS prevention and treatment. [16]

- **Vouchers or output-based incentives.** While the evidence is not conclusive on a large scale, vouchers have been shown to be practical methods of transferring payments directly to patients while also reaching underserved groups (e.g. commercial sex workers and adolescents).[17],[18]

- **Liberalizing policies governing products.** Since many provider networks and franchises depend heavily on products (e.g. contraceptives, ARVs, etc.), liberalizing policies and laws that regulate products, such as registration, importation and taxation, is another form of financial support to the private sector.[19]

Challenges for Implementing Public/Private Partnerships

Despite identifying a number of innovative public policy options for expanding access to and improving the quality of reproductive health in the private sector, several challenges exist that constrain the effective public - private partnerships. These include the following:

- **Minimal understanding of the private health sector.** In many countries, there is limited information on private providers, such as the number and different types, what services they provide or do not, and who do they serve. Conducting an assessment or type of mapping exercise of the private health sector can be a useful exercise in many settings.[20]

- **Lack of political will and support to include the private sector.** In many settings there is a element of mistrust between the public and private sectors. Limited information on the private health sector and limited contact between the two sectors further contributes towards this problem. Private sector representatives are commonly not included in important activities such as health planning, revising and updating norms and designing new programmes, such as health insurance schemes, that will directly impact the private health sector. Government organized meetings frequently are scheduled at inconvenient times or are simply too long for private sector providers. Additionally, in many settings there is an unhealthy sense of competition between the two sectors, further creating unease and distrust.

- **Unfair playing field.** Donors and governments often expect higher standards from the private sector than the public. Frequently the performance based contracts or other types of purchasing agreements impose higher levels of quality of care or service performance than are expected from their own public health facilities. Also, the public sector and donors often assume that profit-making groups do not warrant financial support, setting minimal profit margins

185

on contracts to the point that the transaction or opportunity costs are simply too high for the private providers, making the contract simply not worthwhile.

Donors and multilateral organizations can play an important role in nurturing public sector engagement of the private health sector. A paradigm shift in donor policy that includes new terms and concepts redefining health systems to broadly include the private sector and other actors is a first step. Other, more specific actions include the following:[21]

- Earmarking higher proportion of aid to fund private sector, particularly those that target the poor or provide health care services of public goods nature

- "Blending" aid money with commercial financing in order to create and expand sustainable private sector entities

- Support for documentation and dissemination of best private sector practices and government support to private sector

- Invest in the development of public sector capacity to manage pluralistic health systems

CONCLUSION

Social franchises are an important and unique form of private sector initiative. Many issues germane to their development cut across other types of private provider networks clustered around individual private practitioners. The explicit goal of advancing universal access to public health services in general and sexual and reproductive health programmes in particular, especially by underserved populations, sets them apart in many ways. Closer collaboration and cooperation with government is perhaps more essential for private health franchises than for other types of private sector networks. There is a clear role for both government and the private sector to work together in partnership to promote increased access to reproductive health services. While social franchises offer the promise to expand access to priority health services, further evidence is needed to guide the operation of these franchises in the future and to assist in the formation of public policy to ensure quality of care, to advance equity and to secure long-term sustainability of this unique private sector network.

186

Notes

[1] This paper draws on the following the outcomes of a joint WHO and USAID PSP- *One* meeting "Public Policy and Franchising Reproductive Health: Current Evidence and Future Directions - Guidance from a technical consultation meeting, WHO Geneva, 2007;

http://www.who.int/reproductive-health/healthsystems/meeting06.htm

[2] International Finance Corporation, 2007 "The business of health in Africa: Partnering with the private sector to improve people's lives" World Bank Group, Washington, DC

[3] Winfrey et al. Factors Influencing the Growth of the Commercial Sector in Family Planning Service Provision. 2000. POLICY Project Working Paper Series No. 6.

[4] Zellner, S., B. O'Hanlon, and T. Chandani. *State of the Private Health Sector Wall Chart.* 2006. Bethesda, USA, MD: Private Sector Partnership-One Project, Abt Associates, Inc.

[5] Bustreo, F. et al. 2010. *Can developing countries achieve adequate improvements in child health outcomes without engaging the private sector?* *Bulletin of the World Health Organization* 81, no. 12:886-894.

[6] The Unfinished Agenda: Meeting the Need for Family Planning in Less Developed Countries. Population Reference Bureau, November 2004.

[7] UNFPA/UNAIDS/NIDI Resource Flows Newsletter, November 2007

[8] Cleland, J., S. Bernstein, A. Ezeh, A. Faunde, A Glasier, and J. Innis. 2006. *Family planning: the unfinished agenda. The Lancet.*

[9] UNFPA/UNAIDS/NIDI Resource Flows Newsletter, November 2007

[10] Chandani, T., S. Sulzbach, and M. Forzley. 2006. *Private Provider Networks: The Role of Viability in Expanding the Supply of Reproductive Health and Family Planning Services. Private Sector Partnership-One Project, Abt Associates, Inc.,*

[11] Stanworth J et al. *Franchising as a source of technology transfer to developing economies.* Special Studies Series No. 7, ed. International Franchise Research Center, 7. Westminster: University of Westminster Press, 1995.

[12] Montagu, D. 2002b. *Franchising of health services in low-income countries. Health Policy and Planning* 17, no. 2:121-130.

[13] Montagu, D. 2002a. *Franchising of health services in developing countries. Health Policy and Planning* 17, no. 2:121-130.

[14] England R . Experience of contracting with the private sector: A selective review *Issues Paper - Private Sector.* DFID Health Systems Resource Centre, 2004.

Liu, X., D. R. Hotchkiss, S. Bose, R. Bitran, and U. Giediion. 2004. *Contracting for primary health services: Evidence on its effects and framework for evaluation. Partners for Health Reformplus Project, Abt Associates Inc.*

[15] WHO. 2006. Special Theme Issue: Contracting and Health Services. *Bulletin of the World Health Organization* 84, no. 11:841-920.

[16] Wang, L., J. Liu, and D. Chin. 2007. Progress in tuverculosis control and the evolving public health system in China. *The Lancet* 369, no. February:691-696.

[17] McKay, et al. 2006. Lessons for Management of Sexually Transmitted Infection Treatment Programs as part of HIV/AIDS Prevention Strategies. *American Journal of Public Health* 96, no. 6:7-9.

[18] World Bank, ""A Guide to Competitive Vouchers", Washington, D.C., 2005

[19] IFC, 2007, op.cite.

[20] Chakraborty, S. and A. Harding. 2003. Conducting a Private Sector Assessment. In *Private Participation in Health Services*, edited by Harding, A. and A. S. Preker World Bank).

[21] IFC, 2007, op.cite.

Part II

Chapter 4

Health insurance coverage and
contracting in developing countries

Valérie Schmitt &

Christian Jacquier

INTRODUCTION

Extension of health insurance coverage worldwide remains a topical issue, seeing as a large portion of the world's population still lacks adequate health coverage. The strategies for extending coverage have changed over time, and today a new and promising approach involves what is referred to as "articulated systems". The definition of such health insurance schemes is that they rely on a range of stakeholders and sources of funding (e.g., governments, local communities, insured persons, international partnership and businesses). Therefore, this type of system not only implies contractual relationships between beneficiaries and social security systems, or between social security systems and health care providers; but between all actors involved in financing and running the system: i.e., local government, insurers, NGOs, local associations, etc. With the emergence of articulated systems, contracting is becoming a centrepiece among the strategies and initiatives to facilitate access to health care in developing countries.

In this chapter we begin by giving a brief overview of the different strategies for extending health insurance coverage, followed by a presentation of what is referred to as "articulated systems" and the potential they have in terms of contracting. Then we give a more detailed description of the contracting mechanisms used within the framework of articulated insurance schemes, with a typology and several examples.

1. CHANGING STRATEGIES FOR EXTENDING HEALTH INSURANCE COVERAGE

1.1 Definition of health insurance coverage

Health insurance coverage comprises a series of measures and mechanisms to protect individuals and their families from the financial consequences of illness (and, by extension, maternity).

A range of financial and economic factors justify establishing health protection schemes. In particular, health protection contributes to the fight against poverty – both directly, by providing financial protection and thus preventing households affected by illness from falling into poverty; and indirectly, by virtue of their positive effect on economic performance and productivity.

There are also health-related reasons for establishing such schemes at the national and international level. Health is increasingly considered as a global public good, and the international community therefore carries a global responsibility to monitor health and prevent epidemics, including by helping states with insufficient resources to improve health care delivery.

Finally, health protection is warranted from a rights perspective, as access to social security and health care are two fundamental human rights.

1.2   Exclusion from coverage

An estimated 86 per cent of the population in developing countries have no health insurance cover, compared with 37 per cent in middle-income countries. The majority of uninsured persons are also among the most vulnerable to disease because of their living and working conditions: informal economy workers and their families, and rural populations.

1.3   Strategies for extending coverage

Many strategies have been developed in the past to extend health care coverage and health insurance cover, and it is up to individual countries to design their own extension strategies and the most appropriate mechanisms in accordance with their economic and institutional development and cultural-historic context.

There are two major groups of mechanisms aimed at mitigating the financial impact of illness and maternity:

1. Mechanisms that finance treatment and provide a certain range of health services free of charge for all or part of the population (e.g., the most deprived, the elderly, women and children). This first category includes (1) universal systems providing free access for the entire population or a certain age group (e.g, the elderly, children or women of childbearing age), irrespective of income; and (2) social welfare schemes that provide free access to a range of health services for the poorest parts of the population;

2. Mechanisms that involve promoting structured health care consumption through   implementing contributory health insurance schemes and subsidized insurance premiums for the poor. This second category includes social insurance schemes, commercial insurance schemes, mutual health insurance schemes and microinsurance schemes.

1.4   Towards an articulated system

It is obvious today that neither of these strategies alone can drastically increase health insurance coverage for the uninsured. A growing number of countries have opted for schemes that combine insurance with other mechanisms (e.g., subsidized premiums or free access to certain services), and that rely on multiple stakeholders (e.g., community-based schemes, social welfare entities and government programmes) and a mix of sources of funding (e.g., direct or indirect contributions by insured persons and employers, taxes and social transfers). These are known as "articulated systems". They have already been adopted by several countries in Africa (Burkina Faso, Ghana, Rwanda and Senegal), Latin America (Colombia and Uruguay) and Asia (India and China). The value of this approach – if it is properly coordinated – is that it can facilitate effective development of health insurance cover in the informal and agricultural sectors over the comparatively short term.

1.5   Responding to the crisis by providing a social safety net

The economic and financial crisis has shown that social protection is indispensable for economic stability. Not only does social protection shield households from being plunged into extreme poverty, it also helps to limit the contraction of aggregate demand and prevents lasting recession. Universal social protection seems crucial to reversing the current crisis and preventing potential future ones.

In a context of limited resources, such social protection would necessarily be basic, at least to begin with. Over time, wealth redistribution is nevertheless expected to have a positive impact on domestic consumption and hence on growth, and it should therefore be possible to raise the level of social protection gradually. This has been understood by China, where social protection is being extended to the entire population, starting with universal health insurance coverage by the end of 2010.

The United Nations system and the Bretton Wood institutions recently decided to join forces and act in unison to find a way out of the crisis. Among the nine joint projects these institutions have proposed, the goal of introducing a basic social safety net in all countries is a major step towards universal health coverage. The social safety net will probably be implemented through country-specific systems involving multiple stakeholders and mechanisms.

2.   Articulated Systems and the Need for Contracting

2.1   Basic social health protection

Articulated systems form part of a national strategy for extending social protection that includes options for a basic state-sponsored health care package for all. Since covering all health services for the entire population appears unrealistic in the short term, the focus must necessarily be on a certain number of priority services with a high cost-benefit ratio, especially primary and preventive care. The new systems are used to "disseminate" this welfare package for health to the entire population.

2.2   The need for multiple sources of funding

Although this is a "basic" package, it cannot be financed by households alone. According to WHO recommendations, the total cost of the package is in the range of US$30-40 per head per year depending on the country. It is estimated that families working in the informal economy are generally able to contribute much less (just over US$7 per head per year in sub-Saharan Africa). From the moment the package is approved, financing must therefore also be guaranteed.

Some of the cost may be borne by the state in the form of subsidized health services and/or subsidized insurance premiums. Other, "innovative" financing models could be designed at the national level: for instance, state subsidies financed through taxes or new, specific levies (e.g., the hydrocarbon tax or the national lottery in Colombia) and/or private subsidies, for instance from large companies (e.g., Tata or Arcelor Mittal in India) in the context of corporate social responsibility.

While such national solidarity is necessary, it will nevertheless be insufficient in low-income countries, and it is therefore essential to provide for additional solidarity mechanisms at the international level. The view of health as a common global public good warrants establishing sustainable mechanisms in the health area. International solidarity may comprise official development assistance, new so-called "vertical" global funds (e.g., the Global Fund, GAVI or UNITAID) or the new "diagonal" approach, which has been piloted successfully in Rwanda. Other stakeholders are willing to participate in such a solidarity effort, including civil society, the welfare economy sector, the general public (e.g., the Clinton Foundation in the United States), national insurance scheme contributors (which in Luxembourg subsidize the mutual insurance contributions of poor people in Ghana under the "Global Social Trust" [i] launched by the ILO), and migrant workers (vis-à-vis their families "back home").

2.3   Multiple stakeholders as a prerequisite for operation

Beyond the issue of financing, the functioning of these articulated systems often relies on multiple stakeholders, with a view to making use of their respective comparative advantages as well as to developing synergies. While technical management is best carried out by a professional management entity, it is generally useful to entrust activities related to communication, awareness-raising and education of the target population to local community organizations (i.e., mutual-type and cooperative societies).

2.4   Contractual relationships with care providers

Since the aim of the articulated systems is to facilitate access to health care for members or beneficiaries, they have an ongoing relationship with care providers. In addition to contractual relationships with health care facilities (discussed below), it is also vital to conclude agreements with health sector regulatory bodies (e.g., ministries of health and national health authorities) which play a key role in harmonizing and streamlining contracting practices: standardized regulations for approval of care facilities, standardized agreements, health care mechanisms (e.g., third-party payment or reimbursement) and benefits (i.e., services covered and level of care), etc. This approach helps to simplify the supply side of health care delivery to members, and guarantees that providers respect the rights of the insured.

2.5   The need for contracting in order to formalize linkages

The articulated systems involve multiple stakeholders, each of which fulfils a specific role within the system. They draw their funding from diverse sources, and rely on a range of social protection mechanisms (insurance, assistance, etc.). They can only function on the basis of contractual relationships where all parties effectively honour their commitments. With the emergence of articulated systems, contracting becomes a centrepiece of strategies and initiatives to facilitate access to health care in developing countries.

2.6   Summary of functions and possible stakeholders

Articulated systems involve a series of functions (e.g., management, administration, relationship with care providers) which may be performed by different stakeholders. The table below summarizes the overall functions, describes some of them in detail, and provides a list suggesting possible stakeholders performing those functions.

Table 1: Functions and possible stakeholders in an articulated system

Function 1: Management, coordination and regulation of the system
Possible stakeholders: • Ministry of Health or Ministry of Social Security; • Governing board or national council for social protection (e.g., comprising representatives of members, associates, shareholders, social partners and the Government);

- The system's General Assembly (comprising representatives of the insured parties, associates, shareholders, social partners, the Government, etc.);
- Regulatory commission.

Function 2: Administration: identifying insured persons and classifying them by level of vulnerability; carrying out marketing, distribution and awareness-raising; registering insured persons and beneficiaries; collecting membership dues where applicable; running the information and management system; managing relations with care providers; carrying out budget and financial management, fraud prevention and control; performing technical supervision of the number of beneficiaries covered, payment of contributions and service usage; establishing performance indicators and managing funds collected and financial investments

Possible stakeholders:

- Local authorities (i.e., departments and municipalities);
- Social workers;
- Ad hoc-service (for the system for targeting vulnerable persons);
- Tax and duty authorities;
- Social security funds, public and private insurers, mutual organizations, cooperative societies, community organizations, social welfare programmes and NGOs;
- Health care facilities;
- Professional management bodies such as third-party administrators;
- Suppliers of information and management systems (for software and information flow networks).

Function 3: Health care delivery within the framework of a guaranteed benefit package: developing the benefit package; establishing a network of approved providers; negotiating transparent rates; selecting and establishing arrangements for paying providers (e.g., third-party or capitation); negotiating procedures for patient reception and treatment; establishing a referral system between different levels of the health pyramid; improving and guaranteeing quality of care; adapting the supply of treatment to ensure that the package is delivered effectively (e.g., infrastructure, equipment, supply networks for medicines and consumables, staff (e.g., training and incentives)); and carrying out promotional activities, prevention and education, as well as patient monitoring.

Possible stakeholders:

- Ministry of Health;
- Technical and financial partners in the health sector;
- Public- and private-sector health facilities at different levels of the health pyramid, depending on the scope of their decision-making powers;

• Central purchasing agencies for medicines, pharmaceutical laboratories;
• Funds involved in delivering health care to the poor or restructuring health facilities;
• Care networks.
Function 4: Financing of the system's start-up and operating costs
Possible stakeholders:
• Households;   • Central government (Ministry of Finance and the various other ministries involved: health, labour, family, agriculture, etc.);   • Local authorities (departments and municipalities);   • National partnerships, e.g., with other social protection schemes, the private sector and funds;   • International partnerships, e.g., with global funds, bilateral and multilateral cooperation, insured persons in other countries and civil society.
Function 5: Financial equalization and consolidation
Possible stakeholders:
• Funds for equalization between social protection schemes;   • Reinsurance entities/the State (as a last resort).
Function 6: Inspection, oversight and control
Possible stakeholders:
• Regulatory authority (e.g., insurance control commission);   • Experts and external auditors;   • User committees.

3. Contracting mechanisms used in "articulated" insurance schemes

3.1 Definition of contracting and typology of contractual relationships in "articulated" insurance systems

Contracting is the coordination of all stakeholders in performing the functions listed above. It comprises a set of contractual relationships that define the responsibilities of the various parties.

Establishing contractual relationships and monitoring compliance facilitates the smooth running of schemes, and thus the achievement of their objectives (i.e., delivering a social protection package to the entire target population). Contractual relationships are also a sign of the transparency and efficiency of the system as a whole, and the health sector in particular.

It is possible to distinguish between the following contractual relationships: between the "insurance entity" and the insured; between the "articulated system" and care providers; and between the various stakeholders involved in financing and running the articulated system.

3.2 Contractual relationship between the "insurance entity" and the insured

Definition of the conditions for risk transfer through contracting

By signing an insurance contract an insured party transfers the risk of medical expenses incurred in the event of illness to the insurance entity. By assuming this risk the insurance entity commits to pay for the cost of health care in the event of illness. The contractual relationship between the insurance entity and the insured person defines the precise conditions under which this risk transfer occurs: the guaranteed benefit package; the level of treatment; the approved health facilities that the patient is authorized to attend or where he or she may be hospitalized; membership arrangements (i.e., individual, family or group); cost of coverage and amount of contributions payable by the insured person (where applicable); conditions for qualifying for subsidized rates; etc. This contractual relation should in principle work to the benefit of all, although there are reasons that might induce each party to try to use the system at the other's expense. Information asymmetry between the insurer and the insured could give rise to this temptation, and contracting must therefore anticipate such potential aberrations and try to guard against them. The most common potential aberrant practices are adverse selection and moral hazard.

Guarding against adverse selection

Insurance companies calculate insurance premiums on the basis of a risk portfolio comprising "good" and "bad" risks. Premiums roughly amount to the average cost incurred by an insurance entity to insure an average person. Nevertheless, all insured persons have their own characteristics and some already know at the time they sign an insurance contract that they will require medical treatment in the near future, based on information they have about their own health (e.g., medical history, chronic diseases, planned surgery or childbirth in the coming months). For this category of people, signing an insurance contract can be a good deal. This is called "adverse selection". If an insurer accumulates only "bad risks", this may undermine the viability of the system. A good way to counter adverse selection is to give priority to automatic or mandatory membership for a group of persons (e.g., employees of a company or cooperative society or the entire population of a country).

Guarding against moral hazard

When insured persons visit a medical facility they are the only ones who know whether or not they feel sick. Since they know that they are covered they may be inclined to seek medical treatment more often than necessary, consume more drugs or ask for more medical tests. This change in behaviour generated by having insurance coverage is known as "moral hazard". To counter this risk of overconsumption, insurers define the medical services that are covered in the contracts concluded with insured persons. Insurance contracts comprise a certain number of clauses concerning the scope of coverage, such as negotiation of reference tariffs for services covered (i.e., approved tariffs); lists of services covered and authorized/approved health care providers; exclusion of the medical procedures that are most susceptible to moral hazard; limits on the amounts of coverage (e.g., through co-payment, deductibles and ceilings); prior agreements on costly and non-urgent medical procedures; and a mandatory reference system regulating access to more expensive, high-end medical treatment.

3.3 The purpose of contractual relationships between the "articulated system" and providers

Defining the conditions for "purchasing" medical treatment

To honour their commitments vis-à-vis insured persons, "insurers" must guarantee that the insured and beneficiaries of a scheme have effective access to health services covered by the guaranteed benefit package. This means that there must be certain number of health facilities close by, or that the insured can be treated in accordance with the terms of their contract in the event of illness.

This gives rise to different scenarios: (1) Either insured persons pay out of their pocket for expenses and are reimbursed by their insurer upon submitting an invoice (reimbursement scheme); or (2) the insured do not pay for the services covered by the insurance scheme (except co-payment where applicable) and their insurer pays the provider directly (third-party payment scheme).

In the first case the insurer is not required to set up a network of approved providers. This gives the insured and beneficiaries greater freedom of choice. On the contrary, in the second case it is absolutely essential that a network of approved providers paid directly by the insurer be established.

In both cases insurers may establish reference tariffs (or fee ceilings) as a basis for calculating coverage. It is thus in the interest of the insured to use health facilities that apply the pre-negotiated rates in order to obtain maximum coverage.

198

The second case (third-party payment) contains two options: either the insurer pays the bill issued by the health facility each time the services are used, or the insurer pre-negotiates an annual fee known as "capitation", which is paid to the provider for each member and is supposed to cover the average cost of health service usage by the scheme's subscribers within the facility's catchment area.

In all cases, and especially with capitation contracts, it is in the interest of insurers to negotiate standards that govern the interface with patients and the quality and availability of the health care services delivered to their members. This typology of relations is reflected in the following diagram:

Figure 1: Relationships with health care providers

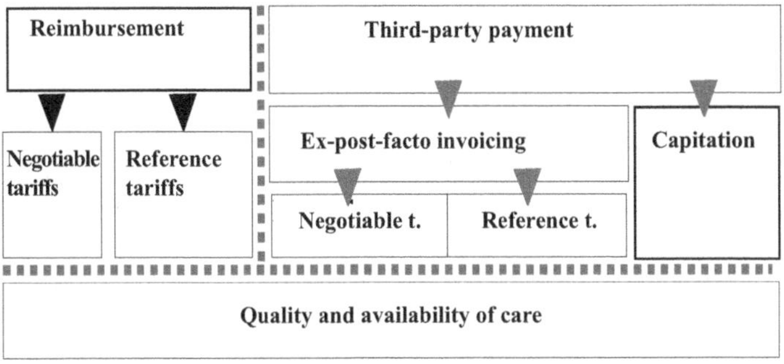

Contracts between insurers and providers govern the relationships between the two parties. The contractual relationships usually fulfil the following functions:

Formalizing the establishment of a network of partner providers

Health insurance schemes normally only cover treatment in a certain number of selected, accredited and approved health facilities. This is particularly relevant under the "third-party payment" system. It is the aim of contracts or agreements entered into with providers to make it easier for patients to be received and treated (e.g., through third-party payment procedures, or standard invoicing under the reimbursement scheme), to ensure a flow of high-quality information about the medical treatment received by the patient, and to guarantee certain standards of medical practice (e.g., drug availability, adequate presence of health workers and adherence to treatment protocols).

Example 1: Colombia

In Colombia, the operators of the subsidized health insurance scheme (called ARSs) are required by law to set up a network of partner health care providers (HCPs). Within this network, 60 per cent of ARS revenues must come from public HCPs. The remaining 40 per cent are contracted out to external private or ARS-owned HCPs. Network HCPs are subject to prior approval by the Government (*www.acreditacionensalud.org.co*). Hospitals are classified according to their level of technical facilities (1 to 4), linked to certification criteria concerning human resources, occupancy rates, financing, medical procedures, the organization of services and access to treatment (e.g., emergencies, triage, outpatient services and admissions). Before certifying an HCP, the ARSs carry out inspections to ensure that a certain number of requirements are met (it must be verified that the hospital – taking into account its technical facilities – can deliver the services covered and guaranteed by the subsidized scheme). Sometimes not all requirements are met. If a hospital is located in an urban area where it competes with other health facilities, the ARS may turn to another HCP; if it is located in a rural area where it holds a monopoly position, the ARS has no other choice but to implement a quality-improvement plan. This was the case with the SER mutual organization SER which, through its foundation (SER Foundation), completely restructured the Carmen de Bolívar public hospital. It was in SER's interest to invest in this hospital, because the quality of health care services had been so poor that subscribers to the scheme preferred to seek care in Cartagena (2.5 hours away by road), which posed many problems (e.g., concerning accessibility of treatment) and incurred considerable cost to the insurer (numerous public and private health facilities in Cartagena). The rehabilitation of the hospital has helped guarantee the availability of quality care closer to the community.

Paving the way for negotiation of rates or the introduction of performance-based payment arrangements

The process of designing a health insurance scheme starts with the developing the package of services covered and calculating the cost of that package. Normally, the level of coverage provided by the package must be weighed against the capacity to finance it. To reduce the cost of the package, however, it is possible and desirable to cut costs and increase efficiency on the supply side, by negotiating rates with central drug purchasing agencies; cutting down on overstaffing, possibly compensated by salary increases for the remaining staff; introducing performance-based payment; billing of certain services at marginal cost; and increasing the utilization rate of the services.

Example 2: Yeshasvini

In the Indian state of Karnataka, Professor Dr Devi Shetty has started two microinsurance schemes: One, Yeshasvini Cooperative Farmer's Health Scheme, covers hospitalization (including highly specialized surgery) and ambulatory care delivered by a network of 320 hospitals; the other, Arogya Raksha Yojana Health Insurance, is aimed at facilitating access to basic health care in villages. The common denominator of the two projects is tightly negotiated hospital and surgery fees (priced at marginal cost under the Yeshasvini scheme) and drug prices (negotiations with Biocon Pharmaceuticals and other drug companies under the Arogya Raksha Yojana scheme).

Performance-based payment involves linking part of the payment that providers receive to health outcomes. This is done to encourage medical professionals to adhere to "standard" practices in order to ensure quality health care throughout a territory (regardless of where a physician works) and eliminate differences in clinical practice. Such standardization also helps to contain the cost of health care services (for public and private insurers). Another aim is to increase the overall quality of health care services delivered to patients, but this is more difficult to achieve. In performance-based payment measurable indicators are used, and it is therefore only possible to recognize the quantitatively measurable aspects of medical practitioners' work (e.g., prescription of treatment in accordance with good practice recommendations; prevention and patient education); by contrast, it is difficult to place a value on diagnostic skills or the ability to choose the right treatment in complex clinical settings, etc.

Performance-based payment has been widely used in the United States (for about a decade) and in the United Kingdom (since 2004), and was recently introduced in France (Social Security (Financing) Act, 2008). It also appears to be used by a growing number of health insurance schemes in low- and middle-income countries (e.g., Rwanda, the Philippines and Haiti). Obviously, the mechanisms are often implemented through contracting in these instances, too.

Defining third-party payment arrangements

To set up a third-party payment arrangement with a health care provider insurers have to reach an agreement with that facility about which services should be covered and the related fees; and define the procedures and mechanisms for exemption from payment of reimbursable medical fees up front, as well as for ensuring that invoices are paid after treatment – i.e., to verify the identity and insurance status of patients as well as their benefit package; calculate the co-payment fee and the amount covered by the insurance entity; and issue the invoice. All these administrative procedures must be specified in the contract. Integrated information systems enable providers to consult the database of insured persons and beneficiaries in real time, and issue invoices to insurers online.

A third-party payment system has a real comparative advantage for the insured, as it considerably reduces financial barriers to health care (patients pay only the co-payment). This also means, however, that it is more vulnerable to abuse and overconsumption, or overprescription by providers. These are things that can imperil schemes' long-term viability or lead to a rise in costs per head and thus to higher premiums. To reduce the risk of abuse, contracts may explicitly lay down defined rules and procedures, such as adherence to treatment protocols for prescription, or the requirement to consult insurers' medical adviser prior to expensive interventions or before incurring costs that are associated with a risk of overconsumption or overprescription. It is then in the interest of insurers to set up a claims monitoring mechanism that will make it possible, for instance, to monitor the utilization of health services per member and per provider and thus identify potential abuse in real time.

Example 3: TPAs in India

In 2001 a regulation issued by IRDA (the Indian Insurance Regulatory and Development Authority) provided for the creation of health-sector companies known as TPAs (Third Party Administrators), which function as intermediaries between health insurance schemes, insured persons and providers. Acting on behalf of the insurers, TPAs develop and coordinate health provider networks and manage the pre-authorization of treatment and claims procedures (i.e., claims verification and payment of bills issued by providers). On the other hand, it is the insurers' responsibility to pay for the services provided (i.e., paying hospital bills or reimbursing patients). The TPAs core function is to offer third-party payment services through a network of health providers in India: Third-party payment accounts for 50 per cent of all claims managed by TPAs. TPAs were able rapidly to develop efficient information and management centres that comprise databases of all insured persons, claims processing software (for each contract), call centres and medical expertise (especially for analysing hospital admission files). This expertise helps keep transaction costs low. TPAs are paid a percentage of premiums, which are negotiated with insurance entities. They are entitled to work with several insurance entities at a time, and the insurance companies may use more than one TPA. In March 2009 India had 27 TPAs.
Source: *http://www.irdaindia.org*

Facilitating agreement on capitation contracts

Providers and insurers negotiate a fixed annual payment for each enrolled patient to be paid by the insurer to the provider in advance at the start of a given period (e.g., at the beginning of the year). This amount is supposed to cover the average expected health care utilization per year. Providers receive the same per capita

202

remuneration regardless of the number of visits per covered person in the course of the year, and therefore "win" when the covered persons consume less than expected and "lose" in the opposite case. Capitation contracts enable insurers to transfer part of the risk associated with fluctuations in the utilization of health services to medical providers.

Providers will obviously do their utmost to "win", and will therefore be tempted to keep the utilization of services by patients at a minimum, for instance by spacing out consultations. This contributes to lowering the quality of care.

This means that it is important to establish a system for information exchange and follow-up with providers in order to verify that the numbers of anticipated and actual visits match, and to readjust the capitated amount if necessary. It may also be useful to release capitation funds in several instalments over the course of the year, and to make the release of the final portion contingent on the disclosure of full information on health service utilization.

Example 4: Sky in Cambodia

Among the many models already in place, the Cambodian micro-health insurance system Sky (started by the association GRET) is particularly interesting. Sky has concluded capitation contracts with 51 health centres and 11 public hospitals. The contracts define the capitated amounts and impose minimum quality guarantees (24-hour reception, non-discrimination between insured and uninsured persons, commitment to delivering quality care). A special mechanism has also been developed to penalize noncompliance with quality benchmarks. The amount of capitation, i.e., the average monthly per capita cost of health service utilization, is calculated in advance and paid monthly to health care providers. A review after 6 months allows for a mid-term assessment in conjunction with health centres, and adjustment of the capitated amount during the year if necessary. The contracts are renegotiated every year based on information obtained through following up how covered persons use health services, in addition to other, more qualitative information. Frequent exchanges with representatives of health facilities and the operational health district help to strengthen the quality of the care that providers deliver. For the insured, capitation contracts have the same advantages as a third-party payment system (exemption from paying reimbursable medical fees up front at the time the health care service is used), but claim management procedures are less complex: No invoices are issued and providers are not paid each time an insured person uses health care services. Capitation is also a safeguard against overconsumption and overprescription. *For more information, see: http://www.sky-cambodia.org/* or the GRET document on capitation entitled: "Principes et modalités de la capitation" (Principles and practice of capitation), Marielle Goursat, August 2009.

Defining health care quality standards

Contracting of health care providers must facilitate better quality of care and transparency of billing practices, and thus improve the management of the health sector. Contracts also provide a framework for the expected quality of services, i.e., standards for the reception of patients, updating of treatment protocols, etc. Establishing an information exchange system is also crucial for identifying and responding rapidly to potential abuses.

Implicit contracting in integrated models

Other models for contracting health services exist, including the integrated model in which health insurance schemes and health facilities form part of the same organization. Integrated models can involve internal agreements between several entities ("insurers" and health care providers) within one and the same organization, but this is not always the case.

Example 5: Grameen Kalyan – internal agreement

This model was adopted by the not-for-profit company Grameen Kaylan, founded in 1996, for the purpose of providing access to health care for employees and customers of the Grameen Bank, a major microfinance institution in Bangladesh (with 7.34 million borrowers in 2007, of whom 97 per cent are women). Grameen Kaylan comprises a network of 38 health centres and "satellite clinics" (held once a week in remote areas), a system of referrals to secondary and tertiary care, and a network of community health workers offering preventive and health education services in home settings. Grameen Kaylan has also developed a health microinsurance scheme to facilitate the utilization of health care services and increase the turnover of its centres. Some 300,000 people had been enrolled in the scheme by 2007; enrolment is open to both members and non-members of the Grameen Bank. Non-members simply pay a slightly higher annual premium of 150 taka (i.e., US$2.18) instead of 120 taka (i.e., US$1.74) for a family of up to six. *More information: http://www.grameenkalyan.org/*

Example 6: Bwamanda – absence of formal agreement

The same approach was adopted by the Bwamanda health insurance scheme in the Democratic Republic of the Congo (DRC). Since 1969 the Bwamanda centre for integrated development (CDI-Bwamanda) has coordinated all economic, health-related and community-based activities in this part of the DRC. In 1986 CDI-Bwamanda set up a mutual society to remove financial barriers to secondary health care, thus simultaneously improving the financial situation of the hospital. Starting out with some 31,000 participants in 1986, the scheme had a growth in membership to 114,465 in 2004, i.e., at a penetration rate of 64 per cent. There was a notable increase in the number of beneficiaries in 2004

---

because fees at the primary care level were no longer the same for members and non-members, as had been the case in the past. Insured persons benefit from a third-party payment arrangement (exemption from payment of reimbursable medical fees up front) in all health facilities in the area (health centres and hospitals) and only pay a deductible of 20 per cent of the cost of treatment. The insurance scheme is one of CDI's activities; running local health units is another. Very broadly speaking, the CDI functions as a "central bank" that centralizes revenue and spreads expenses. Membership contributions are paid into the mutual organization's account at this "bank", and every month claims payments owed to health centres and hospitals are transferred from the organization's account to that of the health facilities through a simple bookkeeping entry within the CDI. Although the relationship between the mutual organization and health facilities is not subject to a formal agreement, there is tacit a understanding to the effect that the CDI acts as guarantor (i.e., an internal accounting operation between the account of the mutual organization and those of the health facilities).

3.4 Types of contracts between articulated systems and health providers

Standard agreements

Health insurance systems are free to negotiate and sign as many specific contracts as the number of providers they have chosen; for the sake of efficiency and equity (between the insured parties), however, attempts are made to standardize contractual relations and frame standardized agreements for each type of provider.

Figure 2: Standardized agreement defined by the health insurance system

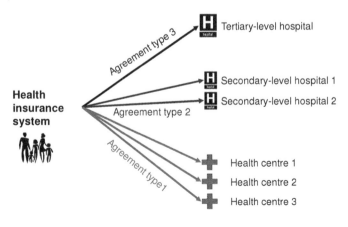

In areas where several health insurance systems enter into agreements with the same health facilities, the latter may find it difficult to manage a multitude of agreements containing dissimilar provisions (e.g., concerning the services covered; rates negotiated; standard of care and financing arrangements (i.e. third-party payment or reimbursement schemes)). This was the case, for example, with the Saint Jean de Dieu hospital in the Thiès region of Senegal, which opted for one standardized contract applicable to all mutual organizations with which it had partnerships. As a result, the mutual organizations of Thiès felt the need to coordinate better among themselves to negotiate the conditions for hospital access for their subscribers.

Figure 3: Standard agreement determined by the health care provider

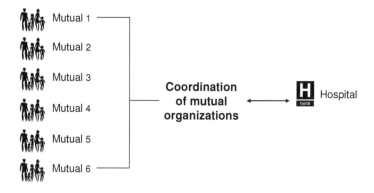

Care networks

Likewise, TPAs (Third Party Administrators) in India enter into contractual relationships with networks of health care providers to make it easier to establish third-party payment mechanisms (e.g., for hospitals, general practitioners, laboratories, pharmacies and dental clinics). Consequently, the beneficiaries of both public and private insurance companies and microinsurance schemes that work with TPAs have access to providers that are members of the network as well as to the third-party payment mechanism.

Figure 4: Care networks

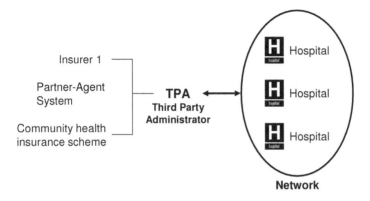

Framework agreements

Contractual relationships may also link several health insurance systems and a number of health care providers that are organized in unions or federations. In such cases, the group of mutual organizations and the group of health care providers will together devise a framework agreement that sets out the main guidelines and regulations governing the relationship between the health insurance systems and the providers.

Figure 5: Framework agreement

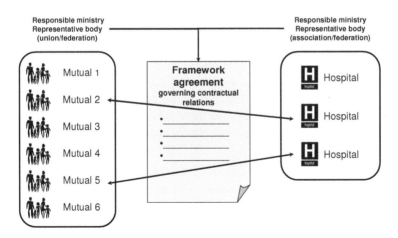

Such agreements may offer a comparatively flexible outline for contractual relations, which must then be specified and negotiated individually between health care providers and health insurance systems. In other cases, they may determine all the contract arrangements. Insurance entities that enter into the framework agreement thus automatically recognize all health care providers that are party to it, and accept the contractual relations established by the agreement. By the same token, health facilities that sign the agreement consent to maintain the specified contractual relationship with all insurance entities that are party to the agreement.

In either case, framework agreements have several advantages: First of all they help to harmonize contractual practices (through common arrangements) and facilitate negotiations (when certain aspects have already been negotiated under the framework agreement, subsequent discussions of each individual contractual arrangement are made easier). By moving negotiations to a higher level, framework agreements involve entities that have a higher capacity to negotiate and thus protect local stakeholders who sometimes lack the skills for conducting complex contractual negotiations or may not have legal personality. The entities representing health insurance systems (e.g., unions or federations of mutual organizations) and health care facilities (e.g., the Ministry of Health, medical associations and hospital federations) also play an important role in monitoring the implementation of the framework agreement by its signatories.

Difficulties in developing contractual relationships

In many countries it is nevertheless difficult to develop contractual relationships between health insurance systems and health care providers, for various reasons.

(1) Certain health insurance systems (e.g., community-based schemes in Asia and mutual insurance schemes in Africa) are not subject to any specific legislation or code, and have no official status. Any agreements they may enter into with health care providers therefore have no legal standing, and the legal remedies available in the event of non-compliance with the obligations the contracts specify are limited. As a result, health facilities may be suspicious of them and demand substantial financial guarantees (i.e., deposits). Similarly, certain public health care providers do not have legal personality and cannot manage their activities independently, and therefore depend on a supervisory authority as the only body authorized to sign agreements.

(2) It can be difficult for health insurance systems to enforce the implementation of undertakings that providers have committed to in the contracts, given the poor quality and limited availability of health care services. Improving the quality of care is thus a prerequisite for implementing such agreements.

208

(3) A bewildering variety of contractual practices can sometimes emerge. If these were harmonized, negotiating and managing contractual agreements would be made easier.

To overcome the difficulties mentioned above, state intervention at various levels seems indispensable:

- Establishing a legislative and regulatory framework for the activities of health insurance systems and carrying out certification and monitoring of their operations (i.e., ex ante and ex post facto oversight);

- Creating a favourable context for the establishment and operation of health insurance systems (including investment in upgrading public health facilities and amending the status of those that do not have legal personality);

- Establishing a framework for contracting, i.e., a reference framework specifying the main stages of the contractual process; the minimum content of agreements; fundamental principles (such as adherence to negotiated fees; nondiscrimination between patients; and confidentiality of medical records); the commitment of the parties to, inter alia, remuneration arrangements (e.g., fee-for-service reimbursement or lump sum); payment tools and mechanisms; financial guarantees; oversight procedures and mechanisms; mechanisms for monitoring compliance with the agreement; evaluation mechanisms; conflict settlement provisions; etc. ILO/STEP is supporting the implementation of this kind of contracting framework in Senegal.

3.5 Contractual relations between stakeholders involved in financing and running articulated systems (some examples)

Articulated systems rely on a range of complementary stakeholders, and are based on the subsidiarity principle. Contractual relationships are crucial for guaranteeing and streamlining their operation. These may deal with the financing of the system or different administrative functions such as targeting and enrolling beneficiaries or collecting membership contributions. Some of these functions, based on real-life examples, are described below.

Identifying and mobilizing one or more sources of financing

As mentioned above, workers in the informal economy or the agricultural sector who are excluded from official social security schemes are often unable to afford the premiums for a basic health insurance package. Subsidizing premiums is therefore vital. This can take different forms: financing through the central or regional state budget (e.g., in India); financing through special taxes (e.g., in

Uruguay and Colombia); redistribution from other social security schemes (e.g., Colombia), financing through international funds (e.g., Rwanda and the "diagonal approach"); subsidies from private-sector conglomerates as part of their corporate social responsibility (e.g., companies in Jarkhand state, India); international taxes such as those advocated by UNITAID on air fares; financing by migrant workers (i.e., cash transfers to finance insurance premiums, which is part of the pilot project set up by ECOLABS in West Africa); or international solidarity (e.g., the "Global social trust" through which voluntary contributions from insured persons in Luxembourg are used to finance a social protection package for vulnerable groups in Ghana).

In Colombia, the subsidized health insurance scheme is financed by several complementary sources, with 41.1 per cent contributed by the Solidarity Fund (FOSYGA). This fund is replenished principally through transfers corresponding to 1.5 per cent of all contributions under the contributory scheme (or 12.5 per cent of the total payroll of companies). The Solidarity Fund also receives contributions through the family allowance funds (known as "compensation funds") and a range of taxes: a tax on owning weapons; taxation of yields from financial products; and revenue from fines imposed on employers for employment tax evasion (i.e., nonpayment of social security contributions). The subsidized health insurance scheme also receives substantial funding (up to 48.1 per cent) from general taxation (i.e., VAT and taxes) and local and departmental resources (up to 10.8 per cent), by way of taxes on alcohol and tobacco, "health" lotteries, local taxes, gambling, contributions from specific companies (e.g., the coffee industry), and financial products. *Source: Gestarsalud, Colombia, October 2008.*

In Rwanda, the national health insurance system is organized on three levels: local branches of mutual organizations, district-level mutual organizations and a national "risk pooling" fund. Members enrol (by way of family membership) with the local branch of a mutual organization in a primary-level benefit package (health centre package) or secondary- and tertiary-level benefit packages (district or referral hospital package). The total cost of the package (primary and hospital care) amounts to 2,000 Rwandan francs (RF) (US$3.54) per person per year; RF 1,000 (US$1.77) is paid by the insured party and RF 1,000 comes from state subsidies (i.e., partial subsidy). Destitute persons, orphans and persons living with HIV/AIDS are exempt from paying premiums (i.e., full subsidy), thanks mainly to external (i.e., donor) funding. In reality, the financing system is more complex and illustrated by the diagram below: Local branches of mutual organizations are mainly financed by contributing members (RF 1,000) and through donor subsidies (which are mainly used to cover the premiums for destitute persons). District-level mutual organizations are funded by the local branches (10 per cent of their premiums revert), the national "risk pooling" fund, local (i.e., district) government; and donor grants. The national "risk pooling" fund is financed by the Rwandan Government (RF 1,000 per person), solidarity contributions from other health insurance schemes (statutory and private) and donors (especially the Global Fund). *Source: Mid-term evaluation of the Global Fund to Fight HIV/AIDS, Tuberculosis and Malaria (GFATM) 5th Round Project on Health Systems Strengthening, 2007.*

Figure 6: Funding framework – Rwandan health insurance system

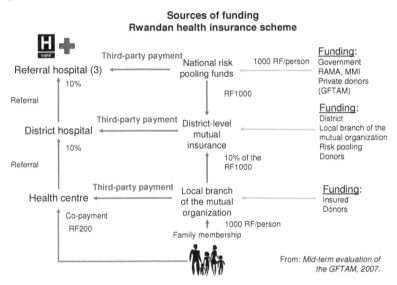

In India, the central government has designed a new subsidized health insurance scheme for below-poverty-line households called RSBY (Rashtriya Swasthya Bima Yojana), which is being implemented progressively at state level. The package covers hospitalization and travel expenses up to 30,000 rupees (Rs) per family (five persons) per year, i.e., approximately US$616. The premium under this scheme is Rs 750 per family per year (approximately US$15.4), 75 per cent of which is financed by the central government and the remaining 25 per cent by the state government; the insured only pay a registration and annual renewal fee of Rs 30 (US$0.6). The running costs of the scheme are borne by state governments. The aim of the scheme is to cover the 300 million persons in India who live below the poverty line in just over one year (between April 2008 and August 2009). Coverage has already been extended to 5.5 million families. *For more information see: http://www.rsby.in*

Targeting beneficiaries

So long as a health insurance scheme subsidizes the premiums for only some of its members or provides different levels of funding or coverage on the basis of vulnerability criteria, eligible beneficiaries must be identified. This is a complex and potentially expensive process requiring a nationwide survey. In the two examples below (Colombia and Rwanda), the identification process was carried out by state institutions (ministry or local government).

In Colombia, beneficiaries are targeted by the DNP (National Planning Department) through a proxy means test called the SISBEN survey. The survey includes questions about education, housing, health condition, living conditions, vulnerability, the number of household members, etc. The findings make it possible to classify families by level of vulnerability and identify beneficiaries of various state-run social programmes (e.g., for education, conditional or unconditional cash benefits or housing allowances), including the subsidized health and social security schemes. SISBEN surveys are conducted every 6 to 7 years on average; between surveys, the database of vulnerable persons is updated on a case-by-case basis. *For more information see: www.sisben.gov.co*

Under the health insurance scheme in Rwanda, the poor and very poor are identified at the community level. The information is then passed on to the department and then the district, and is authenticated by municipalities. *Source: Mid-term evaluation of the GFATM, 2007.*

Enrolling and registering beneficiaries

Linkages with local authorities and civil society organizations that are in direct contact with the target population facilitate enrolment and registration of beneficiaries. Strictly speaking, this is a contract-based approach, even if these arrangements have not been examined from the point of view of contracting so far.

The basic idea for setting up the subsidized health insurance scheme in Colombia was to introduce a new stakeholder – the insurance entities of the subsidized scheme (ARSs) – between hospitals and local government units. These are private entities (insurers, mutual-type organizations and family allowance funds) that maintain contractual relationships both with local government units and health care providers.

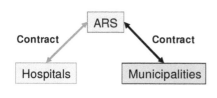

This relationship should ensure a use of funds that is both efficient (fees negotiated between ARSs and

212

hospitals) and transparent (ARSs are obliged to provide comprehensive follow-up information).

Municipalities organize health insurance enrolment campaigns at least twice a year, and enrolled members are free to choose their insurance carrier. The contracts subsequently concluded between the municipalities and the ARSs are based on the number of subscribers, and specify the monthly subsidy payable to the ARSs to cover these persons. *Source: Ministry of Social Security, Colombia, November 2008*

The Rashtriya Swathya Bima Yojana (RSBY) subsidized health insurance scheme for persons living below the poverty line in India also involves a series of contractual arrangements between different stakeholders in the programme: central government, state governments, agencies working with implementing the scheme (e.g., NGOs and cooperative societies), insurers and care providers. State governments are required to choose a scheme operator (implementing agency) charged with targeting beneficiaries, issuing membership cards (smart cards), collecting membership contributions contracting with health care providers, etc. A technical unit at the Ministry helps state governments design the insurance schemes at state level; finalizes the technical and financial apparatus; supports the implementation of the schemes; and monitors and evaluates their implementation. Standard contractual agreements (Memorandum of Understanding) are available on the RSBY website (*www.rsby.in*).

Figure 7: Organizational chart – RSBY in India

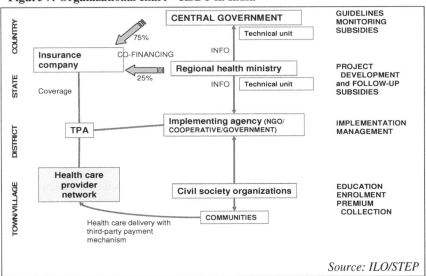

Source: ILO/STEP

213

Collecting contributions

Linkages with organized groups (e.g., cooperative societies, microfinance institutions and NGOs) facilitate the collection of premiums and guard against certain risks such as adverse selection and opportunistic behaviour (especially when group membership is encouraged). Piggybacking on these groups also helps reduce the cost of collecting premiums and makes it easier to establish payment arrangements adapted to the needs of the target population.

In the Philippines, the GTZ-supported KaSAPI project run by the health insurance corporation PhilHealth, which was launched in 2005, is aimed at extending health insurance coverage to workers in the informal economy. Its objective is to boost enrolment among informal economy workers through strategic partnerships with organized groups (i.e., cooperative societies, microfinance institutions, NGOs and rural banks), many of which serve informal economy workers, as well as to reduce the risks associated with the earlier programme PhilHealth Organized Group Interface (POGI), which required informal economy workers and their families to enrol individually. Under DaSAPI, at least 70 per cent of the members of each partner organization must enrol in PhilHealth. This reduces the risk of adverse selection and makes enrolment easier. Preferential rates are available to encourage group enrolment, with the size of the discount varying in proportion to the numbers enrolled. Contributions are collected by the "group" at a convenient time for the insured (i.e., regular payment of small amounts) and transferred to PhilHealth periodically (i.e., annually, biannually or quarterly), something that also suits the insurance scheme. After two years, at the end of the third quarter of 2008, KaSAPI had more than 21,000 subscribers (i.e., heads of households) from 19 organized groups (e.g., NGOs and microfinance institutions). For more information see: ***http://www.hssp.ph***

A similar approach was adopted under the Yeshavini scheme in India, where partnership with the Karnataka State Cooperative Department has helped cut operating costs. Publicity is handled by the Karnataka State Cooperative Department and therefore costs the scheme itself nothing. Likewise, enrolment and collection of contributions are administered efficiently by cooperative societies and cooperative banks, so this costs the scheme nothing, either. This close involvement of the cooperative sector resulted in the enrolment of 1.6 million beneficiaries in Year 1 (2004) and a steady increase in numbers thereafter (in 2007-2008 the scheme covered 2.4 million people). In addition to this operational partnership, the Karnataka state government finances a substantial portion of the scheme each year (between one third and one half), as insurance premiums are insufficient to cover the costs. Finally, the Karnataka state government participates in decision-making as a member of the Yeshasvini Trust Board of Trustees. *For more information see: http://www.yeshasvini.org/*

When microfinance institutions set up microinsurance schemes they often develop synergies for collecting contributions. That is the case for the MS-PAMECAS mutual health care organization in Senegal, which was established under the PAMECAS savings and credit network and is open to PAMECAS members and their families only. To enrol in MS-PAMECAS, applicants must be members of a network savings and credit bank, have a savings account, pay a registration fee of 1,000 CFA francs and commit to transferring a monthly premium of CFA 250 per enrolled person to the savings account. By the end of 2006, the mutual organization was operating in 35 savings and credit banks of the PAMECAS network. *Source: www.microinsurance.org*

Similarly, the VimoSEWA community-based health insurance scheme works in close partnership with SEWA bank to facilitate process of collecting contributions. VimoSEWA offers its members two options for paying their contributions: (1) annual payment and (2) blocked savings deposits equal to approximately 20 times the yearly premium. Under the second option, members open a blocked savings account with SEWA and the interest on the savings covers the annual contribution. This arrangement helps to guarantee that contributions are paid regularly, and cuts collection costs. In 2005 renewal rates under this arrangement were 100 per cent, compared with just 41 per cent under the direct annual payment option. However, when market interest rates drop or VimoSEWA increases premiums, members are required to top up the blocked savings account accordingly; furthermore, the poorest beneficiaries are unable to save and block such a sum. *Source: www.microinsurance.org*

Carrying out prevention and health education

In some cases, articulated health insurance schemes may participate in prevention and health education activities on behalf of the Ministry of Health. In the period 1993-1995 in Colombia, for instance, the Government made an effort to organize communities to enable them to play a more active role in their own health care. Some 500,000 families were involved in awareness-raising and training exercises, and 80 community enterprises were set up. The principal mission of these (mutual-type and cooperative) enterprises was to provide promotional and preventive services and access to primary health care. The annual budget per capita (financed by the state) amounted to just 24,000 pesos, and facilitated the supply of a very limited benefit package which covered only primary care: education, promotion, prevention, general consultations and nonsurgical hospital admissions, as well as the most common medicines. The idea of developing a health insurance scheme only emerged subsequently. Public training activities included health-related training (in particular, education, promotion and prevention) and training in management of community organizations (i.e., mutual-type and cooperatives). *Source: Gestarsalud, Colombia, October 2008.*

CONCLUSION

Extending health care coverage is a priority in developing countries, where a large portion of the population (e.g., workers in the informal economy and people living in rural areas), are still without coverage. This need has become painfully obvious against the backdrop of the economic and financial crisis, and numerous national and international projects have been launched to accelerate the extension of health care coverage. The need is so great, and the resources available so scarce, that efficiency is crucial both when a universal health care package is designed and when its delivery is organized (i.e., financing and management). Articulated systems, which are driven by a range of complementary stakeholders under the subsidiarity principle, appear to be an effective organizational model for facilitating access to health care. With the emergence of articulated systems, contracting becomes the centrepiece of policies to extend health care coverage, insofar as it is no longer limited to relationships between insurers and the insured, or between insurers and providers, but instead facilitates the establishment of contractual relationships between all stakeholders in the system.

Notes

[i] The idea behind the "Global Social Trust", which is an international solidarity fund piloted in Ghana with support from Luxembourg, is to encourage insured people in richer countries to contribute a modest monthly amount on a voluntary basis to support the establishment or implementation of social security schemes in developing countries (i.e., subsidizing premiums). This approach is used by other projects currently in development, such as "1 Euro solidaire", which seeks to recruit certain stakeholders in France's welfare economy to this solidarity effort.

International Labour Office (ILO). 2008. *India Social Security Profile.* Available at
    http://www.socialsecurityextension.org/gimi/gess/ShowCountryProfile.do?cid =103 [Dec. 2009] (Geneva, Social Security Department).
—. 2009. *Colombia Perfil de Seguridad Social.* Available at
    http://www.socialsecurityextension.org/gimi/gess/ShowCountryProfile.do?cid =307 [Jan. 2009] (Geneva, Social Security Department).

—. *UN Social Protection Floor Initiative*. Available at
http://www.socialsecurityextension.org/gimi/gess/ShowTheme.do?tid=1321
[Dec. 2009] (Geneva, Social Security Department).

—. *Cambodia Social Security Profile*. Available at
http://www.socialsecurityextension.org/gimi/gess/ShowCountryProfile.do?cid
=376 [Dec. 2009] (Geneva, Social Security Department).

—. *Rwanda Social Security Profile*. Available at
http://www.socialsecurityextension.org/gimi/gess/ShowCountryProfile.do?cid
=300 [Dec. 2009] (Geneva, Social Security Department).

—. Forthcoming. *Third-party payment mechanism for cashless access in health
microinsurance*. (Geneva, Social Finance Programme, Microinsurance
Innovation Facility).

Schremmer, J., Coheur, A., Jacquier, C. et Schmitt-Diabaté, V. 2009. "Extending
health care coverage: Potential linkages between statutory social security and
community-based social protection", in *International Social Security Review*
(Geneva), Vol. 62, No. 1, pp. 25-43.

Web sites

http://www.grameenkalyan.org
Grameen Kalyan, Bangladesh [Dec. 2009]

http://www.sky-cambodia.org
GRET-SKY Health Insurance Program of Cambodia [Dec. 2009]

http://www.acreditacionensalud.org.co
Instituto Colombiano de Normas Técnicas y Certificación (ICONTEC) [Dec. 2009]

http://www.irdaindia.org
Insurance Regulatory and Development Authority (IRDA), India [Dec. 2009]

http://www.microinsurance.org
Partenariat pour la Mobilisation de l'Epargne et du Crédit au Sénégal (PAMECAS)
[Dec. 2009]

http://www.hssp.ph
Philippine Health Sector Reform: [Dec. 2009].

http://www.rsby.in
Rashtriya Swasthya Bima Yojana (RSBY), India [Dec. 2009]

http://www.sisben.gov.co
Sistema de Identificación de Potenciales Beneficiarios de Programas Sociales
(SISBEN), Colombia: [Dec. 2009]

http://www.yeshasvini.org
Yeshasvini Co-operative Farmers Health Care Scheme, India: [Dec. 2009].

Part II

Chapter 5

Local authorities

Jean Perrot

"Contracts are the tangible expression of the decentralization process and this, in return, is the new prerequisite for contracting without symbolic guardianship", Jean-Paul Gaudin, *Negotiation of contractual policies*, L'Harmattan, 1996

Administrative decentralization, i.e. the transfer of responsibility from the major State bodies to legally independent local authorities with jurisdiction over a specific territory, is becoming a reality in developing countries that have thus far been used to a central, or even regional Government, which, through its administration and activities - law and regulations - controlled public action.

In the health sector, deconcentration generally preceded this type of administrative decentralization, based on a technical rationale caused by the priority given to primary healthcare. Nowadays, this situation causes a problem. Health Ministries, which are accustomed to deconcentration, have great difficulty fitting into the mould of administrative decentralization, which forces them to change their organization and behaviour.

Contracting is therefore perceived as a solution, which would enable the rationales to be reconciled by making this redefinition of the relation between the State and local authorities operational. This chapter shows this inevitable development.

1. THE DEVELOPMENT OF DECENTRALIZATION

Before anything else, definitions must be established. In common language, dictionaries generally define decentralization as "the process by which a central body transfers part of its functions to a peripheral body". This definition is, however, insufficient to reflect the diversity of the situation. In reality the process in the above definition differs according to the degree of autonomy granted to the peripheral body. There are generally three different degrees:

- Deconcentration: corresponds to cases with very little autonomy since it relates to the attribution of specific competences to public service agents. These agents remain under the authority of a hierarchical central power. The degree of autonomy is low, particularly because there is no separate legal personality. In English terminology it would be said that deconcentration is the first stage in the process of decentralization; in French terminology there is a clearer distinction between decentralization and deconcentration: deconcentration must not be equated to any form of decentralization.

- "Functional decentralization" or decentralization by service: this process grants another legal personality under public law the control over or management of a public service with a specific sphere of activity. Under French law this primarily regards public institutions. The level of autonomy is therefore greater. A sense of attachment however remains between the State and its deconcentrated services and local communities. This guardianship oversees major decisions and the respect of regulations, but does not interfere with everyday management.

- "Administrative decentralization": this is not only a political but also a technical concept where the responsibility of major public authorities is transferred to local authorities with jurisdiction over a specific territory. It is generally recognized that the representatives of these authorities are legitimately elected. Although the degree of autonomy is great, it is often weakened in reality by dependence on the central Government for budgetary resources.

- Furthermore, it should be added that the term *decentralization* is sometimes used as a synonym for *delocalization*. This understanding will never be used here.

In French terminology the three concepts are separate and correspond to clearly defined situation which will be developed in this chapter. English terminology accepts more readily the use of the word decentralization in a general understanding, the sense of which is explained in this text. Furthermore, the three degrees of autonomy present in French have different names in English: déconcentration = deconcentration, décentralisation fonctionnelle ("functional decentralization") = delegation, and décentralisation administrative ("administrative decentralization") = devolution.

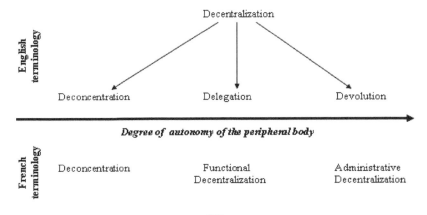

221

Some would add to the concept of decentralization a final step: "privatization", in other words the transfer of activities or health services to private bodies, with or without the aim of financial gain.[1]

In this chapter we will primarily consider administrative decentralization (devolution). Functional decentralization (delegation) will be discussed in a different chapter.

1.1 Deconcentration in the health sector

In and around the nineteen sixties, the central government in the majority of developing countries had to take responsibility for numerous aspects of economic and social life: it was responsible for developing major industries and establishing public services on a large scale, ranging from post offices to railway transport, through rural development and by providing free healthcare and education for the population. This vision of a welfare State, which would perform these tasks increasingly well as economic growth provided the means to do so, lasted until the beginning of the nineteen seventies. The limits of centralism then swiftly became apparent, and in order to overcome them many countries undertook what were known as decentralization reforms, but which in reality were merely devolution measures.

This was the case in the health sector. In 1978, the Alma Ata conference adopted primary healthcare as a strategy for achieving healthcare for all. The health district thus became the frame of reference for the implementation of this strategy. In 1985, during the 35th session of the WHO Regional Commission in Lusaka, African countries adopted a three-tier healthcare development plan, with three functional levels, of which the health district was the linchpin. The health district system was expressly defined by WHO as an advantageous means of establishing primary healthcare.[2] The health district is a more or less self-sufficient element of the national health system. It includes all institutions and individuals providing healthcare at the district level, whether they are governmental, private or traditional. It has sufficient autonomy to ensure that appropriate responses to local health problems can be planned and implemented. This implies that resources are available and that sufficient authority has been delegated; the placement of the district staff under the responsibility of a district medical officer ensures this.

Although appointed and monitored by the central authorities, the district's medical officer enjoys a certain amount of autonomy with regard to everyday management and is not always obliged to undergo *a priori* monitoring. This autonomy, however, remains limited to on-going activities.

This deconcentration relies on the technical considerations of organizing health services. The health district must be seen as a system in the full sense of the word, i.e. i) a linkage between the levels of service delivery and ii) service management. At the same time, health ministries have generally taken these decisions without taking other sectors into account: this is reflected, for example, by an ad hoc division of the health district that does not correspond with any administrative entity. Furthermore, these decisions have generally preceded the administrative decentralization movement, therefore creating a de facto situation from which it is always difficult to go back.

In the context of deconcentration, the allocation of resources remains the responsibility of the central power, while their management is the responsibility of the local level authority. Thus staffing, operating and investment budgets are decided at the central level. The district must apply national programmes, but it defines the methods of doing so. However, with the Bamako Initiative and the creation of management committees, districts have acquired a status akin to functional decentralization.

1.2   Autonomy

Some countries such as Zambia and Ghana have gone a step further and have granted district management teams autonomous status.[3] The district management team also becomes an autonomous agency, which is supervised by an administration council. The director of the agency is responsible for implementing the administration council's policy and managing the day-to-day running of the district agency.

1.3   Administrative decentralization

As well as being a frequent reminder of the organization of certain northern countries that have had a historical influence over certain southern countries, the centralization of powers also corresponded to a time when in developing countries it was difficult to establish local authorities. These conditions have now changed and the disadvantages of centralism are becoming predominant.

Administrative decentralization, which transfers responsibility from major public authorities to local authorities with jurisdiction over a specific territory, whose legitimacy is derived from the election of their representatives, enables decision-making to be brought closer to the community level. These local governments should be more attentive to the specific needs of populations and more committed to finding a rapid and flexible response, since their re-election depends on it. Furthermore, since they are closer to the population, they should be able to obtain public mobilization and participation in local development.

This decentralization does not operate in the same way in different countries. Some have only organized one level of decentralization (generally the municipalities), while others are opting for several levels (municipalities, as well as departments, districts, regions, etc.). Besides having an impact on the division of the responsibilities transferred, this will also have implications for the interaction between these decentralized bodies.

Furthermore administrative decentralization is characterized by its multi-sectoral nature. Decentralized bodies will have responsibilities relating to several sectors: economic (communication, transport, rural development, etc.), social (education, health, employment etc.) and the possibility of defining their priorities with respect to these sectoral fields.

Faced with this decentralization, the role and powers of deconcentrated authorities, as much in the health sector as the general administration, are transformed considerably. Thus deconcentrated State services move from a decision-making role to one of advice and guidance. Such a change is never easy. Since administrative decentralization is specifically a transfer of jurisdiction between two members of the public, it is easy to understand that this process can be a source of conflict between these two persons. Persons having part of their jurisdiction transferred to someone else feel devalued, and if they are not informed of the advantages that this will bring them they may do everything they can to stand in the way of this development. A district medical inspector whose responsibility for managing primary healthcare centres is transferred to the municipal authorities will oppose that change, and more so if he or she is not shown that the reduction of certain administrative obligations will allow him or her to carry out technical tasks that they were unable to do in the past owing to lack of time.

Despite being increasingly effective, administrative decentralization is limited; although it decentralizes the fiscal officer, the decentralization of fiscal authority is generally only partial. As we will see later, the central Government retains the majority of the financial authority and for that reason remains a specific actor above the decentralized bodies.

With specific regard to the health sector, questions should be asked more particularly about this transfer to local authorities. What mandate is given to them? Clearly the answer differs from country to country. In any case two concepts can be maintained:

- Mandate to provide health services: local authorities are given the mandate to ensure the provision of health services: they therefore establish all activities linked with public health, with or without the means of health facilities (clinics or hospital structures). In order for this to happen, the State will transfer public health facilities to them;

- Mandate of responsibility for public health in their sphere of competence: this does not mean a transfer of resources, but rather of responsibility in terms of direction, policy, monitoring, oversight and evaluation. Local authorities therefore serve as an interface between the public (and public needs) and the actors providing healthcare services. The job of the local authorities is therefore clearly more arduous and complex.

The logic behind administrative decentralization however remains the same; if responsibilities are to be given to public bodies, the central level wishes to maintain the possibility of both defining national health policy and harmonizing local practices in order to ensure equity across the population. It is also important to analyse carefully the "decision space"[4] that is in fact decentralized. We can therefore see substantial differences between countries as regards practices, while principles can be quite similar. Bossert (1999) therefore underlines the importance of analysing the "decision space" that the central level grants to decentralized bodies. In order to do so, he proposes to maintain four major functions:

- Funding, for example: what would be the modalities for appropriating and managing revenue from recovered costs, and what would be the modalities for using financial subsidies from the central authority?

- Organization of health services, for example: what type of autonomy would be given to hospitals? What are the modalities for separating provision and purchase of health services?

- Human resources: what are the powers given to decentralized authorities in respect of staff recruitment, and setting contracts and salaries?

- "Governance rules", for example: whether the central level will establish the modalities of civic participation or the composition of administration councils for health facilities.

2. THE LOGIC OF CONFRONTATION

The technical rationale of the health district and deconcentration, which is one of its organizational principles, has generally preceded administrative decentralization reforms. Administrative decentralization will disrupt the balance that was gradually established in the logic of sectoral deconcentration. It introduces new actors who, since they are elected, represent the local interests and have a public healthcare mandate.

The health sector therefore faces two types of rationale:

- The systemic rationale used by health professionals based on technical considerations and for which the health district constitutes the modus operandi;
- The political rationale, where health is only one of the social dimensions for when the elected members of local authorities are responsible.

"How can we reconcile the systemic coherence of the traditional healthcare actors in the health district and the political rationale of actors in administrative decentralization?" This is a question facing many healthcare systems.

2.1   How is the clash between these two rationales expressed?

On the ground, the clash between these two rationales is expressed in a number of ways:

Lack of correspondence of competence between geographical areas

When geographically dividing health districts, Ministries of Health base their decisions on technical considerations relating to optimum population size (for a healthcare facility and a district) as well as the amount of time taken to travel to healthcare facilities. They also seek to make the geographical area of the health district correspond more or less with the geographical area of the other deconcentrated authorities (prefectures, districts, counties...).   Administrative decentralization frequently leads to a different geographical splitting to that of the former deconcentrated entities. It is therefore often the case that the splitting up of the health sector does not correspond, or no longer corresponds, to that used in administrative decentralization. Furthermore, these types of division can develop in accordance with political concerns that do not take healthcare into consideration.

With administrative decentralization, owing to the healthcare-related competences that are transferred, it is almost inevitable that the inconsistency of the geographic divisions leads to confrontations.

The role of the district management team

The district management   team generally does not cope very well with administrative decentralization, since it perceives it as the dispossession of its resources and authority. Since this type of decentralization results in basic health facilities becoming the responsibility of local authorities, the district management team feels that it has lost its authority over these facilities, even if it continues to be responsible for their technical supervision. When this transfer of health facilities also comes with the transfer of the responsibility for healthcare as a whole in the area, that feeling of dispossession is greater still.

The interests of each actor

Administrative decentralization, by increasing the number of actors involved in the area of healthcare, introduces diversity into the interests of those actors. For example, it would be easy to understand that a Ministry of Health might wish to harmonize the practices of actors across a territory, while on the other hand a municipality, since it is not necessarily sensitive to the rationale of solidarity, would whish to always obtain more for its subjects, even if that is to the detriment of the subjects of the neighbouring community. Administrative decentralization is not based on the general interest at the national level, but rather on the law of the majority at each level of decentralization.

Furthermore, the greater the diversification of these public actors, the more possibilities there are for them to form understandings and alliances; there is therefore a risk that political games will take precedence over the general interest.

Global rationale, sectoral rationale

Deconcentration in the health sector follows sectoral rationale: healthcare is organized without reference to other sectors, even if, and this can be problematic, an intersectoral approach is sometimes necessary. Administrative decentralization is based on global rationale. A municipality will want to be able to have coherent and coordinated activities in all sectors under its jurisdiction. Administrative decentralization therefore results in making Ministries of Health reconsider their sectoral approach and become involved in a global approach at the local level. Without renouncing the specific aspects of their technical approach, they thus have to negotiate their place within human activity as a whole. Administrative decentralization therefore results in a certain amount of decompartmentalization of sectoral practices and central administration.[5]

2.2   The institutional context of the health district

This confrontation will take different forms depending on the institutional context in which the health district is found. From a functional perspective, the health district is a system that allows a connection between a local health administration and health service providers, the most important of which operate from health facilities at both the primary (healthcare centres) and secondary (district hospitals) levels. The health district defines the functional relations between all of the elements that comprise it. While there is general agreement on this functional definition of the health district, it is implemented in different institutional contexts:

The health district is an administrative public service under the direct control of the Ministry of Health: in the context of deconcentration, the health district can be seen to have been granted a certain amount of autonomy in respect of day-to-day management in order to simplify administrative and financial processes. The district management team plans the district's activities, coordinates their implementation and provides supervision, etc. In this scenario, public health facilities can have a greater or lesser degree of autonomy: they can be simple administrative services under the direct authority of the health district management, or, conversely, they can be granted autonomous status (for example district hospitals with public institution status). As for private providers, when they have received accreditation or delegated authority, they can have a greater or lesser degree of association with the functioning of the health district: for example, they can be involved in defining the health district development plan.

In this scenario, administrative decentralization aims to define the missions that are transferred from the health district to the local authorities: is there a transfer of the task of providing health services or managing all healthcare administration or parts thereof, or all of these elements?

The health district has been granted a specific legal status and therefore constitutes a legal personality under administrative law. The health district is therefore led by an administrative council, the composition of which may vary, but which comprises persons and entities from different backgrounds: for example, representatives of the Ministry of Health, private providers, members of the public, local communities, representatives of training and research institutions, etc. The district manager is under the control of this authority. Here too, the health district can have several functions: healthcare administration, allocation of public funds, supervision or management of public health facilities.

In this scenario, administrative decentralization will no doubt not bring the institutional context of the health district into question. It could, however, lead to more weight being given to local authorities in the health district's decision-making bodies or a transfer of primary public health facility management to local authorities.

3.   THE USE OF CONTRACTING

Owing to administrative decentralization, local authorities are in charge of health related missions. How will they fulfil these missions?

3.1 The role of local authorities in organizing the provision of health services

First of all, certain concepts should be agreed, and consideration must be given to all activities that affect public health. Health facilities, whether public or private, are unquestionably the driving force in this regard owing to their treatment, prevention and promotion activities; however, they do not have the monopoly. Private practitioners (physicians and nurses in liberal medicine, pharmacists, private clinics, and also traditional healers) conduct healthcare activities. Furthermore, some structures, such as social centres, centres for the disabled or nutritional rehabilitation centres, while they do not fall within the prerogatives of the Ministry of Health, also conduct activities that are closely linked to healthcare. The same can be said for activities such as providing drinking water or sanitary services in schools or communities.

Administrative decentralization carefully defines the areas in which missions will be delegated to local authorities: in this way, administrative decentralization can result in a decision to place centres for the disabled under the mandate of the local authority in one country, while in another a decision can be taken to keep that area in the remit of the central Government.

How will local authorities fulfil these missions? There are two main strategies available to them. The first concerns the structures carrying out activities related to healthcare; and the second is based on conducting specific healthcare-related activities.

The structure approach

The local authority can fulfil its healthcare mission by looking at the structures, i.e. institutions and infrastructures, which carry out activities related to healthcare:

Public structures

Whether on they have established them by themselves or acquired ownership through administrative decentralization, local authorities can establish healthcare activities through public structures. These can be health facilities (clinics, health centres, hospitals) or social structures (social centres, nutritional rehabilitation centres, etc.). Local authorities therefore have a choice between:

- *Direct management:* in this case, the public structures merely constitute departments of the local authority. Financial and administrative management is directly provided by the local authority, even if, technically, a management "board" system is established for the public structure.

- *Autonomous management:* in this case the local authority will have given the public structure autonomous status through a legal personality. However, this autonomous public structure will not be independent. The local authority will exercise guardianship pursuant to the regulations that allow it to do so. Furthermore, this structure will not really be independent from the local authority either in respect of its finances or its human resources. This autonomous structure can overcome this dependence on the local authority on a case-by-case basis and in accordance with informal practices: thus the local authority will take orders for the posting of personnel and will issue operating grants. These relations can however also be formalized through contractual arrangements. After negotiations a contract will be drawn up between the local authority and the autonomous public structure that will set out all the arrangements between the two from a reasonably long-term perspective in order to give the autonomous structure a chance to benefit from coherent management throughout;

- *Delegated management:* the local authority delegates to an external body the responsibility of managing, on its behalf, an activity of general interest with the infrastructures associated with it. Through the contractual relationship, the operator (the entity that has accepted the management role) is responsible for the management of the service it has received; in this context, the operator is responsible for its own acts, and must answer to those who have employed its services. That notwithstanding, the authority is not totally disconnected, since it maintains the overall responsibility. In this regard, if the operator fails, the local authority is able, and in some cases obliged, to intervene and take over the operator's duties.

There are two different types of case according to the degree of involvement of the private entity (the assignee) in the infrastructures and equipment:

- The private entity receives existing resources from the Ministry of Health, such as buildings and equipment, in the state in which they are found, in order to fulfil the public service mission. Generally repair, maintenance and renovation work is provided jointly by the assignor and the assignee, in accordance with the terms set out in the contract. In technical terms, and under French obligations of obedience, the term used is *"affermage"*; under English obligations of obedience the term used is *"lease contract"*. These resources remain the property of the State,

- The private entity is responsible for providing buildings and acquiring equipment. These will be given to the State at the end of the contract (which is generally a long-term agreement). Under French obligations of obedience the term used is "*concession*"; Under English obligations of obedience the term used is "*Build, Operate, Transfer (B.O.T.)* ".

Private structures, involved in healthcare-related activities

The local authority has the possibility, through a contractual relationship, to bind these private structures to ensure that they improve their provision of healthcare-related activities. These contracts can aim to recognize the role played by this private structure and provide certain incentives (work assignments, tax incentives, access to supplies (medicines), absorption of certain operating costs (water, electricity, etc.)); this will be the case with private health facilities, but it can also be with private structures that carry out healthcare-related activities (such as social rehabilitation). These contracts, however, can lead to certain activities: thus the local authority can establish an agreement with a private hospital whereby the latter provides continuous training for healthcare professionals working in public health centres under the aegis of the local authority.

The activities approach

In the context of the mandates given to them by administrative decentralization, local authorities want certain healthcare-related activities to be carried out. Here the activities concerned are clearly set out: social marketing, follow up of people living with HIV/AIDS and monitoring of high risk groups (for example prostitution in a an area with high truck traffic density), street children, awareness raising and prevention among school children, etc. The local authority can use its own services to run these activities, but it can also undertake contracts with actors that will conduct these activities on its behalf.

- The local authority can undertake contracts with establishments that do not primarily work in the field of health. For example, the local authority can establish a contract with a primary school (private or State-run) to run a vaccination awareness-raising campaign.

- It can establish contracts with entities that do not have any infrastructure. For example, the local authority will engage in a contract with a local NGO mandating it to conduct an AIDS awareness-raising campaign among opinion leaders.

The contractual relationship is based on the purchase of services: with the financial means at its disposal, the local authority purchases, through a contract, the provision of this activity from an actor that commits to performing the activity in accordance with the terms set forth in the contract.

3.2   Links between local authorities and the Ministry of Health

Local authorities that have acquired a mission in the health sector in the context of administrative decentralization are not, however, independent; particularly in developing countries. This lack of independence will manifest itself in two ways:

- De facto non-independence: administrative decentralization generally confers areas of responsibility to local authorities, but does not confer the possibility of defining the ways in which they can fulfil these responsibilities. Thus, generally, local authorities will continue to depend on the central Government for their financial resources. Similarly, State public service is not always transferred to local public service;

- Non-independence linked to State supervision. The State, when setting out a national health policy as required under its regalian functions, sets a framework for healthcare that is imposed on actors working in the sector and, as a result, on local authorities; thus healthcare institutions established by local authorities will be obliged to follow the national policy: reference system, typology of institutions and definition of activities at each level. More significantly, through laws and decrees the State can impose certain constraints on local authorities; for example, the local authority must guarantee vaccinations for children, must respect the system for reporting epidemics, etc.

In this environment, local authorities, like the Ministry of Health, cannot live in isolation. Administrative decentralization thus necessarily leads to methods according to which actors will have to regulate their interaction. It is very difficult for these relationships to continue on an informal level: neither will a legal context allow relationships to be formalized in an efficient manner. Contracting therefore offers a possibility to formalize the relationships while maintaining a balance between the two parties. Use of contracts in the organization of relations between the State and local authorities is the result of questions being raised about the mechanisms guaranteeing the supremacy of the State. Negotiated agreements supersede measures of authority in defining objectives and allocating resources. However, just because public actors are obliged to collaborate this does not mean that the relationship will be established without any difficulties; since their interests are often different, the negotiation will take place in an atmosphere of competition rather than frank collaboration.

Through contracting, administrative decentralization gives local authorities a real potential to make their points of view heard and express their needs. In contrast to the law, which is a unilateral act of the State, the contract recognizes local authorities' power of negotiation. Negotiation between public actors therefore has an aim - the contract - that enshrines reciprocal commitments. Decentralized authorities therefore posses a legal document that cannot easily be brought into question and under which the parties make a commitment for the future, which is not possible in classic administrative relationships. These commitments can be specified to a greater or lesser degree, but they always constitute terms of reference in the eyes of contracting parties as well as external actors. It does not matter whether these commitments constitute contractual obligations in law or simple political commitments; the interdependence between the actors will oblige each of them to respect their commitments, since they will need to be able to depend on the commitments made by the other party.

Even if it is generally the central Government that orders and establishes administrative decentralization, it cannot easily relinquish its dominative habits, and will have a tendency in its day-to-day behaviour to take back with one hand what it has given with the other. Under a range of pretexts, particularly harmonization of practices across the national territory, the central Government will tend to want to pilot contracting. It has several options. It can, for example, define the contractual context so precisely and narrowly that it leaves no room for discussion or choice; in this case it is very close to the notion of a standard-form contract in which the contractual terms are set by one of the parties and the other can only accept them as a whole or reject them, without being able to have them modified. In this regard, the right to contract given to local authorities through administrative decentralization is not a sufficient guarantee; the local authorities also need to be in a position to make the most of this right.

One of the positive aspects of contracting in the context of administrative decentralization is that it obliges local authorities to establish coherent projects, in other words projects that define clear objectives and ways of attaining them. This practice categorically breaks away from the "cash desk" rationale, which sees the central Government as a cash cow that exists simply to finance the local authorities' activities without question. From this point of view a contract is considered more restrictive by the local authorities than a traditional grant, in that it compels the local authorities to plan their projects in response to the norms set by the State, to undertake their own financial commitments and to accept the establishment of a procedure for monitoring and evaluating their activities. This move is further strengthened by the development of the notion of results-based management.

Thus contractual cooperation should be seen as a sign of a deep change in relationships between a State that has become frugal, or rather re-focussed on its national responsibilities, and local authorities that have matured. However, there is still a large gap between this vision and reality and the central Government and local authorities have a long way to go.

Although contracting between public actors has a number of advantages, it is not devoid of problems:

- Although administrative decentralization concerns local actors that are independent and therefore equal in law to the central authorities, the relationships between them often remain unequal. Firstly, the central Government has an *in fine* supreme sovereignty that places territorial authorities in a position of inferiority. This inequality is expressed in power relationships. The central Government often remains the initiator of a contractual process: it defines its context and direction, and establishes the monitoring and evaluation bodies. The central Government has the necessary financial resources and can decide whether or not to allocate them to a contract, and therefore has a powerful means of imposing its points of view and influencing the direction of local policies.

- Contracting gives most benefit to the strongest actors, i.e. those who have the greatest resources (particularly financial), the most developed professional capacities and the capacity to develop effective lobbying. Managing relations between public actors by contracting runs the risk of benefiting those with the best resources for developing good projects. It is not generally the local authorities that have these resources at their disposal. Contracting can therefore result in increasing the inequalities between territorial entities.

- Contracting between public actors does not guarantee better local democracy. Although contracting as a result of administrative decentralization in fact enables representative democracy (based on elected representatives) to develop, it does not necessarily lead to a development in participative democracy (based directly on populations and their associations), which is desired and desirable in all approaches in contractual cooperation. These difficulties lead to a number of obstacles: lack of availability or interest of users, obscurity of administrative jargon and technicality of contractual procedures, weak representation and lack of real authority for community organizations.

- The contract is a new form of relationship between actors, but as a result it is also a new form of distributing public funds. The actors will therefore adapt to this new rule of the game. Since projects and contracts are now required, ways of responding to this new rule of the game must be established. The most qualified and the fasted to adapt will therefore win; these are not necessarily those who need to the most.[6]

- The contractual relationship between public actors is based on a rationale that is not a market rationale. It concerns an agreement where prices are not necessarily the main determining factor. These negotiations and agreements are based on a range of mechanisms. The criteria for judging whether a contract is

234

valid for its final recipient (the population) are difficult to set. As a result various degrees of ineffectiveness, poor judgment of priorities, and even corruption, can easily infiltrate these contractual processes. Agreement of political views has a role to play: it is often easier for a municipality to obtain a contract with the State if it has a mayor with the same political leanings as the central power. We can also witness illegal practices; anyone who detains the authority to sign contracts has a real power that could be monetized.

Furthermore, in the context of administrative decentralization, local authorities become responsible or jointly responsible for drafting and piloting local health policies. In this regard, the planning of health districts, which was the prerogative of the Ministry of Health and its deconcentrated authorities (the district management team) can no longer ignore administrative decentralization. Here again, public actors are driven to come to an agreement. Contracting therefore becomes a vital tool. The issue is no longer specific contractual arrangements as it was in the previous case, but rather to define the local health policy, and its implementation, coordinated by different local actors, including the private sector.

Contracting therefore constitutes part of the structuring of territorial policies. It is not simply the consolidation of specific contractual arrangements, but rather the definition of a context for collaboration established in agreement with the actors involved at the local level. This is far from the commercial type of contracting based on an exchange of services and therefore on an act of purchasing. Furthermore, this type of contractual relationship undoubtedly enables State activities to be redefined; these activities are no longer centred around monopolistic provision of health services, but rather on the organizational function of the health system through various means at its disposal: regulation, incentives and adjustment.

Specifically, the agreement that public actors must reach, if possible with the collaboration of private actors, is akin to the notion of a "plan-contract". These contracts establish a stable relationship between the State and the territorial authorities that are signatories, based on the definition of programmes of action and the acceptance of norms for the behaviour of all parties. Under the contract, the public authorities specify the norms of their relationships with each other by defining their objectives, commitments and a certain number of organizational rules.

All of these issues can be covered in a single contract; known as an "objectives and resources contract", i.e. contracts that define both the objectives to be achieved and the means and resources that will be put to use to do so. In some cases, a distinction is made between "objectives contracts" and "resources contracts". An objectives contract will place particular emphasis on the district development policy and the role of each actor; the health district development plan or strategic plan can be seen from this angle, as an objectives contract. Under this understanding it is no longer an indicative plan, but rather a contract connecting the different actors who have freely decided to sign it. Resources contracts, which are based on objectives contracts, provide more explicitly for the operational relationships between the actors, and emphasize the resources, in particular the financial resources, which will be used in the context of the contract. The contract itself therefore provides a context for each of the specific contractual arrangements that must be signed for the implementation of each activity.

3.3   The relationships between local authorities

In the context of administrative decentralization, it is common to see that the geographical areas of local communities do not correspond with the technical definitions made by Health Ministries. Thus a local community, except in large cities, covers a smaller area than that of the health district. Let us take the example of a health district where the district hospital is within the territory of the largest local community, but that authority has a smaller area than that of the health district. When administrative decentralization placed that hospital under the responsibility of that local authority, the other local communities and health centres for which they are responsible must establish ways of accessing the district hospital. Thus the local authorities of the district must reach an agreement on the establishment of links between the health district's health facilities. The resulting contractual relationship enables the systemic rationale of the health district to be recovered.

Furthermore, local authorities can also agree to run joint activities:

- For example, they could agree to establish an inter-communal nutritional rehabilitation centre. The centre's status would demonstrate the involvement of all of the local communities participating; the centre's status could therefore also be considered as a contract binding together the local communities. Furthermore, the local authorities could decide to manage the inter-communal centre themselves, or to delegate its management to a body that would accept that responsibility.

- They could decide to conduct targeted activities. For example, several communities could form an association for the effective elimination of mosquitoes in an area that covered several local communities. Their agreement can be formalized by a contract stating their respective responsibilities in this regard. Similarly, they can agree to choose a joint operator with whom they will jointly establish a contractual agreement.

236

In this regard, administrative decentralization pushes local authorities to develop contractual relations with the central Government and, as a result, the Ministry of Health, and it also invites local authorities to strengthen their relationship with each other. This horizontal contracting allows the geographical areas of political entities to be adjusted in accordance with the technical considerations of the health sector.

The plan below summarizes the options presented in this chapter:

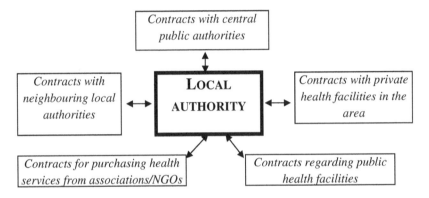

CONCLUSION

Nowadays Ministries of Health can no longer and must no longer ignore the administrative decentralization that is occurring. Without renouncing the specific elements of their technical approach they must consider the implications of global decentralization. These Ministries still do not have the resources and capacities to drive these developments and provide for solutions. Furthermore, the Ministries responsible for piloting global decentralization often tend to be unaware of the technical realities of these (line) Ministries and the generally weak relationships between all these Ministries is an obstacle for developing a coherent approach.

Furthermore, the central level, as guardian of the general interest of the population, has considerable difficulty in avoiding to accentuate its role as the "principal" as defined in the agency theory. With the means it has at its disposal (mainly incentives and sanctions) it will try to influence the "agents", in other words the decentralized bodies, in order to make them respect its objectives; for example depending on its preference for primary healthcare, the central level can force municipalities to allocate a minimum percentage to this level of healthcare (as is the case in Colombia and Senegal, for example). Thus the decision space that is left to these decentralized institutions could vary greatly from country to country and the strength of the relationship between the central authorities and the decentralized bodies.

However, the most recent development of partnership research based on contractual cooperation reveals new horizons and allows one to think, without being naive, that a negotiation between partners that consider themselves equal even thought they do not necessarily have the same objectives, can result in a form of cooperation that is advantageous to both parties. This contractual approach, particularly between public partners, leads to a considerable change in the development of relations between healthcare actors. Such a change is not easy and consideration must be given to the fact that time and trial and error will be needed to reach a balance and that those responsible should use the necessary techniques to ensure that this approach is established effectively.

Local authorities therefore play an increasingly important role in the area of public health. Their prerogatives come from administrative decentralization and the enactments related to it. At the same time, we can see that necessary though these enactments may be they are generally not sufficient to define operational methods. Contracting is therefore used as a tool for defining the operational modalities. Contracting does not replace these laws and regulations, but rather it completes them.

Notes

[1] Mills, A., J. P. Vaughan, D. L. Smith, and I. Tabibzadeh. 1991. *The decentralization of health systems*. Geneva: WHO.

[2] Resolution WHA41.34 of May 1988 "Strengthening Primary Health Care"

[3] Cassels, A. 1995. Health sector reform: key issues in less developed countries. Journal of International Development 7, no. 3:329-347.

[4] Bossert, Th. 1999. Decentralization of health systems: decision space, innovation and performance . LAC Health Sector Reform Initiative. 17.

[5] Lerique, F. 1997. Contractualisation et politiques territoriales: les politiques de la ville. In *La coopération contractuelle et le gouvernement des villes*, edited by Marcou, G., F Rangeon, and J. L. Thiébault.

[6] This strategy is of course effective between public actors, but it also develops with other actors. Therefore in some countries that have decided to base their partnership with the private sector on contractual relations rather than classic grant methods we can see that these private actors adapt: first of all they organize themselves as legal entities, enabling them to issue contracts and present projects culminating in the signature of contracts. Contracting thus becomes a competitive market.

238

Part II

Chapter 6

The best use of sub-contracting and outsourcing

Abdelali Belghiti Alaoui &

Jean Perrot

INTRODUCTION

An organization is an entity structured around the production of goods and services in order to achieve an objective. Legally, an organization is an independent or autonomous entity, i.e. one with a distinct legal personality.

Two types of organization can be distinguished in the health sector: purely administrative entities that may exist at a central or decentralized level (a central authority or external services), or institutions that provide treatment and services, whether in the public or private sector. Hence private clinics, hospitals, health centres, clinical laboratories, radiology units, pharmacies or even drug distribution structures are all organizations providing treatment and services. However, they are only considered as such if they have legal personality and the capacity to determine their own future and can manage their own resources.

An autonomous organization with distinct legal personality is answerable for its own performance. But in order to achieve high performance it must ensure that its inputs are optimized. The organization's legal status will facilitate or constrain this effort. Control of inputs is therefore a major element in ensuring the survival and efficient operation of an organization. However, production techniques have developed and logistical tools diversified to such an extent that control of inputs and means of production is becoming increasingly difficult. Likewise, organizations are aware that they must procure their primary materials at competitive prices, employ competent staff and monitor the quality of their output. This is only possible when they have recourse to external providers and intermediaries to guarantee their output; hence their interest in subcontracting or outsourcing to alleviate these constraints.

In the health sector, these problems are all the more delicate because the primary materials need to be made safe (consumables, medicines, blood, etc.) and the customer is in a weak position in the sense that he cannot himself vouch for the quality of the service (asymmetrical information). Unable to meet all these requirements using their own resources, health institutions are obliged to make use of outside expertise to provide certain services more efficiently and at lower cost, particularly those that do not involve direct interface with patients.

For hospitals, as for other organizations, it was long held that the delivery of intermediary services by the organization itself was an indicator of efficiency and independence. Efficiency, because recourse to an outside provider would necessarily cost more; and independence, because recourse to an outside provider meant placing oneself in a situation of dependence on an outside agent.

For many years, hospitals themselves provided these services to a certain extent: they prepared certain medicines, kept a vegetable garden and relied on a well for their supply of drinking water, etc. They assumed that they should provide all intermediary services: a clinical laboratory and radiology unit, buildings maintenance, security services, tending the hospital gardens, book-keeping and staff training, etc. Nowadays this is no longer possible.

Health service administrators or managers are not necessarily in the best position to provide the required intermediary services efficiently. All organizations face the choice of providing in-house services or resorting to subcontracting. The purpose of this chapter is to provide an overview of this issue. Part I focuses on the definition of outsourcing and subcontracting. Parts II and III concentrate on the prerequisites for outsourcing and the reasons for choosing it as an option. Part IV considers which areas might be amenable to outsourcing. Part V explores some of the difficulties that might arise, and Part VI dwells on the need for planning of outsourcing within the organization.

1. DEFINITIONS

Subcontracting refers to the means whereby an organization (the commissioning party) entrusts the performance of an operation to an outside provider. This management tool has gradually become the norm for organizations, enabling them to satisfy new production needs and tap outside expertise. Since then, subcontracting has rapidly become one of the most commonly used management tools in private and public sector organizations alike. This has led to the development of the concept of "outsourcing".

Outsourcing is a sophisticated form of subcontracting that involves greater cooperation in the conceptualization and performance of activities, increased accountability for the results and greater specialization as in "facility management"[1] or "information management".[2] Outsourcing is the act of delegating, over a number of years, the management of one or more functions of the organization to an external provider. The long-term nature of outsourcing forms an important contrast with subcontracting, which is normally short-term.

Outsourcing has subsequently become a strategic option for organizations, enabling them to overcome problems connected with lead times, additional production costs and poor service quality, and also to develop alliances or networks with other providers that can potentially improve and consolidate the organization's position.

2. THE RATIONALE OF OUTSOURCING

Using outsourcing, in the form of subcontracting, is nothing new, but formerly it was sporadic and only involved ancillary activities. Today it is regarded as a strategic option and tends to be executed in a more professional manner.

Outsourcing has been defined as "the act of delegating certain functions to service providers outside the organization for a multi-year contractual term".[3] It means arranging for an activity to be performed by an outside provider in accordance with predefined contractual conditions that are binding upon the parties. Organizations that do not possess legal personality or the capacity to delegate powers to a public officer cannot enter into this type of contract and therefore cannot independently decide whether or not to outsource. Thus, although it is an internal strategic option in public-sector organizations, the decision to outsource is closely linked to a policy of decentralization.

For wholly independent organization such as private hospitals, the decision to outsource is entirely at the discretion of the director or manager of the organization. In a public-sector organization, however, the choice is one for political decision-makers, not managers. In a public hospital, autonomous or otherwise, the decision to outsource can only be made by decision-makers. It may be that outsourcing is not permitted: for a long time, this was true in many fields such as catering, laundry, and security. In other areas the decision to outsource is made on a case-by-case basis: the decision-maker determines whether or not to outsource. Outsourcing is sometimes given the go-ahead in certain precisely defined areas (laundry services but not catering, for example), while in still other cases it is permitted and the managers of the organization decide whether or not to implement it.

In the public sector, outsourcing is equivalent to purchasing a service, and as such is governed by the rules on procurement. These vary in flexibility depending on the country, the charter of the institution and its degree of autonomy (public or otherwise), or on the type of services being outsourced (treatment, services, logistics, etc.). These rules are normally formulated at national level and apply across the board to all sectors, unless special arrangements are specified for a particular organization.

In addition, within one and the same country, these rules change over time: there is greater flexibility and transparency, more competition and more accountability. This means that the scope for outsourcing has expanded considerably in recent years.

242

3. REASONS FOR OUTSOURCING

To be strategic, a decision to outsource must always result from a strategic analysis in order to ensure that the outsourcing of an activity or a function is first and foremost a means of attaining a given objective, and then that it is the best choice from among a range of possibilities.

Nevertheless, this best choice will be weighed up against a number of criteria that each organization will assess differently. The most frequently cited criteria are:

- Cost savings: Some organizations may become interested in outsourcing because they hope to be able to reduce intermediary service costs. For example, a central administration may be interested in subcontracting the cleaning of its premises to a private company because it hopes it will save money by not employing its own staff to do the job;

- Better service: For example, a hospital may subcontract security to a private company in the hope that it will be more effective in clamping down on favouritism because it is not so closely involved in local community life. The quality of security will thus be enhanced;

- Bypassing administrative constraints: Specifically, constraints involving human resources and skills shortages and the unwieldiness of administrative procedures. Thus, a hospital that is unable to recruit maintenance personnel could outsource work to a private company that employs people who are not on the hospital's staffing table, thereby bypassing administrative rigidity.

- Focusing on core activity: By recruiting private companies to perform tasks that do not constitute the core activity of the organization, it can hive off energy-consuming activities and thereby concentrate on its central mission. Thus, a hospital will tend to withdraw from all non-medical activities in order to focus on its therapeutic mission;

- Minimizing risk: For example, by subcontracting photocopying work, an organization can transfer risks to the private company responsible for the activity. If the machines break down, it is a problem for the subcontractor rather than the organization. Not every risk is transferable, however (for example, in catering, if there is an outbreak of food poisoning, the hospital will call the subcontractor to account, yet it still bears responsibility in the eyes of patients ... and the law).

Each organization will weigh these criteria differently in the light of its situation and priorities. For example, some organizations with very tight budgets will be more interested in cost savings, whereas others with less pressing budgetary constraints will be more interested in enhancing quality.

4. AREAS OF OUTSOURCING

As a rule, the most commonly outsourced functions are general and support services, followed by logistics, IT and telecommunications. Given that levels of development vary from country to country, these areas will continue to be the most affected by outsourcing for the foreseeable future.

In the health sector, the outsourcing of support or general services has become necessary, first of all because it delivers better service, but also, given the shortage of personnel familiar with health systems, especially in developing countries, it is increasingly difficult to justify personnel requirements for support and logistics functions. Because of their common characteristics, because they are fairly well developed in all countries and because they enable organizations to focus on their core activity, these are the areas most commonly affected by outsourcing.

The areas in which outsourcing is most controversial are those that affect the organization's mission or its core activity. In health care, this means treating patients. Is it possible to outsource this? Most stakeholders and decision-makers would say no, not for technical reasons but because of political considerations regarding the role of the State in the health sector and the importance of a public health service. The debate on this fundamental issue opens different perspectives on the development of health care. It should be borne in mind that:

- First, outsourcing is simply a tool for decision-makers and managers. They decide to outsource in the context of implementing a health policy that defines the "why" and the "how" of outsourcing in terms of satisfying needs or resolving problems.

- Second, outsourcing is a management tool that has to be planned and correctly applied to be effective.

Following this interpretation, it is possible to say that, for a hospital, "everything is outsourceable" or "nothing is outsourceable" depending on the rationale for outsourcing and the possibilities for its effective use that have been outlined. The situation will vary from country to country and hospital to hospital, but the authorities are responsible for creating opportunities and hospital managers are responsible for knowing when to seize them.

Today, some theories (utopian or visionary?) treat institutions (for example hospitals) as a cluster of contracts (a contract node, in economic jargon). These theories hold that the institution's managers handle all the contracts while the institution itself produces nothing directly. Under this arrangement, intermediary services are of course outsourced, but so is the operating theatre (to a group of specialist physicians, for example). The wards are managed by specialized enterprises, and the radiology unit, the clinical laboratory and the pharmacy are all run privately. The role of the hospital management is thus to ensure that all these contracts are consistent and complement one another. The management team thus comprises a handful of individuals. Today this vision is still not a reality. But who would have thought just a few years ago that institutional catering would be handled by private companies outside the hospital?

5. PLANNING FOR OUTSOURCING

Outsourcing is not a magic solution to every problem. Its success depends on planning and the method of implementation. As in any other field, planning for outsourcing originates in the organization's strategic assessment. This assessment may be limited to the principal issues facing the organization and might be backed up by an audit (financial, organizational, or operational) or by an organizational performance analysis. To be relevant, a decision on outsourcing must be justified by the ability to deliver at reasonable cost a solution to at least one of the problems facing the organization. Thus, depending on the nature of the services designated for outsourcing, planning must incorporate the possible reorganization of work and production processes that are connected with the implementation of outsourcing.

Once the decision to outsource has been taken, it is necessary to specify the activities or services that are going to be outsourced, the comparative cost of the operation, the arrangements for implementation (including the contractual arrangements) and monitoring and evaluation procedures. Because the decision to outsource is normally irreversible, planning should not be limited to a single budget cycle, even one that is spread over several years; all the implications that outsourcing will have for the organization (in relation to staff, clients, suppliers and policy) should be examined.

Planning for outsourcing should thus be considered in four phases:

(i) Rationale phase (justifying the need to use outsourcing);

(ii) Implementation planning phase;

(iii) Drafting of contractual arrangements phase;

(iv) Implementation and follow-up phase.

Confronted with a situation, an outsourcing implementation plan should be drawn up. Even if analysis of the situation indicates that a number of areas could be outsourced, it is likely that the organization will not be able to outsource them all at once: it should set priorities based on situational parameters. An example is appended to this analysis to show the value of planning.

6. ISSUES FOR CONSIDERATION

Outsourcing raises certain issues that need to be considered whenever this option is selected.

1. All too often, outsourcing is used to resolve problems that cannot be resolved in house. Frequently, therefore, it does not address the underlying issue because it does not treat the malady. Outsourcing is not a stopgap arrangement. So before asking whether outsourcing is appropriate, it is worth taking the time to find out whether issues can be resolved internally. The mere threat of outsourcing can sometimes be enough to trigger internal improvements. The outcome could be various forms of internal contract arrangement; for example between the hospital management and in-house logistics services.

2. Trade unions are often fiercely opposed to outsourcing, because transferring the existing services at a hospital to outside contractors entails the abolition of posts or the redeployment of staff to posts that do not match their primary qualifications, or even redeployment to other, understaffed hospitals (geographical redeployment). In addition, trade unions believe that outsourcing will weaken their power in the hospital by making use of a more docile, less unionized workforce.

3. The contract or general contractual specification is the core element of any outsourcing arrangement. It outlines in detail the requirements of the contractual relationship. Outsourcing requires that the hospital monitor the contract on an ongoing basis, not just through financial or administrative reporting. It should verify whether results have been achieved, whether quality targets have been met and whether patients are satisfied. Hospitals normally lack qualified staff to perform these tasks. Subcontracting, even at the simplest level, cannot be considered a way of shirking this responsibility. On the contrary, the hospital must monitor the contract and contractors on a daily basis. But certain hospitals often resort to subcontracting to rid themselves of a problem, and the results are disappointing.

4. Contractual provisions: Should the terms of the contract focus on the resources assigned to the task or on the expected outcomes? For example, will a contract for cleaning services define the number of times the cleaner is to make the rounds of the premises and at what time, etc.? Or will the contract specify that the premises should be clean at all times (the subcontractor will determine how best to achieve this result)? Sometimes resources have to be shared (e.g. water and electricity), in which case the contract should specify how these resources are to be regulated. In any event, the contract should include results-based indicators so that services can

246

be monitored. This should prompt the hospital to define its expectations of outsourcing more precisely.

5. Competition: If the decision is made to outsource, a mechanism must be established to encourage competition between potential providers. But very often this kind of competition is not possible because there is only one potential provider at the site. Thus the hospital rapidly risks becoming overly dependent on this provider.

6. Qualifications of potential providers: There are very often no qualified providers in developing countries. Even for straightforward activities such as catering, the existence of companies able to provide such a service at a hospital cannot be taken for granted.

7. The best offer: It is obvious that the conventional approach of accepting the cheapest offer is pernicious because it does not enable decision-makers to determine who would provide the most appropriate service. Action should also be taken to ensure that the selection procedure admits the possibility of negotiation with the potential provider(s). Consequently, this should be permitted under national regulations.

8. Long-term or annual tendering arrangements: It often happens that, because budgets are annual, contracts are signed for one year only. But companies need to know how long they should commit themselves so as to be able to invest in the contractual relationship. The longer a contractual relationship lasts, the more it is conducive to cooperation. Here too, the Code governing public works or supply contracts should permit this eventuality.

9. Confidentiality: Outsourcing raises the issue of the confidentiality of medical information on patients. Sometimes, by the mere fact of their presence in a cancer or tuberculosis unit, subcontracted staff will be aware that certain patients have these diseases. In the most developed forms of outsourcing (payroll, information systems, billing, etc.), subcontracted staff will have access to confidential information about patients, hospital staff and the organization as a whole. Yet subcontracted staff are not bound by a code of professional ethics. They could pass on information to friends, relatives or even a wider public. There are two solutions: either bear this constraint in mind when choosing what areas to outsource, or draw up a charter of confidentiality with outside providers and/or insert a confidentiality clause in the contract.

10. To contrast the advantages of outsourcing in relation to in-house production, the two scenarios should be compared. This is never easy. First of all, in a hospital, it is impossible to compare the two scenarios simultaneously, since both cannot

247

coexist. Thus any comparison must involve different periods of time (before and after), or different hospitals (which are never exactly comparable). In addition, it is important to be able to gauge all the costs (particularly the salary costs of in-house production) and the social costs engendered by outsourcing. As far as benefits are concerned, it is important to consider not just the financial advantages but other aspects of quality and satisfaction as well, particularly as patients perceive them.

11. Reversibility: Once initiated, outsourcing is hard to reverse, even when it turns out to have been the wrong choice. This would involve re-establishing a service or function and re-employing staff. Although reversibility is theoretically possible, organizations tend instead to refocus or enhance their outsourcing arrangements.

12. Outsourcing can be seen as a means to introduce a new activity, whether permanently or otherwise.

13. The development of outsourcing in a given country will necessarily involve regulation of practices. Generally speaking, however, statutes and regulations in this area are inadequate and/or not tailored specifically to the health sector. As outsourcing becomes more and more widespread, the need for ground rules will become more obvious. The purpose of such a framework of reference is not to impose limitations but to protect the public and health workers.

Notes

[1] "Facility management" refers to enterprises that simultaneously provide a range of internal services. For example, multi-technical services covering all aspects of facilities and buildings maintenance and the utilities and networks at these facilities. This type of service provider specializes in areas such as heating, air conditioning, water distribution networks, ventilation, electricity, gas, and telecommunications networks. But it can also handle reception, parks and gardens, minor maintenance, lifts, reprography, removals and installations.

[2] "Information management" is the management by a third party of all or part of an enterprise's IT facilities. This term currently refers to maintenance of computer equipment, project management, information security and even training.

[3] Outsourcing Barometer 2003, Ernst & Young

Part II

Chapter 7

Contracting health personnel

Eric de Roodenbeke & Gilles Dussault

INTRODUCTION

At first sight, human resources recruitment appears to be a matter of proposing contracts that specify employment conditions.. The concept of the employment contract is closely linked to labour law, as defined in each country in relation to the recommendations of the International Labour Organization (ILO). Consideration of the employment contract therefore involves delving into the labour laws in force in each country.

Reducing the scope of human resources contracting to employment contracts is a simplification that would deprive anyone responsible for health policies, of a significant lever for the mobilization of human resources. While labour laws are important, contracting is a powerful additional tool for managing human resources more effectively. In a setting where the shortage of skilled workers[1] is recognized as a major constraint to access to health services, optimizing the use of health personnel is a priority.

Following a brief sketch of the concept of the employment contract, this chapter focuses on the use of contracting procedures to deploy human resources more effectively, in the context of national policies, and of a labour market dominated by public-sector employees in health institutions, which often lack management autonomy..

Another issue is how contracting can contribute to ensuring that individuals devote their best efforts to serving their employer organization, and that the workforce as a whole functions optimally in the pursuit of common objectives. There is a potential tension between the contracting mechanism for maximizing organizational performance and that for optimizing human resources, as incentives to promote the former are not necessarily suited to the latter.

After discussing the importance of human resources in the delivery of health services, and the specificities of the health labour market, this chapter reviews the various employment contract arrangements. The conditions for the use of a contractual tool will be analysed from the standpoint of optimizing human resource management and implementing sector policies. Recommendations on the appropriate use of contracting will conclude the chapter.

1. THE IMPORTANCE OF HUMAN RESOURCES IN HEALTH SERVICES

Jean Bodin (1530-1596), an eminent jurist considered to be one of the founding fathers of economic thought, thought that people are the only true source of wealth.

While this maxim is of general relevance, it is particularly significant in the health sector. Even in countries that make full use of new electronic and information technologies, human resources remain at the heart of health-service delivery.

The importance of this human dimension increases in proportion with the complexity of the organization in which people operate and in which there are numerous relations of interdependence between the various producer categories, offering fertile ground for contracting processes.

1.1   Personnel, a Specific Factor of Production

Staff costs

Human resources deployment absorbs a large portion of total health expenditure. Depending on the country, the proportions vary according to the pay scale and the cost of health products, particularly pharmaceuticals and equipment.

The significance of staff costs can be measured in many different ways. In the case of civil servants and other public-sector workers, this item can easily be measured in the Ministry's budget. In countries where public health care is mostly centralized, staff costs account for between 30 and 50% of all Ministry of Health expenditure.

In hospitals employing highly qualified staff, staff costs may absorb over 60% of the budget. But, while this is the average in OECD countries, it is seldom the case in low- and middle-income countries, given the variability of activities funded out of hospital budgets. In all cases, however, staff costs account for at least one third of total expenditure.

Specific aspects of remuneration

Employment terms for health workers vary according to their qualifications. While salaried employment predominates, physicians are also remunerated on a fee-for-service basis for all or part of their activity.

In the latter case, the relationship with the organization is different from that of those on salary, and the formalization of relations through a contract will reflect this remuneration arrangement linked to productivity. Remuneration arrangements do not constitute a contractual relationship. A contract can be used to specify the services to be paid, the norms (of quality for example) to be met, and the payment mechanism, which may include benefits such as access training or continuing education.

251

While remuneration is often emphasized as a key tool for motivating individuals to perform, its level needs to be considered in the country context and in relation to other countries.

The following model illustrates how high levels of relative remuneration can be considered insufficient in a country with a much higher standard of living.

Figure 1: Health professionals' gross and relative incomes

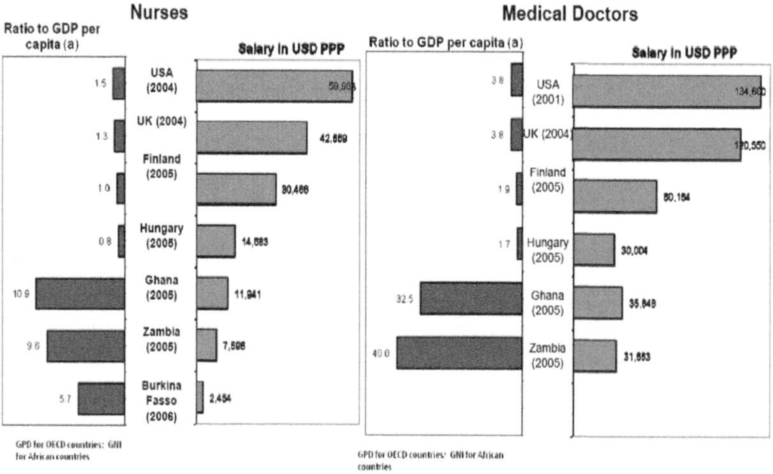

Source: Peter Scherer OECD, OECD-WHO Conference
http://www.who.int/hrh/migration/who_oecd_dialogue/en/index.html

The concept of human capital

Employees' skills constitute a critical asset. Skills result from investment in training and from cumulative practice.

The effective and efficient use of human capital requires that contractual relations are designed within a long-term framework, providing for career development and ensuring skills progression. This is rarely done in low-income countries, due to inflexible public service regulations and poor management capacities.

Contracting provides an opportunity to incorporate such an approach in employer-employee relations. Organizations that are free to contract beyond the minimum legal requirements can utilize this approach when formalizing their career development policy.

252

Skills-mix

While two skill areas (nurse and physician) largely dominate health sector professions, it is wrong to confine human resources development to these two groups. Health services use a wide range of professions and occupations, some exclusively dedicated to health care and can be practised in an institution or in the community, whereas others are less specific, but need some skill to be exercised in health institutions. Some occupations can be practised in health services or in other types of services.

This diversity implies that employment arrangements may vary according to the nature of professional practice, which influences will influence the nature of relations with the employer. The content of contractual relations cannot be the same for those working in different organizations, or for those who carry out very different activities in the same organization.

Accordingly, several types of contract could be considered.

A one-size-fits-all policy is clearly not appropriate, even though all contracts include elements applicable to everyone, such as general rules or common values. Nonetheless, the relevance and scope of a contract will depend on ensuring a good match between the factors it is designed to regulate and the specific situation of the employees.

These considerations suggest the possibility of implementing sets of contracts, each of which dealing with a specific aspect of the employer-employee relationship. No two groups of individuals will have the same portfolio of contracts. In practice, this does not mean binding each employee to so many contracts that he cannot understand what he has to do; moreover, multiple contracts increase the risk of contradicting each other. A balance needs to be struck between the value of implementing several contracts and the need for simplicity and effectiveness, given the transaction costs associated with implementing a contract.

The complexity of organizations

The duration of the relationship is an important factor in the contract, given the human capital investment and specific nature of the skills involved and organizational complexity. The more complex an organization the more likely it will rely on a heavy set of rules. Learning these rules is an important element in the performance of employees, which makes duration a factor to take into account.

Organizational complexity also raises the need to strike a balance between formalization and flexibility of relations between individuals. The bigger the set of rules governing individual activities, the harder the control of their application, unless a large proportion of internal resources are dedicated to this.

In principle, health service users should enjoy uniform service provision, and providers should adopt similar practices. This entails that service provision cannot be left to the discretion of each individual. Benchmarks and pre-defined results can help achieve these two objectives. The former serve to guide practice based on elements recognized as effective. Benchmarks are defined externally on the basis of acknowledged expertise, but some margin of manoeuvre can be granted to take account of contextual factors. Results are relevant at the end of the process; they express what has been obtained by the users; but measuring them poses major difficulties, particularly for practices that contain a random element or when it is difficult to attribute a result to a single or specific intervention.

1.2   A Complex Labour Market

Shortages of health human resources affect most countries to some extent. These particularly acute in the most qualified and specialized jobs, for which the production cycle is long and employment conditions are complex.

These skew the market in favour of health professionals rather than potential employers. Contracting thus becomes a tool to attract such professionals rather than a means of bringing them to adopt certain attitudes and practices. . It does not imply that health professionals can dictate their terms of employment, but that negotiation and reciprocal interest are particularly important in contracting policies as they apply to the health sector. Shortages or deficits of physicians is a general trend, but in some countries unemployment among doctors is a cause for concern. Another recent trend is the higher mobility of health professionals, particularly from poorer to richer countries. Contracting policies need to take these trends into account. Another one is the tendency of highly-qualified professionals to prefer urban practice, particularly in the capital city) Even in a situation of shortage, the possibility of working in the capital city in a well-managed and well-equipped organization puts the employer in a dominant position to negotiate a contract. In contrast, to attract doctors to a difficult or remote region with a weak technical infrastructure requires making conditions of employment attractive. These two extreme situations will be reflected in differences of emphasis in the respective contracts.

The attractiveness of private practice is another factor that should be taken into account. Countries can choose between allowing the private sector to develop in response to market forces and opportunities, and encouraging private practitioners, through contracting arrangements, to contribute to the provision of public health services that meet priority needs. To achieve this, public authorities need to skilfully balance the contracting process with health-care financing arrangements.

Lastly, contracting policies should include appropriate measures to enforce ethical practices and ensure that health professionals are properly paid, with a view to avoid compensatory behaviours, such as under-the-table payments, pilfering, absenteeism, and so on.

A thorough labour market analysis is important to identify the profile of health professionals in different contexts of practice, both in the capital and in remote areas. It would be unwise adopt policies which are not adapted to the particular conditions of the national health labour market.

1.3 External Contracting as an Alternative to Direct Employment

Outsourcing will be discussed specifically in terms of its relevance, limitations and modalities of implementation. Outsourcing does not necessarily involve dealing with a commercial enterprise. Hospitals may pool their resources to ensure that a certain activity is performed by an organization under their control, or a hospital may also sell services to another.

When they receive additional funding, hospitals tend to recruit more staff; but many activities can often be outsourced instead. Ad hoc recruitment to satisfy specific needs masks the potential for reorganization through the redeployment of staff to activities that need to be maintained and/or strengthened. Rather than responding to demand for services by hiring additional staff, existing resources might be put to more effective use by modifying the employment framework, through a negotiated process that results in a contract acceptable to both parties.

In situations where outsourcing is possible, this option can usefully be compared with reassignment of existing staff. The extent to which a hospital has capacity to manage contracting tools will affect this choice. When external supply is available, it may seem easier to choose outsourcing, particularly when dealing with staff employed in a highly protected framework of the public service.

2. A SET OF CONTRACTS TO ORGANIZE LABOUR RELATIONS

In most countries, employment is formalized by a contract specifying the conditions under which paid activities will be performed. Depending on the legal system (i.e. Roman, Anglo-Saxon or customary law), contractual arrangements are not limited solely to employment contracts; in fact, such arrangements cover all collective enterprises, of whatever shape or form, as well as specific relations arising in professional practice. These contracts, which supplement the main employment contract, can cause significant administrative difficulties if they are not part of an overarching framework.

2.1   Private and Public Employment

It is important to distinguish between public and private-sector employment. Workers in the public sector are civil servants directly employed by the government. The civil service defines the nature of their employment, which is directly determined by public authorities. Public service may take many forms, with specific charters distinguishing central government civil servants from those employed by local authorities (or the provincial/regional authorities in a federal state, for example). There may also be specific charters for a given sector of activity, such as in France for example, for the military and health workers; but this diversity does not alter the fundamental principles governing employer-employee relations.

Public service employment is not linked to a specific post but attached to a professional category. While this provides guaranteed employment, civil servants are covered by general employment conditions defined in regulations. The employee does not sign an employment contract, but is in a statutory position (defined by a charter). To make employment more flexible, in recent years, public authorities in many countries have altered the statutory position by moving towards post-based recruitment. If the post becomes obsolete, this can mean termination of a guaranteed job; but these developments do not alter relations with employees, who remain in a law-governed, non-contractual framework.

Public employment obviates any formal possibility of a contractual arrangement based on a collective agreement such as in the private sector. Social dialogue between unions and the public authorities takes place at national level as it can occur in the private sector, but the outcome of the negotiations will generally be enshrined in law. By contrast, the social dialogue in a specific health organization can lead to the adoption of staff employment measures reflecting the specific conditions in that organization. Such agreements cannot overrule laws, but can introduce specific arrangements in areas where legal provisions are imprecise.

The room for contractual manoeuvre available to civil servants will thus depend on how precise the regulations are in the country; and contracting will only be possible if organizations have sufficient management autonomy to translate agreements into action.

Specific sectors of activity cannot negotiate advantages that ignore the rules applicable to workers generally. Thus, in order to analyse the terms of employment that prevail in certain sectors, it is useful to focus on a specific civil service component— particularly when employment is dispersed among a number of autonomous bodies.

The existence of a public institution does not mean that all jobs are civil-service based, because the institution must also implement employment contracts for its non-public-service staff. Depending on the country, contractual relations are established either by reference to a public service charter or in relation to private-sector labour law. When there are numerous private-sector jobs, it is particularly useful to deal with them through a contractual procedure rather than proceeding on an ad hoc basis.

2.2   Collective Bargaining

Collective bargaining with unions is a frequent practice in all countries where a structured social dialogue exists between employees and employers. Collective bargaining aims at defining terms of employment for a group of employees; agreements are an extension of the statutory framework which make it unnecessary for employees to negotiate their terms of employment in a specific enterprise on an individual basis (or prevent them from doing so).

Collective bargaining processes can encompass similar branches of economic activity; and agreements covering workers in the health and social sector are commonplace, just like in sectors such as commerce and metallurgy, etc. Such agreements seek to specify employment conditions and enhance employee protection, even in small organizations. The transaction costs of negotiating surpass the capabilities of the individual participants.

Collective agreements can thus fine-tune terms of employment in certain occupational groups, based on the nature of the job and the responsibilities assigned to employees in a given category (agreement covering executives in the service sector, supervisors, etc.).

Collective agreements are only possible if workers are represented by a trade union or a professional organization; and it is also important that the employers' representative has a clearly defined mandate. A collective agreement can be implemented through a regulatory framework binding all parties. This combination of a genuine contractual procedure and regulation to impose the result of the agreement is necessary in negotiations. As this implies a majority-based decision-making process, the agreement may not suit all stakeholders, which is why majority rule needs to be imposed.

2.3   Employment Contracts

In most parts of the world, a contract is the normal vehicle to define labour relations in a formal organization. Here we shall merely mention certain principles that are important for the staff in charge of contracting policy within a health organization.

If there are general principles defined by a contracting policy, either nationally or within a health organization, human resource officers need to be aware of them and apply them, or identify exceptions to the general rule.

The employment contract specifies the tasks of a given individual in the post he holds in the organization. The contract may be vague because it is signed for a period which may be indefinite or last for several years. An employment contract is not be expected to specify all the activities to be undertaken in a given period, which forms part of an annual process often associated with employee appraisal.

The contract often specifies how relevant laws are to be applied in a given job. For example, that employees must have a place of work; the contract specifically identifies the place of employment and indicates whether or not it is exclusive.

The main difficulty encountered by large organizations providing health services is in specifying the details of enforcement the contract, without constraining flexibility. For example, he contract may state that the worker will be required to travel within the country and abroad, thus enabling the organization to deploy the worker outside the workplace, indicating the place and frequency of such travel.

It is also important to ensure that all employees in a similar employment situation are covered by the same type of contract. In some countries the principle of non-discrimination is enshrined in the Constitution, thus representing a fundamental rule that promotes equality between individuals in similar situations.

Even if the employment contract is negotiated, the employer is usually the dominant party. Nonetheless, in practice it is the state of the labour market that determines whether the employer or the employee has the upper hand. For professionals in short supply that plays a vital role in the organization, the employer has to make concessions or even raise its offer to attract their services.

In view of the scarcity of certain specialists, tailor-made employment contracts are often used to attract or retain skills that are essential for functioning of the health service. The process is delicate, since a snowball effect can be generated if the special conditions granted to one employee are known by the others. To limit this risk, the details of contracts are not generally made public but only shared between the signatories.

Lastly, recruitment may itself constitute a *de facto* employment contract. The lack of a formal contract reduces the contractual content to respect for regulations and established practices. A contractual link nonetheless exists, formalized by the recognition of an employee-employer relation implied by payment for work done. This *de facto* contract starts on the date such remuneration is first paid. Employee practices then become the "labour contract", which may ultimately place the employer in a less comfortable position than if there were a contract with flexibility clauses. Returning to the workplace example, an employee working for a year in a given location might refuse to travel, invoking past practice to claim that his conditions of employment do not involve travel. Thus the lack of a formal contract should not be construed as handing the advantage to the employer.

2.4 Additional Agreements Associated with Employment

Outside the labour contract or a statutory post, additional agreements can be signed to cover specific aspects of the employer-employee relation, in both the public and the private sectors.

In the public service, for example, in return for free and paid training, employees are often required to sign a commitment to serve for a defined period. This agreement is specific in that it is not linked to the job as such. This type of contract is particularly used in countries experiencing a major exodus of professional workers, or that wish to ensure the geographical distribution of health workers. At the end of the training period, the employee is posted at the public authorities' discretion. This type of agreement is also possible in the private sector, and often includes a requirement to repay the full cost of training, should the beneficiary resign before the end of the period specified in the contract. This is similar to an investor (public or private) seeking to protect an investment, to ensure a return for a minimum period. An agreement of this type has implications for subsequent professional practice, particularly in the private sector. In the public sector, except in situations of major national upheaval, the rules of the game are known before signing the contract stipulating work obligations. In the private sector, if pay is freely negotiated, there is an incentive to sign the future employment contract at the same time as a commitment to serve for a given period in return for the financing of studies. If this is not done, the worker may be in a weak position and forced to accept unfavourable employment conditions later. This is a situation of linked contracts operating over a relatively long period of time.

259

Apart from initial training, continuing education can also provide opportunities for an active contracting policy. Depending on the extent to which it is formalized and on the scope of legal requirements, it is always possible to implement rules to ensure that the benefits of training are capitalized upon. The principle is similar to the case of initial training: anyone who benefits from additional training must offer something in return. As the notion of continuing education is vague, a distinction can be made between training that is needed to adapt to a job or to master a new tool, and training procedures that improve the professional skills of an individual in particular. Contracting will be used in the latter case particularly, because in other situations the benefits of training are perceived directly in the job. Each organization can design the contracts that best suit it, but they can be expected to reflect the principle of sharing the training received or its application. If an individual has acquired new skills, the employer will want to share the skills as much as possible, either by dissemination to colleagues, or through their application, which should be reflected in the contract-. Furthermore, combining the contracting tool with continuing education changes expectations regarding this important, but often neglected, investment.

Apart from training, other opportunities exist for contracting, particularly where fringe benefits such as accommodation are involved. Accommodation might be included in the employment contract or be a statutory requirement, but that does not imply anything about how such accommodation will be used. A contract similar to one between landlord and tenant would avoid difficulties connected with staff turnover, particularly with regard to excessive wear and tear on the accommodation. A company car can also be included in a contract, similar to vehicle rental.

This type of procedure clearly has limits; and it would be excessive to formalize all aspects of the employer-employee relationship. The underlying logic of this approach is to make a person responsible for any benefit received. The absence of rules raises the risk of abuse, which could ultimately lead to the benefits being withdrawn. Contracting is not a matter of bureaucracy or a desire to restrict the benefit granted to employees; on the contrary, the aim is to maintain benefits by ensuring appropriate use. This evokes a rule well-known to economists: anything that is free tends not to be valued and will therefore not be used or managed well. Contracting places a value on what is seen as free, thereby encouraging rational use of the corresponding benefit.

3. THE LAW AND MANAGEMENT DIMENSIONS

Additional agreements associated with employment belong mainly in the legal domain because they govern an essential aspect of social life. Here, we are not interested in contracts from a legal standpoint; but in its economic aspects, along with its organizational consequences. Following a brief outline of the field covered by the law, we will consider the managerial aspects of using contracts linking employees with employers. The contract then becomes a lever to bring employees to give their best and gain satisfaction from their activity, with a view to improving the performance of the organizations.

3.1   Contracts Applying the Law

The employment contract described above generally reflects formalism based on laws. In countries where employment is regulated, particularly via implementation of the conventions signed by ILO Member States,[2] employment contracts reflect the provisions contained in the corresponding texts. The field covered by the contract thus reflects the country's legal environment. In countries where the law is poorly developed and poorly enforced, the employment contract is not very important. The balance of forces between employers and employees is heavily biased in favour of employers, who make their own rules and leave the employee to choose whether to accept them or quit — a choice that does not realistically exist when jobs are scarce Figure 2 uses World Bank governance indicators and shows that use of the law for employment contracts varies widely according to countries and their development level.

More than the employment contract, it is labour law that determines the extent of worker protection and the room for manoeuvre available to employers. The traditional distinction between public sector, where jobs are reputed to be for life, and the private sector, where the employer can lay off workers at will, does not reflect the reality of countries and current trends. First, employment protection in public service is being scaled back sharply as recruitment for individual posts gains ground. In other words, when models of organization render a post obsolete, employment can no longer be guaranteed. Secondly, many countries have set up strong protection for employees in the private sector, making layoffs difficult except in economic conditions that put the enterprise's survival at risk.

261

Figure 2: Rule of Law

The data on chart is sorted in descending order from top to bottom.

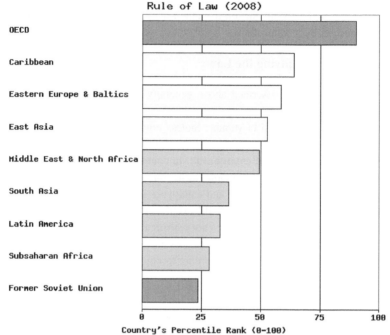

Rule of Law (2008)

Country's Percentile Rank (0-100)

Source: Kaufmann D., A. Kraay, and M. Mastruzzi 2009: Governance Matters VIII: Governance
Indicators for 1996–2008
Note: The governance indicators presented here aggregate the views on the quality of
governance provided by a large number of enterprise, citizen and expert survey respondents
in industrial and developing countries. These data are gathered from a number of survey
institutes, think tanks, non-governmental organizations, and international organizations.
The WGI do not reflect the official views of the World Bank, its Executive
Directors, or the countries they represent. The WGI are not used by the World Bank Group
to allocate resources.

Country's Percentile Rank (0-100)

90th-100th Percentile   50th-75th Percentile   10th-25th Percentile

3.2 The Contract as a Human Resource Management Tool

While taking account of international conventions and the legal environment prevailing in the country, contracting can be used to improve human resource management. Effective human resource management is a decisive factor in health service organization and provider performance, but it is clearly not sufficient alone; the best doctor willing to work to the best of his or her abilities cannot provide health care without diagnostic tools or a supply of medicines. Similarly, the availability of medical technology and full access to medicines is not enough when health workers are unwilling to give their best. In countries with a strong regulatory environment and a robust rule of law, employment contracts cannot encompass all dimensions of each individual's employment, so additional tools need to be used. For example, it might be useful to specify the various actions that need to be undertaken to ensure that assignments are fulfilled. Such actions evolve through time and need to be formalized for the operational unit where the employee works. Moreover, the complexity of the actions in question determines how they should be described. All this can be formalized in a contractual framework.

The employment contract governs relations between the employee and the employer and might specify hierarchical positioning through a job profile. The relations between those working in a team where collaboration is important for achieving the expected result can be formalized contractually.

Lastly, the employment contract may include a clause on remuneration linked to specific results, such as sales figures in the commerce sector.

These comments illustrate the various contractual options for human resources that are available to managers. It is not possible to formalize everything in a contract, due to transaction costs that can become prohibitive and therefore counterproductive. The risk of over-formalizing actions and relations between individuals may become obstacles to innovation and efficiency.

Before selecting priority areas for contracting as a tool to enhance performance, it is important to ensure a good match between the management model and tools intended to improve the performance of human resources. Like any proactive tool, contracting exists within a context; when it is unfavourable, the tool cannot be expected to produce results. Three broad models of organizational management can be distinguished, with hybrid forms.

Hierarchical management is a familiar model in military institutions. It is also present in a more moderate form in government and in business. The issuing and execution of an order is the essential part of this mode of management in organizations where human resource performance is considered secondary to

263

respect for procedures. Contracting is not seen as needed in such organizations; it could even be argued that contracting which involves a stage of dialogue between all stakeholders is a potential threat to this form of management.

Consensus-based management leaves room for dialogue but also preserves a strong chain of command, based on the principle of time for discussion and time for execution. Here, the search for consensus or even majority agreement is not a goal, but consultation before a decision is formalized is seen as useful. This type of model is open to contracting, given the dialogue between the participants to identify the solution that best meets the organization's stated objectives.

Participatory management is based on the systematic mobilization of all stakeholders in decision-making and execution, prioritizing consensus rather than optimal performance. By definition, contracting is superfluous in this model, as consensus is supposed to exist. Contracting will have its place if the participatory process involves only some of the participants, owing to representation systems.

Table 1 summarizes the situation in different organizations and the opportunities for human resources contracting.

Table 1: Situation in different organizations and the opportunities for human resources contracting

Management model	Role of human resource performance	Opportunity for contracting
Hierarchical	Weak	Limited
Concerted	Important	Very significant
Participatory	Medium	Significant

In organizational practice, it is not uncommon to find arrangements that borrow partly from each management model, based either on the personality of the decision-maker or reflecting the components of the organization.

The management model taught in schools in Western and richer Asian countries is not necessarily applicable/applied in health organizations in low-income countries.

The management model can vary from one organization to another and can evolve over time. Convincing managers to use a contracting process might be viewed as a first step towards adopting a consensus-based management model, which would lead to an increased focus on human resource performance.

If contracting is used solely to promote one aspect of human resource management, it will yield only limited results. In particular, it would be harmful to restrict the use of contracting to the introduction of financial incentives linked to the health institution's activity.

4. THE DOMAINS OF CONTRACTING

When contracting is used to support human resource management, a number of lines of action need to be identified, and the contractual approach needs to be built around them. This approach will make it possible to implement a contracting policy guided by the governing authority or by a representative organization of the country's health institutions, or those of the region or professional category. This sector approach entails significantly lower individual transaction costs. Moreover, a minimum degree of uniformity in the choice of the object of contracting will facilitate comparisons between stakeholders and thus lead to improvements in their practices and results.

4.1 Individual Development

Contracting concerns aspects that optimize individual performance in the short and long term. It forms part of a framework in which employees are not viewed as having a "unique use" but as an asset with a potential to be maximized, whether they are highly skilled personnel and fulfil more mundane tasks. In a complex organization, in which many different tasks are performed, knowledge of internal practices and of the social fabric is almost as important as individual technical skills. Contracting which takes individual development, will then apply both to the annual work plan and to the career plan.

Systematic implementation of an annual work plan makes it possible to formally define what is expected from the employee in terms of activities and outcomes. This type of approach is used in most large organizations, as part of the individual performance appraisal process. It involves a contract, because the actors negotiate and reach agreements on a number of provisions, and the results are reviewed at the end of the specified period. Monitoring during execution can allow for an initial agreement to be corrected. There are numerous configurations of this principle that are easily accessible in studies on human resource management. Nonetheless, one recommendation is to choose an approach that is compatible with the management system currently in place. Intensive use of information technology tools will facilitate the adoption of a detailed procedure; but with manual management, it is best to opt for a minimal provision. In all cases, it is necessary to specify, for each post, the activities expected in relation to the job description, and guidelines on volume or quality will accompany the description. The annual work plan can be implemented either independently or in conjunction with all other elements of human resources contracting. Human resources contracting is a flexible approach that can be based on one or more of the components described in this section; a single contract covering various dimensions of the expected performance is preferable to multiple ones. The work plan will form the backbone of the contracting process, by linking what is expected from the worker in the short term with medium-term perspectives.

The introduction of career plans makes it easier to retain health workers and enhance their professional potential . Studies on human resource performance show that a durable support framework that gives security to staff by offering prospects for development based on the results obtained, is more effective than emphasizing short-term results, which threathens job security if these are not achieved. This form of management can yield short-term results, but it produces rapid worker "burn out" with serious social consequences and a high collective cost. It is not adapted to the health sector. If the ethical point of view and general economic conditions fail to convince decision-makers, then the human resource crisis in the health sector needs to be invoked. The relative shortage of health workers generates a favourable environment for professional practice[3] in the context of long-term professional relations. The contractual approach is particularly useful to link various actions, such as training-related activities, ensuring that skills progression is matched to responsibilities within the organization. The career plan can also provide explicit opportunities for progression in terms of acquiring professional skills through practice. Developing a career plan is not synonymous with moving up the responsibility and pay scale; it also means a professional track that offers a diversity of experiences. For a nurse, this could mean moving from one unit to another after a given period of time, or from one type of practice to another. Viewing individual development only in terms of progression within a hierarchy associated with a rising pay scale leads to a dead end, even if the employer has streamlined the staff age pyramid. In addition to opportunities for progression, it will be possible to offer a motivating alternative for those who do not have the aptitudes required to obtain a higher post.

4.2   The Enterprise approach

In any organization, it is hard to optimize individual performance and involve each person in the overall institutional dynamic. A sense of belonging to an organization, and of sharing its culture are proven factors for individual and collective success.

Ensuring adherence to this enterprise approach requires clarity as regards the organization's purpose and key values. Often, mission statements are little more than unconvincing "politically correct" generalities, , or are so ambitious that employees do not recognizes themselves in them.[4] Employees can only identify with the established objectives and values if these are consistent with actual practice.

If an organization is serious about its stated objectives and values, then it is important prior to recruitment to check that the candidate for a job subscribes to them; and, during recruitment, it is appropriate to sign a contract in which these values and objectives are accepted. Then, in the annual work plan, provisions can be included requiring workers to uphold these objectives and values in their job.

The enterprise approach can also be reflected in a link between the results of the enterprise and the employee's level of remuneration. This is effective in commercial sectors that have high growth potential, but it is not well suited to health services that do not aim to maximize sales or profits, let alone their stock market price. It is preferable to pursue an approach that links the individual's pride in their employer's reputation; but this is only possible if the worker feels included in the life of the enterprise and the latter develops social activities that promote strong internal cohesion.

In countries where social between workers and employers is difficult, conditions for creating an enterprise approach are not favourable. This explains the place currently occupied by all forms of performance incentives to ensure that the employee's contribution to the enterprise is translated into individual benefit.

4.3   The role of incentives

Dimensions of the Incentives Process

By introducing incentives, the employer rewards a given conduct or result. The worker considers that this reward makes it worthwhile to adopt a particular conduct or produce a specific result. The contractual logic is fully applicable in such cases. The same instrument will produce different effects in different environments. While incentives mechanisms can be universal, specific incentives are not. Even within a country or sector of activity, the effects of an incentive will vary according to the worker's position and his personal attitude towards the stimulus. It will also vary with the passing of time.

The range of incentives is wide, which means that a combination of different types of incentives will produce an even more uncertain effect than using just one.

The results obtained by a given instrument in one country should therefore be considered with caution before implementing it elsewhere. Adopting an incentives approach is by definition uncertain from the outset. This uncertainty will diminish if a preliminary survey is conducted. The impact of an incentive may be simulated and tested. When an incentives approach is formalized in a contract, changing the incentives is both costly (the previous contract needs to be renegotiated) and risky (if one of the parties benefits, renegotiation will create a sense of bitterness and a desire to get even). Discrete choice experiments[5] can be useful as a form of testing the potential success of specific incentives.

When considering the use of an incentive, it is important to know whether it is of a long-term nature or associated with a specific event or intent. The formalization of the incentive in a contracting process will depend on this.

Types of Incentive

Incentives may be included in the legal terms of employment or they may be the outcome of a collective bargaining agreement. In the latter scenario, the room for manoeuvre is limited; but numerous incentives can be implemented outside a pre-established framework. The range of incentives that can be implemented nationally or locally is limited only by imagination. Nonetheless, incentives can be assigned to three major categories, and the organization's management can choose those that seem best suited to their objectives. While the effect of an incentive may not be identical everywhere, the conditions for introducing it will be set out in a contract at the organization level. This does not mean tailor-made contracts for each employee. Different ways of introducing incentives can produce the same effect; while the effect may be identical for the employee, it is not the case for the employer who will use different forms of organization.

NIGER: Introduction of contracting in relation to a performance bonus

One of the four areas of human resource policy involves the introduction of a target-incentive contract designed as follows (AMPS Conference, Douala, June 2007).

- Set up a performance score scheme:
  - for each operational unit (district, hospital, etc.),
  - based on the extent to which commonly agreed objectives are achieved;
  - measured at year-end by an independent team.
- Introduce an annual performance bonus in the contracting framework:
  - agreed upon among the entire district team,
  - based on the performance score achieved over the past year
  - to be paid over the next 12 months.

The contractual approach is based on the principle of collective reward for results achieved, measured by a score covering various performance dimensions.

268

Direct financial incentives

As an addition to basic pay, direct financial incentives mainly represent a premium or bonus that depends on the results achieved. Often this type of incentive is explicitly included in employment contracts for jobs in the commercial sector (insurance agents, salespersons, etc.). In some countries this type of clause is also used with health workers, if there is performance-based pay.

Direct financial incentives may also extend to fringe benefits that can make the job more attractive, such as housing, transport or clothing allowances, etc.

They can also be made available in the form of complementary insurance coverage, particularly in countries where social insurance is provided mainly by the private sector (health insurance, family allowances, old-age pensions, etc.)

In all cases, direct financial incentives involve a monetary contribution by the employer and savings for the employee. A distinction needs to be made between incentives based on results at work and those that are applied systematically to a category of workers or a particular situation (subsidies). The former seek to elicit a higher return, while the latter aim to retain workers by making their life easier.

Indirect financial incentives

This category of incentive includes benefits in kind for employees. They cost the employer as much as direct financial incentives, although they do not entail purchasing a service, but are organized directly by the employer. Examples include provision of transport or meals, which differs significantly from the payment of a transport or meals subsidy, because the introduction or withdrawalof such benefits operate within a different time frame. Accommodation belonging to the health institution made available to certain staff is another example.

What characterizes indirect financial incentives is the investment that the employer has to make to implement them. Health organizations in isolated or less attractive areas that cannot attract staff need to offer such incentives in order to remain competitive or just to function.

Non-financial incentives

Employers can organize their employees' work time to enable them to manage their personal life more effectively; and this clearly represents a strong incentive, particularly when employees have to cope with significant family constraints. Ongoing vocational training and promotion policies also provide opportunities for implementing non-financial incentives. There again, implementation arrangements can vary, in terms of days off, flexible working hours, authorizations of absence with ways of making up lost time. These methods are not yet widely used because they require work planning capacity to reconcile these arrangements with organizational objectives and constraints, particularly in public services large organizations also have bargaining power to obtain benefits for their staff, such as preferential access to social or cultural services. Non-financial incentives aim to make the job more attractive without incurring a major cost to health institutions. Small health organizations have fewer options in this regard than larger ones.

4.4   Contracting health professionals from foreign countries

All countries in the world experience some type of imbalance in their supply of health workers, of which shortages are the most visible form. The incapacity to fill all available positions or to supply services to populations which are prepared to pay for them is a common phenomenon. In poor countries, the cause can be that there are not enough workers available or willing to accept available positions. This may be because the production of health workers is insufficient, because the country looses workers to emigration, to premature death (as in the case of HIV-AIDS high prevalence countries), or because trained workers are not willing to work in the health sector or to accept the working conditions offered. This is often the case when workers refuse to work in remote, isolated or poor areas. In most instances, shortages can be attributed to a mix of causes. Accordingly, policy-makers would do well in considering various options to address the problem. One obvious option is to train more personnel or "scale-up" the production, which many countries have started doing recently (Dussault et al. 2009). These include rich countries, like England, France, Canada, but also many poor countries in Africa and Asia. This option requires the capacity to augment the production, in terms of infrastructure, trainers, and even of adequately prepared students (Dussault et. al 2008). It is costly and produces results after a time lag, which can be as long as 7-8 years in the case of specialist physicians. Another option is to reduce attrition rates, by offering working conditions and remuneration which will keep workers in the health labor market. This supposes a good knowledge and understanding of the factors which contribute to attrition and a capacity to adjust policies in accordance to these factors. A third policy option is the creation of packages of incentives to attract and retain workers in zones and services which experience shortages (WHO 2009).

Some countries have used and are still using a fourth option that consists in contracting foreign workers to fill positions for which not enough nationals are available or willing to accept. This can take various forms:

1- Promoting an open door policy: this strategy can be observed in rich countries where demand for health services grows more rapidly than the supply of health workers. This was the case of Britain in the late 1990's, until about 2005, which "imported" workers (doctors, nurses, dentists) from India, the Philippines, English-speaking Africa and the Caribbean mainly(Buchan 2007). The process consisted basically in recruiting potential candidates through agencies who actively solicited candidates on behalf of national health organizations. Contracts are then passed on an individual basis.

This process became strongly criticized lately (Chen et al. 2004) and pressure to adopt rules of "ethical recruitment" mounted. Codes ethics were adopted, but their effectiveness has yet to be evaluated (Buchan et al. 2009). In England, the code specifies the countries from which recruitment is not appropriate, and specifies under which conditions recruitment can take place. At the same time, England increased the number of entrants in medical and nursing schools and has gradually become more self-sufficient; as a consequence, the number of immigrant health workers has declined radically (Buchan 2007) Other rich countries have had similar policies of attracting foreign workers to compensate the difficulty of recruiting internally. This is the case of the USA, of Canada which recruited from from the Caribbean and South Africa, of Germany (http://www.dw-world.de/dw/article/0,,3190640,00.html), from Eastern European countries, of Ireland (Humphries 2008), and France (Cash, Ullman 2008). In the latter case, doctors have been recruited from French-speaking North and Sub-Saharan Africa for many years to work in public hospitals, without being granted the right to practice outside these institutions. More recently, there were efforts to recruit from Romania to fill positions in underserved geographical areas, in spite of France having globally enough physicians to cover the needs of its population. Poor countries obviously do not have this option; they are rather source countries from which richer countries can draw personnel. The loss of professionals who are already scarce can have severe negative effects on access to care in the "exporting" country as is illustrated by the case of the Philippines (Brush, Sochalski 2007).

2- Promoting cross-border mobility and contracting personnel who works in the country, but still lives in another one is another policy option. Many Spanish physicians and nurses living close to the border of Portugal were contracted in this manner, particularly during the 1990's and early 2000's when working conditions and pay were better in Portugal. Typically, these workers would cross the border everyday back and forth. In other cases, health workers are contracted for short periods of time, after which they return to their country of origin.

3- Negotiating bilateral agreements is a more formal option that requires negotiations between interested countries. England signed an agreement with Spain in the early 2000's and recruited about 700 nurses. It also has an agreement with the Philippines (Prometheus in print). Portugal has an agreement with Cuba and with Uruguay for the recruitment of family physicians. Poorer countries are the ones who are more likely to use this form of contracting through formal agreements. It is the case of Guinea Bissau, where the Faculty of Medicine is staffed mostly by Cuban trainers to compensate the absence of national qualified staff. In Mozambique, a country of 19 million inhabitants, out of a total of 820 physicians in 2007, 217 were foreigners, a majority of them from Cuba, many of the others from Eastern Europe (Tyrell et al. 2010).

The practice of "importing" health workers is a symptom of a country's difficulty in meeting its demand for services (let alone its needs). This is often due to the absence of planning mechanisms and to the lack of priority given to improving access to services. While mobility of health workers cannot be constrained, since it is a human right to move freely, the question can be raised of "self-sufficiency" as a policy objective. The ideal situation of equilibrium between demand and supply, or the even more ideal one of equilibrium between need and supply is clearly out of reach. But this should not deter countries from planning better their workforce and to avoid dependency of foreign health workers, particularly when these are imported from countries with high levels of unmet needs (WHO 2008).

5. STAKEHOLDERS IN CONTRACTING PROCESSES

Labour policies are closely related to politics and therefore involves a broad range of stakeholders, particularly in contexts of a well developed civil society. Clearly identified social partners will engage in a social dialogue in the context of rules accepted by the parties involved.

5.1 The Role of Senior Management and Executives

Senior management oversees human resources contracting policy in two ways: first, since the development strategy of any organization is based on strategic choices necessitating the mobilization of human resources, it might be advantageous to embody the desire to mobilize human resources by means of a contractual approach that prioritizes the various levers described above, combined to reflect priority issues. For example, when the objective is hiring specialists, the incentives will differ from those require to strengthen nursing teams. If the aim is to reduce staff turnover, then the approach will be based on factors that promote individual development and the enterprise approach.

The other aspect systematically present in the contractual approach is human resource management. It is preferable, but not essential, to link this concern to the development strategy. Health organizations that are not under intense pressure to develop will seek to make the most of their resources, including human ones.

For the first aspect, oversight will be the responsibility of management in close collaboration with the governing authority; whereas in the second case, responsibility will rest with the human resources department.

Management will play a major role in all cases, in gathering the information required to guide decisions, and to monitor and measure the results achieved in relation to the processes adopted.

If the contracting options are chosen by senior management, it will be important for supervisors to buy into them. They must therefore be included in and recognized as a party to the contracting process.

5.2   Decision-making and coordination bodies

As soon as an organization gains an institutional memory, decision-making is handled through established mechanisms, and there is no reason why human resources contracting should be excluded from this. Often, staff issues are handled not only through a hospital's decision-making and coordination bodies but also through ad hoc mechanisms. Strategic alternatives will be debated and adopted at a more general level. The mechanics of implementation will be discussed in the ad hoc staff bodies, and finally the detailed formulation of contracts will be dealt with among the parties.

The boundary line between what needs to be discussed by the ad hoc bodies and what needs to be done by the management team is not easily determined and is largely left to the discretion of managers. Contextual factors will guide the choice of approach. Overuse of ad hoc bodies tends to slow down the process because they meet periodically and clearly seek consensus rather than striking out in new directions.

5.3   Staff Representatives

If a form of staff representation is in place, it is essential to involve it in the contractual process. Generally speaking, this representation operates in the relevant bodies, but it is also preferable to engage in dialogue upstream in order to identify obstacles to the implementation of a contracting process, and to overcome these without distorting the objectives in view.

Depending on the type of staff representation, the rationale for contracting may not be appreciated at first, since it implicitly differentiates between employees (according to post, category, results, family situation, etc.). For organizations that promote egalitarianism, it is hard to accept that incentive-based contracts will benefit one group more than another. On the other hand, when the parties represent professions, it is clear that their concern will be to promote these professions alone, unless they have to deal with the repercussions of a contractual agreement indirectly (for example the introduction of new working arrangements that give a greater role to nurses).

The notion of dialogue should not be confused with seeking consensus. Dialogue makes it possible to explain the motivations underlying a process and the objectives pursued. While agreement is clearly preferable, it is not essential for the introduction of a contracting process. Fierce opposition, which could go as far as instructions to boycott contracts, will wreck the contracting process. Management will then have to choose whether to impose the process by exercising its decision-making power, or to back down if the issue is not vital for the future of the organization.

Social dialogue is not improvised; it is the outcome of continuous practice based on mutual respect between stakeholders. When social dialogue does not exist, it will be hard to introduce a contracting process, because the dialogue needs to be built when the agreement is negotiated. In the absence of social dialogue, it will take much longer to bring the process to a conclusion than if social dialogue is well established.

6. IMPLEMENTATION OF THE CONTRACTING PROCESS

6.1 What needs to be taken into account

Contracting cannot cover everything. When embarking on human resources contracting, it is advisable to stake out a defined area and not stray outside it. The most damaging approach is to engage in human resources contracting on a piecemeal basis. That does not mean that nothing should start until everything has been foreseen. But, when adding a new dimension, it is useful to review what is already in place and ensure overall consistency.

Limiting the field of intervention will focus attention on the benefits for employees and for the employer. While these benefits will not be the same for all, they must nonetheless exist for everyone. The benefit relates not only to the object of contracting, but also to the advisability of embarking on a contracting process. Given the importance of the contractual relationship for human resources management, it might be worthwhile implementing economic and managerial contracting as opposed to full-blown legal contracting.

The discussion of the content of contracting entails defining the role that will be assigned to each party. Given the complexity of health organizations, a review of the different stakeholders and their respective roles will be needed to ensure implementation without upsetting the contracting mechanism. Contracting is more than a simple agreement between an employee and an employer representative; account needs to be taken of staff representatives and the various levels in the chain of command.

The notion of delegation, as a link in the decision-making chain, has a specific role to play. The delegation process thus needs to be formalized and its nature and scope clearly defined. This formalization is especially important when evaluating outcomes and liability for actions taken to obtain this result.

6.2   Performance measurement aspects

The goal of achieving a specific result and improving performance underlies the contractual process. But, in the case of human resources, what performance criteria should be used? Without providing a definitive answer to this question, we propose six key dimensions of performance. As with more general considerations, proposing several dimensions presupposes that they will be weighted. It is unwise to embark on this path without background knowledge; but it may be best to deal with the weighting issue as part of the contracting process itself, so as to produce a weighting that is acceptable to the main parties. Contract performance and monitoring will yield information to review the initial weighting.

- Quantity or volume: This is an obvious criterion that makes it possible to seek to improve productivity by recognizing and rewarding the amount of work done. Merely measuring time spent on the job will not be meaningful because physical presence says nothing about the work actually done. Instead one should measure a quantity delivered in a given time, such as the number of consultations held per hour. In the case of jobs that involve fairly simple activities, it is easier to quantify a result, like measuring the number of sheets folded, the number of m^2 of floor cleaned, etc. For activities involving caring for people , the quantitative approach has its limits. It would not be very appropriate to evaluate the results of a nurse's work by the number of injections given! This measure also needs to recognize difficulty; and "case mix" adjustment is used to take account of the nature of patients and the pathologies treated.

275

- Quality: This is the counterpart of quantity, because producing volume is only of interest if the work is well done. This measurement can use two approaches; to refer to a quality standard (percentage of prescriptions complying with the treatment protocol), meaning that everything in compliance is good; or measuring quality improvement. Measurement is more difficult when not related to some benchmark.

- Compliance with deadlines: This criterion takes account of the time element. Committing to an appointment within a certain time frame can be an excellent performance criterion, but its implementation will have consequences for methods of work. Moreover, the adoption of a sole criterion such as meeting deadlines can have serious consequences for quality, if in order to meet the deadlines, consultations are shortened with the attendant risk that patients will not be properly diagnosed.

- Rational use of resources: this relates to the efficiency of the service provided. In some cases, this concern may conflict with the volume criterion, because cases can be dealt with faster when a lot more consumables are used. This notion of rational resource use is also relevant in executing the service budget; but it is harder to apply to each individual employee.

- Measurement of effort: while acknowledging that individual capacities differ, this criterion takes account of a positive attitude. Effort can also be measured in terms of initiatives above and beyond activities specified in the work plan. Encouraging individual employees to give their best is an important engine for improving results.

- Conduct: This is a particularly sensitive dimension in the area of health care. Behaviour may be what is expected under current social norms (punctuality, respect for others, etc.), but it may also reflect a way of interacting with patients and their families. Direct measurement is not easy here, for while performance failures generally trigger complaints, highly positive behaviour is not always easy to observed.

These six criteria are not exhaustive, and the aim is not to cover the entire field of performance measurement; they provide a sound basis for a contracting process with staff. The relative importance of each of the criterion will vary according to the job and post.

6.3 Reconciling the Individual and Collective Dimensions

Promoting human resources contracting in health services includes an assessment of the risk of exacerbating individual strategies to the detriment of group cohesion. It is known that the sum of individual actions is not a collective action, but, on the contrary, the potential of the collective result can be reduced if the individual result is emphasized. The single relationship between physician and patient is not really valid today, since patient care requires participation by multiple professionals who themselves must be supported by an administrative and logistic organization.

As the following diagram shows, an individual performance-based remuneration process can take account of the context, thereby ensuring that this performance makes a positive contribution towards achieving the overall objectives.

Figure 3: Linking remuneration to broad performance approach[6]

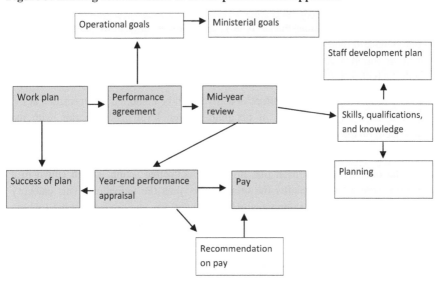

An individual performance agreement will be implemented in relation to the post and indirectly in relation to the skills needed to accomplish the task.

It is also important to recognize the result achieved by the team to which the individual belongs.

While the principle is simple, it is not easy to apply, since team boundaries vary, particularly in complex hospital organizations. Some teams operate within a

277

health-care unit, others possibly within a department, others at the establishment level. Can a formula be found to prioritize individual commitment to the objectives pursued at each level? The principle of incentives linked to group results, common in private-sector industry, is unsuitable for the public health sector.

The sense of belonging to an entity that is well regarded by the public, and the pride that comes with it, depend on an effective communication strategy based particularly on brand image, rather than setting individual commitment in a contractual framework based on results.

Conversely, there are real possibilities for incorporating a human resources dimension into a results-based contractual approach at the unit level. The link between individual action and collective outcome is very clear for the members of the unit. While the size of the unit may vary, it is important to ensure a certain degree of continuity in individual practices, as well as clear objectives and possibilities for close communication between team members. This type of approach nonetheless presupposes a decentralized budget system and assumes that human resources management policy produces a degree of stability among individuals in their units. If turnover is very high and if a large proportion of staff work in mobile teams, then efforts to engage each individual in a collective process will not be feasible.

To encourage collective effort, objectives will be identified and measured at the unit level. This may consist of obtaining a high level of satisfaction with the treatment on the part of patients and the family; but it may also involve optimization of resource use or improvement of productivity, etc.

Introducing an approach that prioritizes collective action is well suited to a form of reward that benefits the group rather than the individual. This category includes all actions that improve workplace conditions, an indivisible benefit whose effects are felt by each team member. It is also possible to introduce forms of reward for all beneficiaries (group training, day off to attend an event, etc.).

While contracting is promoted to encourage each individual to improve performance, it can also be used to reward collective effort. So how these two processes are linked? Some thought should be given to the issue of how to reward individual contributions to collective results without rewarding those who are not pulling their weight.

Individual contracting occurs quite specifically around actions linked to a specific job. For a laboratory assistant, the manner in which he performs tests will be the most important consideration, and the work thus performed will be part of the organization's overall objectives. For the laboratory team as a whole, results can also be evaluated by considering the laboratory as a production unit. There is no need to develop a complex mechanism to measure individual contribution precisely; but steps will be taken to ensure that everyone is pulling their weight, and that there is not too much divergence between a positive and a neutral or negative attitude. Laboratory management staff will be responsible for assessing whether individual contribution to the collective result is as expected. It is also possible to implement a collective self-assessment system to avoid aberrations associated with individual evaluation.

6.4   Coordinating Contracts with Human Resources and between human Resources and Institutions

Contracting for organizations differs from individual contracting. The range of incentives is broader for institutions that for human resources, because there is more scope for contracting. Te benefits expected by individuals are closely linked to individual behaviour, whereas institutions combine this type of approach with considerations relating to public goods.

RWANDA: Health services production premium and target-incentive scheme for employees.

To sustain access to health services, Rwanda has carried out several experiments to encourage health-care providers to boost their output. This initiative was tested in health centres before being extended to hospitals.

- Specify the expected results
    - Increase activity at the point of service
    - Prioritize free actions that are important for treatment delivery (e.g. antenatal care)
    - Do not restrict transfers to the higher referral level
- Adopt arrangements for monitoring outcomes
    - List of documents to be produced
    - Arrangements for checking veracity
- Introduce dual contracting
    - Results-based remuneration arrangements (between the health centre and the donor)
    - Mechanisms for rewarding staff (between the health centre and staff)

The contractual approach is based on a productivity bonus with a choice of areas in which it is desired to mobilize staff. Implementation is a lengthy process (source: Bruno Meessen ITM)

- Establish models (roles, flows, indicators, prices).
- Draft model contracts.
- Mapping of funding for hospitals + coordinate funds for specific programmes
- Inform decentralized levels.
- Evaluate compliance with preconditions
- Train decentralized levels and support start-up
- Monitoring
- First disbursement

The objectives pursued are different because the development and viability of an organization are different from the individual perspective of professional practice. While the concept of a career plan can be used to retain individuals in the long term, the core issues addressed in an individual contract need to be expressed in annual terms. For an organization, while an annual cycle is used to mobilize funding, the related strategy looks to the medium and longer term. A short-term contract can be used to mobilize individuals, but less so organizations.

Criteria for measuring performance are complex if a holistic approach is required; but this complexity is greater in organizations than for individuals. Six key criteria can be used to measure individual performance, whereas many more results need to be measured for organizations to avoid the perverse effects of performance indicators (i.e. the strategy of only improving the result measured by the indicator to the detriment of the others).

Lastly, this type of human resources management is not neutral in respect of the possible introduction of contracting, whereas in the case of institutions, contracting can be introduced irrespective of the form of management, since the object of the contracting is more far-reaching.

It is not necessarily desirable to ensure that a contracting process is in place at the institutional level before implementing the same process for human resources; but the contracting process and its accompanying instruments clearly need to be mastered. The existence of a contracting policy at the national level is a generally desirable starting point, to avoid contracting on a piecemeal basis.

Human resources contracting is more likely to be successful if it follows a process of take-up within the organization in which:

- Employees are involved in defining objectives
- Performance parameters are agreed upon with the employees
- Employees are associated with the results achieved
- Employees commit to the initiative over the long term

While contracting is possible in any organization, it is nonetheless sensitive to the economic, social and legal environment.

Limited exposure to market forces will not be favourable for any form of contracting that links employees to results.

If the organization has limited scope for providing incentives, particularly because of very limited resources, this will reduce contracting opportunities, or at least require an additional effort of imagination to avoid resorting to solutions that are easy to adopt initially, that link employee performance to direct or indirect financial incentives.

Lastly, both in the area of human resources and at institutional level, poor governance and inadequate mechanisms to ensure accountability greatly reduce the scope for contracting. Passive citizenship reduces the demands made on health staff in fulfilling their activities.[6] In this case, the ambitions of human resources contracting will be moderated; and it will be necessary to progress through the six criteria for measuring human resources performance using an approach based on those results that are easier to improve.

CONCLUSION

Possibilities for human resources contracting exist in all scenarios, but the implementation stages need to be carefully selected for each context.

Bearing in mind the particular sensitivity of the human dimension and the risks of labour union action, it is wise to test measures before implementing them.

In view of this sensitivity, it is preferable to start in areas where improvements can be effected quickly. Attacking areas that are considered important, yet where the chances of achieving success are less certain, could risk creating long-term problems for the contracting process, because, in the event of failure, it is always easier to blame the tool rather than acknowledge that the process was badly implemented.

Although it is important to clearly coordinate contracting processes at the institutional level and with respect to human resources, one approach cannot replace the other. A process focused on human resources might have some impact on an institution's results, but in an indirect and incomplete way. Similarly, an institutional process could affect the behaviour of workers but in a limited and often very specific way.

From the very outset, therefore, an institutional approach needs to be combined with an approach designed to mobilize human resources.

Notes

[1] See World Health Report 2006: Working Together for Health, WHR 2006, WHO.

[2] See http://www.ilo.org/ilolex/french/convdisp1.htm

[3] http://www.whpa.org/ppe.htm

[4] For example, an organization might be mandated to participate in reducing inequality and poverty .... but setting this as an objective to reduce poverty in the world could lead to a belief that it can do this alone, which is not credible.

[5] Reference: Discrete Choice Experiment
http://www.who.int/hrh/migration/hmr_expert_meeting_lemiere.pdf

[6] http://appli1.oecd.org/olis/2002doc.nsf/43bb6130e5e86e5fc12569fa005d004c/00934faacdd51ec bc1256b72003c6810/$FILE/JT00128656.PDF

[7] Jaffré, Y. and J-P. Olivier de Sardan. 2003. *Une médecine inhospitalière. Les difficiles relations entre soignants et soignés dans cinq capitales d'Afrique de l'Ouest.* (Paris: Karthala).

For further information:

Brush B, Sochalski, J. (2007). International Nurse Migration: Lessons From the Philippines, *Policy, Politics, & Nursing Practice*, Vol. 8, No. 1, 37-46

Buchan J. (2007). International recruitment of nurses: policy and practice in the United Kingdom: *Health Services Research* 42 (3 Pt 2):1321-35.

Buchan J et al. (2009). Does a code make a difference: assessing the English code of practice on international recruitment? *Human Resources for Health*, 7(33).

Cash R., Ulmann P. (2008). Projet OCDE sur la migration des professionels de santé, *Le cas de la France.* OECD health working papers no.36 (http://www.oecd.org/dataoecd/13/10/41437407.pdf)

Chen, L. et al. (2004), Human resources for health: overcoming the crisis, *Lancet*; 364: 1984-90

Day C. Taking Action with Indicators. London, HMSO, 1989.

Dieleman, M. et al. The match between motivation and performance management of health sector workers in Mali? *Human resources for health*, 4:2

Dussault G., Codjia L, Kantengwga K, Tulenko K (2008), Assessing the capacity to produce health personnel in Rwanda. *Leadership in Health Services*, 21(4): 290-306 [http://www.emeraldinsight.com/10.1108/17511870810910092].

Dussault, G. et al. (2009), *Scaling up the Stock of Health Workers*, International Council of Nurses, Geneva, 48 p. (ISBN:978-92-95065-64-2)

Ferrinho P. et al. Dual practice in health sector review of evidence, *Human resources for health*, 2:14

Francis, H., Keegan, A. (2006), The changing face of HR: In search of balance. *Human Resource Management Journal*; 16(3): 231–49

Harley M. The measurement of health services activity and standards. In: Holland W, Detels R. Knox G, eds. *Applications in public health*. Oxford Textbook of Public Health. Vol. 3: Oxford, Oxford University Press, 1991: 145-157

Harris N D. *Service Operations Management*. London, Cassell, 1989.

Hornby P, Forte P. (1997). Human Resource Indicators and Health Service Performance. *Human Resources for Health Development Journal*. 1(2): 103-118.

Hornby P, Forte P, Ozcan S. Report on a Pilot Study in the Use of Human Resource Performance Indicators. Centre for Health Planning and Management, Keele University, December 1999 (unpublished document, available on request from Centre for Health Planning and Management, Keele University, Darwin Building, Keele, Staffordshire ST5 5BG, UK).

Humphries,N., Brugha,R., & McGee,H. (2008). Overseas nurse recruitment: Ireland as an illustration of the dynamic nature of nurse migration. *Health Policy 87*(2): 264-272.

IGAS *Rapport sur rémunérer les médecins selon leurs performances: les enseignements des expériences étrangères*, Paris Juin 2008

Jenkins L et al. *How Did We Do?* London, CASPE Research, 1988.

Ketelaar, K, Manning,N, Turkisch E. *Performance-based Arrangements for Senior Civil Servants - OECD and other Country Experiences*, OECD Working Papers on Public Governance 2007/5

Liu, X., Mills, A. The effect of performance-related pay of hospital doctors on hospital behavior: a case from Shandong, China, *Human resources for health*, 3:11

Ministère Français des finances, La démarche de performance : Stratégie, objectifs, indicateurs. Guide méthodologique pour l'application de la loi organique relative aux lois de finances du 1er août 2001, Paris Juin 2004

Mullen PM. (1985). Performance indicators - is anything new? *Hospital and Health Services Review*. 81 (4): 165-167.

NHS Management Executive. *Health Service Indicators Handbook*, 1994 edition. Leeds, NHSME, 1994.

Nigenda G, Gonzalez L. Contracting private sector providers for public health services in Jalisco, Mexico :perspectives of system actors, *Human resources for health*, 7:79

283

OCDE ; *Comment Gerer La Performance Individuelle --Rapport National Du Royaume-Uni ;Régir la performance dans le secteur public,* Colloque de haut niveau co-organisé par l'OCDE et l'Allemagne, Berlin 13-14 mars 2002

OCDE: *Relier la performance aux niveaux de l'organisation et des individus ;Régir la performance dans le secteur public* Colloque de haut niveau co-organisé par l'OCDE et l'Allemagne, Berlin 13-14 mars 2002

OECD (2008) *The looming crisis of the health workforce :How can OECD countries respond?* Paris. OECD

Ozcan S. *A study of the potential for performance indicators to improve management motivation.* Centre for Health Planning and Management, Keele University, March 2000. (unpublished document, available on request from Centre for Health Planning and Management, Keele University, Darwin Building, Keele, Staffordshire ST5 5BG, UK).

Soeters R, Griffiths F. (2003) Experimenting with contract management : can government health workers be motivated – the case of Cambodia. *Health Policy Plan*;18:74-33

Tyrell A et al. Costing the scaling-up of Human resources for health: lessons from Guinea Bissau and Mozambique, *Human Resources for Health*, accepted 2010

US office of personnel management A Handbook for Measuring Employee Performance: Aligning employee performance plans with organizational goals. Washington DC, Sept 2001

Woo-Sung PARK (2000). Transformation and New Patterns of HRM in Korea. Korea Labor Institute, Seoul, Korea

World Health Organization. *World Health Report 2000: Health Systems – Improving Performance.* Geneva, WHO, 2000.

World Health Organization. *Public hearings on the Draft Code of Practice on the International Recruitment of Health Personnel: summaries of contributions.* Geneva, Copenhagen (http://who.int/hrh/public_hearing/comments, accessed 19 November 2009).World Health Organization (2009). *Increasing access to health workers in remote and rural areas through improved retention: Background paper for the first expert meeting to develop evidence-based recommendations to increase access to health workers in remote and rural areas through improved retention: draft.* Geneva, WHO (http://who.int/hrh/migration/background_paper.pdf, accessed 22 November 2009).

Part III

Chapter 1

Performance incentives for health care providers

Jean Perrot, Eric de Roodenbeke, Laurent Musango,

György Fritsche & Riku Elovainio

INTRODUCTION

It is generally agreed that, all things being equal, the health of a population will be better when the country's health system performs better. Notably, since the 2000 WHO World Health Report, a lot has been written about how to measure health system performance. But what we are interested in is rather to question the determinants of this performance. It is not easy to answer this question, but we can agree that elements such as the definition of a clear health policy, presence of a structured and coherent organization of health services and presence of a good regulatory framework can contribute to the performance of a health system. But, we should also not forget that institutions (health care administrations and health providers) and persons working in them are important determinants of health system performance. The better the latter perform, the better the entire system will perform.

This document will not treat the performance of a health system, neither in terms of a comprehensive assessment or a full analysis of its determinants. But it will examine one of its determinants in particular, namely the performance of health care providers and, more marginally, of the health administration. More specifically still, it will examine how these health care providers can be encouraged to enhance their performance and, thereby, contribute to the performance of the health system. To that end, it will be necessary to:

- Define and assess this performance, i.e. the results expected from a health care provider;
- Analyse the factors and mechanisms that encourage health care providers to perform better in order to design mechanisms that act on these factors and mechanisms.

For a long time, the logic has been that differences in results achieved by health care providers were explained:

- By differences in resources. If more resources were devoted to these health care providers, better results would automatically be achieved;
- By differences in the level of effective command and control based on a system of sanctions;
- By differences in the professional conscientiousness of staff working in health facilities.

Yet, the reality is often different. With similar resources, health care providers obtain substantially different results. Besides, quite often, available resources are deemed insufficient for achieving good results. Furthermore, 'command and control' as an operational principle is increasingly less accepted by various actors, and in addition is not a guarantee for achieving the best possible result.

Facing these observations, a new strategy was gradually developed over the past years, based on the use of incentives, which encourage health care providers to do more and better. Therefore, incentives had to be defined that would get health care providers to consider intensifying their efforts so as to achieve better results. It is this logic - "incentives" lead to an increase in effort, which in turn leads to improved results – which we will be analysing in this part. This is a logic well known in the business world. The merchant knows that by working more and better, (s)he will boost his (her) income: the incentive is obvious. In the health sector, notably in the public sector, this logic is still new. It is, therefore, important to analyse with much attention how it can be implemented. Performance incentive mechanisms are more complex than they appear, both at the level of concepts and in the operational modalities, all the more so, since there is a lack of documented experience. This document will attempt to present these issues so as to provide field actors, both the incentive providers and incentive beneficiaries, with the tools for understanding why these methods are currently being implemented in many countries.

1. DEFINITIONS AND CONCEPTS

The term "performance" is a concept, which, initially, appears quite simple. Yet, when looking up this term in a general dictionary, you find the following two definitions:[1]

- *"Result obtained in a specific area by someone"*
- *"Remarkable exploit or success in any area"*

The difference is essential. In the first case, "performance" is a synonym of "result", whereas in the second case, only good results will be described as "performance". This is the difference between a 'deed' and a 'feat'.

The concept of 'a result', which clearly maintains close links with the concept of 'performance', must itself be specified:

- The result may be judged in relation to a maximum value considered as the best attainable result: for example, in the educational system, a mark is given in relation to perfect success (in as much as one can agree on what constitutes a perfect paper in philosophy). But it can also be appreciated in relation to the best result known so far: for example, sportsmen compete with each other for a world record... which changes over time.

- The result may also take into account the individual characteristics of the actors: for example, for a world-class athlete, running 100m in 11 seconds is not a good performance today, whereas running it in 20 seconds may be an excellent performance for a person with disabilities. All things being equal, a well-equipped hospital may perform surgical operations to resolve more complex health problems than a poorly-equipped hospital.

- It is important to take the environment into account. Take, for example, the case of two equivalent health facilities, one of which is established in a rich district and the other in a poor district. If we consider as a performance indicator the monitoring of pregnancy then, in that case, all things being equal, it will probably be easier for the first health facility to obtain good results than the second one, since, the socio-economic status of mothers influences their behaviour in the use of health services. Same applies to a comparison between a health facility in a poor rural environment and another facility in a privileged part of the capital city. The socio-economic and cultural aspects are important and they are imposed on the health care providers.

Hence, the notion of performance implies showing interest not just in the result, but relating it to other results obtained in a specific area. This is the approach adopted in the 2000 World Health Report (page 25), where performance is defined as: **given the resources at its disposal**, these are the results that the health system should be able to attain. Looking at the results actually achieved, the comparison of the two indicates its level of performance. If it exceeds what one legitimately expects from it, then it can be considered performing well. If it is less than expected, then it can be considered under-performing. Performance is a relative notion. One cannot ask Chad to do as well as Switzerland in terms of results, but one can see how, given its resources, Chad compares to countries that are in a similar situation.

Hence, in this chapter, "performance" and "result" will often be used as synonyms. However, we should keep in mind that the notion of performance implies placing the result in its context.

Result and performance

Although often used as synonyms, the words "performance" and "result" relate to different concepts. The word result is used to describe the measurement of an attained situation. In order to define a result, a measurement scale, a measurement instrument and an indicator have to be established.

When it comes to performance, a qualification on a scale of results is added to the concept of result. Moreover, the concept of performance allows the measuring of a combination of results that have contributed to a performance.

The concept of result is often related to a quantitative measure: number of patient visits, rate of nosocomial infections; whereas the concept of performance will aim to include qualitative dimensions. Instead of focusing on the "more", one prefers the "better".[2]

Measuring performance can thus be based on qualitative instruments and surveys providing a notion of a global result.

2. DETERMINANTS OF PERFORMANCE OF HEALTH CARE PROVIDERS

To understand how a health care provider can be encouraged to change its behaviour and improve its performance, it is necessary to understand its behaviour, i.e. to analyse the determinants of the provider performance. Hence we start with a general thought, which consists in that the performance of a health care provider, i.e. the results obtained by this health care provider, depend on the one hand on factors associated with the demand from the populations living in its catchment area, and on the other hand, the personal characteristics of the supplier:

Results achieved = f (Demand, Characteristics of the Supply)

2.1   Factors associated with demand

If the focus is on the volume of the activity, it is obvious that the results achieved by the health care provider will be better if the demand for his or her services will be higher. Yet, this demand depends on many determinants, including:

The environment in which the demand is made. For example, a heavy rainy season may affect visits to a health care facility, since the access roads are cut off for several months;

The income of the population. It is known that a poor population, with very low income will express low demand for health care services, especially when the provider charges a fee-for-service. This income of course depends on the socio-economic status of the person, but it may also evolve over time, depending on external factors as is the case during unfavourable climatic conditions in a given region;

The perception of the quality of health care providers. Individuals will be less willing to consult a health care provider, if they know that the services on offer are of poor quality. To a certain degree there is interplay between supply and demand; all things being equal, a weak demand can be due to a low quality supply.

289

Cultural factors: in some contexts, especially in Africa, one can observe a lower than expected frequency in the use of health care services for certain illnesses for which the western medicine is believed to be ineffective.

These factors determining demand are very important. Some of them can evolve over time (for example, the revenues of a population) whilst others are elements that one cannot change (the climate for example). In identifying these factors, it is obvious that there are some that can be changed through appropriate action (e.g. the revenues of certain population groups), whereas others cannot be changed (e.g., one cannot act on climatic conditions).

2.2   Factors associated with characteristics of the supply

The results achieved by a health care provider will also depend on its characteristics. These include:

The human and financial resources: to carry out an activity, a health care provider needs resources and the level of these resources will affect its results. For example, it is quite obvious that, all things being equal, if a nurse does not have enough dressings, she cannot adequately care for patients who need them. If an X-ray unit has no films adapted for certain examinations, it cannot perform these examinations, or will poorly perform them, by using less appropriate films;

The know-how, which reflects individual competence in the control of the production process within an organization. This know-how depends on individual capacities or the organizational set-up brought about by these capacities. Know-how may be improved, particularly through investment in knowledge and through practical experience (investment in human capital). But, one should also accept the fact that there are inequalities in the capacity to master know-how. Investment in human capital may partially improve this situation. At the level of an organization, the differences in the individual know-how may be compensated by the establishment of protocols. Training, providing protocols and transfer of know-how contribute to improved performance. Hence, knowledge of how to dress a wound will impact on the result of nursing care, and the knowledge of how to adjust X-ray machine settings will lead to better X-ray exams.

The efforts[3] made are linked to several determinants:

[Efforts = f (sanction, level of professionalism, relative remuneration, work value, context, incentive …)]

Sanction: it presupposes a wrongdoing. For example, the person does not provide the minimum work expected or his behaviour harms the functioning of the organization that employs him. A higher authority (the manager) may then sanction him. The sanction may take various forms and can be gradual: warning, indictment, transfer, dismissal, etc...;

Level of professionalism: it refers to the desire of the employee to perform tasks assigned to him, ensuring that he does it to the best of his ability. This value may find its source in religion or in other social systems, and it also stems from professional training;

Relative remuneration: all things being equal, an employee will correctly perform his task if he considers that he is well remunerated; otherwise, he might not do it well. What is important is not what is objective but what is subjective (the employer may judge that he is paying a good salary, whereas the employee might feel that he is inadequately remunerated for the work done);

Work value: this refers to the importance that the individual attaches to the paid work that he is doing in competition with other social activities – family life, social relations, personal development ...). Work value gives social and personal satisfaction that exceeds the accomplishment of tasks compensated by remuneration.[4]

Context: a person rarely works alone. There are other employees in the institution in which he works. The behaviour of these other employees will have an effect on his effort. Hence, a person who sees that his colleagues have a tendency of regularly coming late to work without any sanction being imposed on them will also tend to arrive late, for he does not see why he should dissociate himself from the others. The context is different from the environment, for it makes reference to behaviour of individuals within a given group;

Incentive: it is the granting of compensation, a bonus, an allowance, a grant to individuals or institutions depending on the results achieved. This incentive may be financial or non-financial. This is the determinant we will focus on in this document.

The components of effort are not independent variables. The nature and intensity of the relations however are difficult to establish and to model. The nature of social relations and in particular social constraints affect the intensity of the effect of these variables on effort. For example, in a totalitarian State, sanction will play a more preponderant role than in a State where the protection of individuals is highly developed.

Let's take an example: *You need some information and, to get it, you need to go to an information centre of the Ministry of Health - the office hours are 8am-12noon and 2pm-5pm, there is a break between 12noon and 2pm.*

- *First Situation*: *you arrive at 9:30; you observe that the person who should inform you is not there. A security guard informs you that he has not yet arrived. You come back at 11:30: the same person tells you that you are not lucky, for the person who can inform you just left! You should, therefore, come back at 14:00; he should normally be here!*

- *Second Situation*: *you arrive at 11:55. The person who can inform you is around, but he tells you that he closes at 12:00 and cannot inform you within such a short time; he will resume work at 14:00.*

- *Third Situation*: *you arrive at 12:00. The person who can inform you should be going for his break, but, understanding that you have come from far, he kindly receives you and informs you diligently and competently. You leave at 12:30. The person who informed you then goes for his break with no other formality.*

- *Fourth Situation*: *you arrive at 12:00. The person who can inform you must go for his break, but understanding that you have come from far, he kindly receives you and informs you diligently and competently and mobilizes colleagues to answer questions that are beyond him. You leave at 12:30. The person who informed you then goes on break, but he does not forget to note that he has worked for an additional thirty minutes, which should be paid to him or requests you that you complete his "appreciation book" (which is used to establish the service bonuses).*

This example can be represented by the following figure:

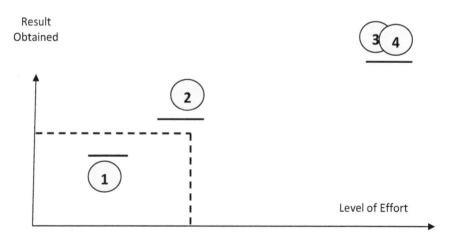

Situation 1: corresponds to the situation in which employees and their institutions make a "**minimum effort**" and, consequently, obtain poor results. Only extreme sanctions may be imposed, and that is why staff will make a minimum effort. On the other hand, even common sanctions are not applied, even if provision is made for that. In fact, it is practically impossible for officials to apply them for various reasons: the unions are powerful, the group pressure is very strong, habits are ingrained, the manager himself is frequently in situations where he himself should be sanctioned, etc. Similarly, dedication is very low. For both the staff and the institution, dedication is not a shared value. Consequently dedication is not a factor that could encourage the employee to make an extra effort. Inadequate accomplishment of one's task is not considered a serious offense. If the employee does not correctly accomplish his task, it means that there are good reasons that take precedence over this task. For example, if the person does not get to work on time, it is because he has to take care of his family, find additional revenue, or it is because he lives far away from his workplace and finding a means of transport is not easy, etc. Work is not valued, as individuals prefer to mobilize their energy for other social activities. Besides, the person feels that he is inadequately paid and, therefore, reduces his efforts to a level commensurate with the remuneration. Finally, the institution has no mechanism to recognize those who fully accomplish their tasks. Generally speaking, we are dealing with organizations where liability is virtually non-existent. This often reflects situations of weak governance in which the public interest is of little importance and in which civil society is weak.

Situation 2: corresponds to the situation what is generally presented as "**normal effort**". Activities to be performed are defined by the hierarchy. The staff or institution will respect this norm for one or several reasons:

- The use of sanction is possible and, consequently, the staff or institution has interest in carrying out the planned activity;
- Level of professionalism is an acknowledged value: the sense of public service, duty or devotion is expression of the level of professionalism. The staff or the institution will consider it normal to produce the necessary effort to attain the required result. The terms of reference are defined and what is demanded is accomplished. But, there is no reason to do more;
- Remuneration is considered acceptable and the person is not compelled to spend his time on other activities;
- The work or activity is considered important by those who carry it out; they therefore give it due priority.

For example, in a hospital staff is present during the required working hours. They perform the tasks that are defined in their job descriptions. They perform these with honesty, mobilizing their technical skills and using resources made available to them. They fill out the files as expected. They work with colleagues they have been asked to work with, and they address clients respectfully. BUT NO MORE! They will not initiate efforts to improve their skills; they will not try to find out how they can do better. They will make no particular effort towards users, etc. This is the attitude described as "being present behind one's desk": waiting for the client and serving him correctly; but without anticipating the client's needs. For example, if the mother has not brought her child to the health centre to be vaccinated, the employee of this health centre will not attempt to find out why she has not brought her child, he will not try to mobilize means to try to vaccinate that child. In this situation, the concept of 'time required for this activity' is important, for it is expected that the remuneration paid corresponds exactly to this level of effort.

Situation 3: corresponds to the situation in which employees or their institutions consider that it is normal to make all possible efforts. This is another notion of 'level of professionalism' that goes beyond the idea of making only the necessary efforts to meet what is demanded. This specific level of professionalism does not define itself any longer by accepting a level of effort that is about sufficient to reach result. This specific level of professionalism judges normal to do whatever it takes to get a maximum result. The level of professionalism and work values are, therefore, highly valued. We can find this situation when individuals have a keen sense of duty and devotion: serving the State, serving one's neighbour. It goes beyond the mere exchange of a product (one's work) against remuneration in order to accomplish an activity. The notion of time devoted to work or activity to be provided becomes less important in the relationships between providers (those providing a service) and purchasers (those receiving a service, or clients, or those paying for others to receive this service).

For example, the health staff of a hospital will consider that they should seek to improve their skills and to stay abreast of technical developments, they will look for ways and means to improve their performance in the tasks entrusted to him, they will try to see how they can improve the documentation which is required of them, and they will attempt to provide additional support to clients/patients who are felt to be in need of this. By this attitude, one leaves his desk and anticipates the wishes of the client.

Situation 4: corresponds to the case where the staff or their institutions are prepared to **"make an effort beyond the normal"**, as long as they are compensated for this additional effort. Level of professionalism is replaced here by incentives. Performance improvement is facilitated by the use of incentives. It is the incentives that will encourage the staff or their institutions to maximize their efforts. It is in their interest to do so.

For example, the health centre of a particular zone has vaccinated 50% of the children in its catchment area, and this 50% corresponds to those that have come to the health centre themselves. They are received and vaccinated correctly once they come to the health centre. However, the health centre is prepared to make special efforts (outreach activities, sensitization campaign among local authorities, etc.), as long as it gets an additional budget to do so when reaching coverage rates beyond 50%.

NB: it is worth recalling that the libertarian provider payment practice falls within this fourth category. Indeed, the practitioner paid on a fee-for-service basis will earn a lot more if he works more (supposing that he does not perform useless acts) or when he has attained an outstanding reputation. However, he will frequently concentrate his efforts on activities where he can ask to be paid for his services, which excludes a number of preventative activities, when these activities are either not paid, or poorly remunerated.

What is the situation today?

There are very few cases where one finds himself in situation 3. It may, however, be present in certain circumstances:

- Religious contexts: in many religions, the believers should make maximum efforts to serve their neighbours; the compensation will be an immediate or subsequent, internal or social recognition;

- Humanitarian NGOs: the staff, like the institutions themselves, find it normal to maximize their efforts; they are guided by convictions, the realization of which will give them personal gratification;

- In the public sector, there is another value system, which considers that the civil servant must always do the maximum; he is at the service of the public; this rationale is based on social recognition;

- Some Marxist offshoots (Stakhanovism, for example) pushes individuals towards a certain ideal, the accomplishment of which is compensated by collective recognition;

- Certain forms of paternalism: the employee will do everything possible for his employer, for he is indebted for the efforts made by the "good" employer.

Some NGOs operated for a long time according to this logic. They could obtain from those with whom they were working maximum output without having to use incentives. Today, some of them tend towards situation 2: devotion to the cause is no longer strong enough to naturally attain situation 3. Other NGOs work with staff or institutions that do not operate according to this logic. They cannot get the latter to adopt behaviours that would lead to situation 3.

Situation 3 is the most interesting for the employer, for he obtains a higher result without making particular efforts in terms of remuneration or incentives. But, these situations are finally quite rare in reality, since they presuppose that work value coupled to level of professionalism are the main drivers of level of effort.

The normal situation would, consequently, be situation 2, which is generally at the basis of the definition of public service: you have a job that is placed within a legal regulatory framework and you should comply with these legal regulatory requirements. However, there is no reason why you should do more than what is requested of you (e.g., if you are legally required to work 8 hours a day, you have no interest working for an additional hour, for nothing is offered to compensate for this effort which exceed service obligations). In this situation, the work provided is assessed in its quantitative (you are present at the time you are supposed to be) and qualitative (you do your work according to the rules of your trade or prevailing procedures) aspects. You are there to accomplish correctly an assigned task. Ministries of Health pretty much subscribe to this situation. In some countries, the Ministry of Health would be happy to see its entire staff and all its institutions attaining this level. However many Ministries of Health slide towards situation 1, notably when the hierarchy is weak or when the social pressure does not promote work value. This is also true when workers feel that they are inadequately remunerated.

In the face of slipping standards, and to reverse this downward trend, some people are resorting to the use of incentives in order to attain situation 4. Certainly, this situation is more expensive for the financier, since it requires putting in place a mechanism for providing these incentives and supervising them, but it helps to maximize the level of effort of staff and their institutions. Maximizing efforts means working faster (accomplishing a task with greater efficiency), working longer and working better. Such an approach implies making formal the relationship between effort and compensation. Hence, some actors, believing that staff should maximize their efforts, but observing at the same time that situation 3 has no chance of occurring naturally, will therefore tend to turn to situation 4, i.e. using incentives to maximize efforts. Hence, they will obtain a result comparable or higher than the one obtained in situation 3, but at a much higher cost since the financier has to set up a mechanism for organizing and measuring performance and distributing performance incentives.

The use of incentives to enhance performance becomes interesting when the results obtained are higher than the costs incurred. This statement seems obvious in a classical market situation where supply meets demand. It is less obvious for services that are linked to public goods. In this case, it makes more sense to improve the quality of service and to determine its marginal cost in order to decide whether or not to finance an additional expenditure to pay for the incentives.[5] When one takes a long term perspective, there is no doubt a risk of getting used to incentives, thereby creating a situation where the staff and their institutions will always ask for higher incentives for the efforts they are prepared to provide. It is, therefore, necessary to institute a mechanism for reducing, over time, the risk of diminishing returns for the incentive. It is in this spirit that organizations use the prize list system to compensate the employer who achieves the best result. There is constant competition between individuals to be included on the prize list. This will be all the more true if the inscription on the prize list is accompanied by a specific bonus and if the mechanism is set up in a transparent manner and based on objective criteria for measuring the results.

3. THE LOGIC BEHIND THE PERFORMANCE INCENTIVE

3.1 Admitting failure of the classical approach

For a long time we adhered to the hypothesis that, all things being equal (e.g., in a constant environment), the performance of an institution will be better if factors of production were present in greater number and of a better quality. According to this approach, called "input-based" approach,[6] the health care provider would achieve better results as long as it has sufficient and well-trained staff, adequate equipment, state-of-the-art technologies, drugs at affordable prices which are delivered on time, and efficient and easily-accessible (geographically) infrastructure, etc.

Preconditioned on this availability of inputs good results would be achieved because an adequate combination of these inputs would help attain the best possible result. In the classical production logic, it is command and control that will facilitate the achievement of such a result. Commands are given in linear and hierarchical fashion. The all-knowing hierarchy knows the objectives to be attained and the best way of combining inputs. The command can use sanctions to ensure the respect of orders. This operating procedure is valid for both the public and private sectors. You do your work: all your work, nothing but your work. As we shall see later, there are other mechanisms that can lead to an optimal use of inputs.

The results of this approach are not always as poor as is too often said, notably in health systems where methods are not too limited by a lack of resources. On the other hand, in poor countries where funding constraints are considerable, it should be noted that those few resources available produce results that are often insufficient, given the immense needs of the populations. To attain the objective of improving results, the traditional strategies, based on the supply of inputs and hierarchical command and control as a means of ensuring the optimum combination of these inputs, are quite inefficient. Furthermore, health service providers with equal resources and working conditions do not produce equal results (identical inputs ≠ results); resources are thus not the only determinant of health service providers' result.

3.2 A new approach: incentives

Therefore, let us change our strategy in a radical fashion by the use of *incentives*. The latter would become our strategy for enhancing performance. Incentive is defined as *the interest one has in doing better*. Incentive mechanisms, therefore, presuppose two types of actors:

- There is, first of all, the *incentive provider*: This is the institution that has become aware of the importance of encouraging health care providers to improve upon their performance, and which has identified that the best strategy for doing so consisted in the use of incentives, and which has the necessary resources (notably financial resources) to carry this out. This incentive provider will chiefly be the Ministry of Health. But it may also be a development partner, who will operate through the Ministry of Health (e.g., the World Bank which might incite the Ministry of Health to introduce performance incentive mechanisms), or a partner that is capable of acting directly (e.g., an international NGO, which provides support through performance incentive mechanisms). It may finally be health insurance institutions, which institute performance incentive mechanisms with health care providers they deal with. The aim of these institutions is to encourage the latter to enhance their efficiency in terms of services they render to their clients. Given the fact that the incentive is generally monetary, some people prefer to use the term "purchaser". It is also possible to use the term "financing agent" which is used in the OECD accounting system and which refer to institutions and entities that purchase or finance health care services.

- There is also the *incentive beneficiary*: it is the health care provider (hospital, clinic, health centre, community health worker cooperative, etc.), who is being encouraged to change its behaviour and, consequently, improve its performance. But, the incentive beneficiary could also be the health administration, notably the local administration, which is being encouraged by the incentive provider to adopt a new behaviour in order to enhance its performance. The target of this approach is thus the institution: it is the institution that will need to improve its results. The implementation strategy is frequently, but not uniquely, as we shall see later on in this chapter, based on incentivizing staff working for these institutions. There is some experience with incentive schemes directly targeting staff; whereas such an approach might yield some results in pilot schemes, it might be challenging to scale this up.

The agency theory

Facing incentive schemes, economists resort to the agency theory, which defines the agency relationship as a contract under which an organization (the principal) - i.e. the incentive provider - engages another organization (the agent) - i.e. the incentive beneficiary - to perform, on its behalf, any task entailing a delegation of some decision-making power to the agent.

The first important notion of this theory is to take into consideration the fact that the two parties may have diverging interests:

- It is in the interest of the incentive provider (the principal) to ensure that its agent (the incentive beneficiary) maximizes its efforts to attain the best possible results;

- For the incentive beneficiary, it is in its interest to minimize its efforts to receive the rewards.

The purpose of the incentive, which will be defined in a contract, will be to reconcile the interests of the two actors, who from the onset do not have the same objectives, to get them to pursue the same objectives.

The second important notion of this theory lies in the difficulty for the principal to assess the effort of its agent so as to offer a fair remuneration for this effort. It should, moreover, be underlined that one cannot observe the effort, but only the result of the effort. The agent, therefore, has some information the principal needs (particularly on the process of production) but for which the agent has a disincentive to make overt. It is due to this notion that the principal will be putting a particular emphasis on measuring results, to pre-empt under-achievement by the agent.

Issues related to Terminology

The performance incentive, as used in a health systems context, is described differently by different people. The differences between these descriptions are often only a question of terminology, as the different terms used have basically the same semantic structure.

They are mostly structured as follows:

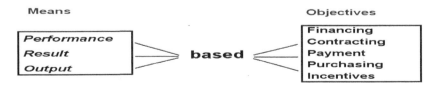

299

What is interesting to note in the logic of the current terminology, as above, is that it reverses the logic. Concerning the performance incentive, the objective of the action should be the performance (or the result, or direct realization) and the different tools used to influence performance should be considered as means.

Strategy		Objectives
Incentive	*for*	*Performance*

The reversed logic of current appellations could find its origin in the fact that they reflect the point of view of the donor: the objective of the latter is to disburse and channel the funding; there are several ways of dealing with the issue and one of the methods consists in establishing a link between financing and performance.

One of the terminologies is in line with basic logic: *Pay for Performance (P4P)*. However, the fact that the latter includes only the payment concept (which may cover the financing of inputs as well as the incentive for direct achievements), whilst excluding the other non-monetary aspects of the incentive, makes its use problematic.

Finally, it should be noted that the terminology currently used has not conceptualized the logic of *performance incentive* and that, in reality, there is a consensus around the term Performance-Based Financing (PBF), at least concerning the health systems in developing countries. This terminology has been adopted in a generic sense in most publications.

3.3 Incentives for demand and supply

To get the incentive beneficiary to improve its performance, the incentive provider has, at his disposal, two main types of strategies:

Actions on demand, essentially on individuals, but these may also be communities. This presupposes that the population (notably the poorest, but there may be other determinants) do not consult health care providers because they do not have the means or because they do not see the interest in doing so. Incentives will rely on tools that will encourage these populations to use health services and, thereby, increase their demand for the services of health providers. These tools may be:

- A policy that is based on price differentiation depending on the medical history or the nature of the individual. These price related incentives may be applied in both ways, by charging the target persons a lower price, or by fixing penalties for those who have access to services considered excessive (e.g., those who directly consult the specialist physician, without first consulting a general practitioner);

- The voucher system prioritizes the pro-active identification of a target population whereas the preceding mechanism is limited to the care provider. Here, a financier - the Ministry of Health, a development partner or a health insurer - distributes to the target populations vouchers they can use for either accessing freely, or against a reduced fee designated health services. This free access or fee reduction boosts greater demand for health services by the designated population. There will be an increased utilization of health services due to increased demand.

Experiences based on voucher systems

Since 2006, the KFW has been supporting a voucher programme in 3 rural districts and in the outskirts of Nairobi. It is aimed at assisting poor families to have access to quality maternal care and family planning services. The KFW is financing similar programmes in Uganda and Tanzania.

These programmes have been established in Nicaragua for prostitutes, drug addicts, homosexuals and young people at risk, in Indonesia to facilitate access of poor women in rural areas to private midwives, in India and Pakistan, etc.

- Insurance or user fee exemption schemes: by encouraging the populations to subscribe to insurance schemes or by financing the exemption from user fees, the financiers will encourage populations to use health care providers. Since the population knows that use of health providers will no longer result in catastrophic expenditure, these populations will hesitate much less to seek care. Hence, the institution of voluntary health insurance schemes, unless a major gate fee is introduced, will result in an increase in demand for the services of health care providers. Similarly, under the poverty reduction programme, payment for subscription to a health insurance scheme by a financier (development partner, for example) will result in an increase in demand from this population group.

- Conditional cash transfers: these mechanisms consist, for a financier (Ministry of Health or development partner) in giving money to a target population (usually the poorest) conditional on achieving certain socially beneficial activities. These conditions may concern health or education. The financier will request that the beneficiary of the aid sends her children to school, that she ensures that they are vaccinated, or that she uses mother and child health services when pregnant. These conditionalities will encourage these population groups to visit health facilities and to send their children to school.

This financing of the supply of health services through demand will have an effect on the performance of health care providers. Indeed, generally, this implies an increase in the volume of services consumed, accompanied by better equity in the use of these resources. There is certainly an improvement in the supply of health care and, therefore, of its performance (and consequently of the performance of the health system), but it is the financing of the demand that has led to the improvement of the offer and not the direct funding of the supply. It is of course not appropriate to talk about performance of the demand, but performance of the supply induced by the demand (which is different from the concept of supplier-induced demand);

Actions on the supply of health services. Through appropriate incentives, the incentive provider acts directly on the health care provider by encouraging him to change its behaviour and practices in a positive sense. Through this action, the incentive provider incites the health care provider to enhance its efficiency and its effectiveness. Later on we shall see that this logic can be translated into different types of approaches.

Actions on supply and demand. There have also been actions taken simultaneously on supply and demand. A development partner can put in place an intervention that has an element targeting the supply of health services and another targeting the demand. In some cases two development partners can be present in the same geographical zone, one acting on the supply the other acting on the demand. There are also schemes in which the incentive financier acts on the supply in order to motivate the health care provider to increase its results and, consequently, the provider will act on the demand in order to increase its outputs (supplier-induced demand in a positive sense). These measures can be either agreed between the financier and the provider, or they can be implemented as a creative initiative by the provider.

An example of simultaneous action on demand and supply (certain health centres in Rwanda)

The incentive financier (the Ministry of Health) pays 2500 FRW, about $5, to the provider (health centre) for uncomplicated deliveries; the provider purchases second hand baby clothes for each new born for 500 FRW and keeps the rest as net reward from the incentive. Moreover, women who come for an antenatal checkup during the fourth month of pregnancy are offered a soap bar and water purification tablets. These in kind incentives have their advantages but they can also create some problems; there is in particular the risk of resale of gifts received.

Some health centres pay Traditional Birth Attendants (TBA) FRW 500, for each referred delivery and in addition to that, for 10 referred cases the TBA receives an annual subscription for the community based health insurance.

The logic of performance incentive of health care providers may be summarized as follows:

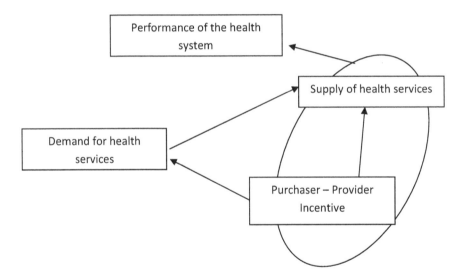

In this document, we have limited our attention to supply-side incentives for health providers (the yellow circle above), also implied by the title of this manuscript.

4. PERFORMANCE INCENTIVE IMPLEMENTATION MECHANISMS

The logic is now established: through appropriate actions, the incentive provider will try to get the health care provider to improve his performance. The incentive provider proposes[7] these incentives, but, of course, he cannot impose them. The health care provider, for his part, has an option i.e. he will react to these proposals by adapting his behaviour. Obviously, his reaction will depend on the interest that these incentives arouse in him. If the latter are substantial, it will be in his interest to make efforts to improve his results. If on the other hand he finds these incentives inadequate he will only make very little effort and, consequently, will increase his results only marginally.

Generally speaking, the performance incentive scheme will be made operational following three stages:

Stage 0: Before any action is taken, a decision on whether to use performance incentives has to be made. The diagram below indicates that the financier could use the classical strategy which consists of providing the necessary inputs to the health care provider and using either 'command and control methods' or relying on the providers values in order to attain a desired level of performance. Here, the strategy consists of using incentives, and the path to increased performance is based either on regulation or through contracting.

Results and Performance

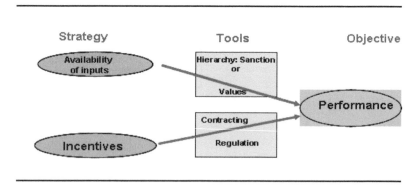

Stage 1: This stage is composed of two phases:

- Phase 1: Setting up the rules of the game. Every performance incentive scheme needs a set of 'rules of the game' which define its objectives, the

304

domains covered by it, a credible performance measure, the modalities of attributing incentives, the exclusion rules, etc. These rules of the game can be defined unilaterally by the financier and such being the case the public authorities will establish an official text that applies to everyone. But more often, the rules of the game will be established in consultation with providers and development partners. These rules of the game will be recorded in what is often referred to as an "Implementation Manual".

- Phase 2: Formalizing the agreement between the purchaser (incentive provider) and the provider (incentive beneficiary): there are two types of tools that the incentive provider can resort to:

  - **Regulation-contracting:** in this case the incentive provider will define the rules of the game, in consultation with the health providers who will be covered under the scheme. This consultative approach will lead to a consensus that is more or less solid. But it is important to realize that it is the incentive provider that will unilaterally make the final adjustments and finalize the implementation manual. Generally, the health care provider will be free to participate in the scheme, but as these mechanisms do not generally provide for negative incentives, it is always in the interest of the care providers to participate even if their chances for gains are low. This adherence may be expressed in different ways: by a letter from the health care provider indicating its desire to participate or through a contractual arrangement;[8] in all cases there is some form of contractual relationship because some form of agreement has been reached and formalized. However, this agreement is not based on negotiation but simply on acceptance of the rules of the game as defined by the incentive provider. This support may appear hypocritical in some cases. Indeed, in many cases where this regulation is established by the State the latter becomes virtually mandatory as public health providers cannot exempt themselves from the established regulation;

  - **Contracting**: in this case, the rules of the game are defined through negotiation between the incentive provider and the health care provider; they constitute the purpose of the contract. The agreement is, therefore, complete and can be specified in each contract, unlike the case mentioned above.

The use of regulation or contracting is a choice of which every decision-maker must be aware. As we will see later, the use of contracting is a common approach used in the pilot phase by development partners. On the other hand, the going to scale, i.e. scaling up the performance incentive strategy for the entire country, leads

305

near automatically[9] to the use of regulation. Indeed the rules of the game must therefore be the same for all actors and only the State may impose this regulation.

The rules of the game will define all necessary technical and institutional aspects of implementing performance incentives and will be elaborated upon below. But it also defines in the first place what the objective of the performance incentive scheme is. We can distinguish two different models which differ significantly:

- The objective of the performance incentives is to install an incentive-based regular provider payment mechanism. This situation is referred to as a service purchase arrangement. The incentive financier purchases a defined set of services from the provider. This incentive based financing constitutes a (substantial) part of the regular budget of the provider. In this approach the gap in time between the effort provided and the settlement of the incentive payment will be short: the payment will be monthly or quarterly. This arrangement is a genuine provider payment method;

- The objective of incentive scheme is to install a bonus system that has no direct linkage with the general budget of the provider. The bonus system introduces a supplementary funding which is not strictly needed for running the provider's activities. The use of this bonus will happen outside of the general budget of the provider.[10] The payment of the bonus will occur relatively seldom, for example once a year. This gap in time between the effort and the reward is a factor that reduces the effectiveness of the incentive and it is thus preferable to reduce this gap as much as possible; although a wider time gap does have the advantage of reducing the cost of monitoring.

In reality, these two models are rarely found in a pure form, there are often intermediary situations:

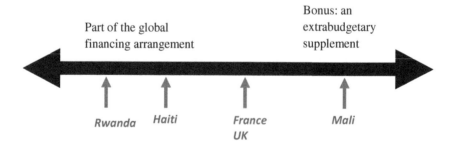

Another major distinction can be made between schemes that cover all or most of the providers' activities and those that cover a limited set of activities. The schemes that cover all or most of the activities of a health care provider have the objective of increasing the overall performance of the institution, although some activities can be emphasized through the choice and weighting of indicators. Other schemes target from the outset only certain activities: for example the European experiences described above, or the HIV/AIDS services related incentives in Rwanda.[11]

Stages 2 and 3: Having analysed the tools that enable the incentive provider to act on the behaviour of the health care provider, it is now necessary to know how this incentive mechanism is put in place. Two successive phases may be distinguished:

- Stage 2: it concerns the distribution and attribution of the incentives. Operationally, the situation is presented as follows: the health care provider starts his operations and after a certain period of time, one observes what happened. By relying on the rules of the game (defined by the regulation or contract), the reward for the activities of the health facility can then be calculated. The results observed are converted into incentives, which the incentive provider must pay to the health care provider. This amount is generally called "an allowance" or "bonus" for on the one hand it constitutes only a part of the budget of the health care provider and, on the other hand, of course varies depending on the results attained by the health care provider. The reward is generally financial; but it can also be compensations in various forms: trophy, best health centre label, etc.[12] At the end of this phase, the health care provider/manager[13] has a sum of money, which he will have to use.

Mali

Incentives can be other than financial. In Mali, the quality service label, the *Ciwara d'Or*, is awarded on the basis of a set of criteria fixed by community representatives and care providers. The criteria define strict norms governing the services offered by the health centre, the equipment and material. They also require the presence of adequate health staff as well as the effective participation of the management committee of the health centre. Before awarding the prize, the quality supervisory committee organizes a competition between community health centres (COMHCs) to encourage them to improve the quality of their services. The *Ciwara d'Or* quality label is awarded jointly by the team in charge of quality supervision in the health area, the local administrative and political authorities and the National Health Department at the COMHC, which would have obtained the highest score in terms of provision of quality health services."

- Stage 3: the use of the reward. During this phase, the health care provider will use the financial amounts he has received as remuneration for his performance. Two types of uses may be observed: individual or collective. In the first case each employee of the health institution will receive part of the reward: salary bonuses, specific training, etc. In the second case the reward is collective. It may for example be the refurbishment of the room for staff on duty in a hospital, the acquisition of specific equipment, which could not be acquired on the regular budget, etc. We can also have a combination of the two. For example, the reward could partly be used as bonuses to staff and partly for increasing the current operational budget of the health care provider. In all cases, it presupposes that this use of the reward will result in a motivation which in turn will enhance the performance of the health care provider. One may wonder whether individual incentives are more effective than collective incentives or vice versa. Of course one can opt for a combination of the two types of incentives: part of the reward going into individual incentives (e.g., bonuses to staff) and another part used to finance incentives that cannot be individualized (e.g., the purchase of a television set for the room for staff on duty in the hospital).

Moreover, the health care provider may strategically decide to compensate not individuals directly but service units instead. Hence, because such a service unit might have performed better than another – e.g., contributing relatively more to the overall health facility performance improvement – the health care provider may decide to allocate a greater part of the performance bonus to the former and less to the latter. The issue of whether or not to individualize incentives can be posed at this lower organizational level, with the head of the unit deciding to use one or the other. Taking this intermediate level into account will be all the more opportune if the health institution is complex. This is the case when the results achieved do not depend on a single person, but on the interaction of several people and teams. The result of team work will be better than that of individual efforts.

Whether they are individual or collective incentives have their advantages and disadvantages. Individual incentives reward the individual effort but results in lower levels of cooperation. Yet, the latter may be a factor of efficiency (for example, team work is absolutely necessary in the operating theatre). Collective incentives (or per team) enhances the value of the result of the team but will result in phenomena known as the "illegal passenger", namely that it is in the interest of the group individual to minimize his efforts and take advantage of the effort of others.

The process of implementation of the performance incentive may be summarized as follows:

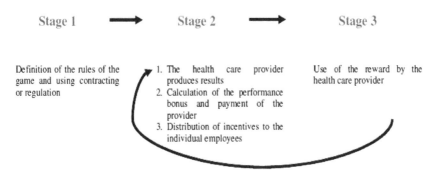

It is important to take into account the three stages of the incentive mechanism. Stage 1 defines the rules of the game and will be valid as long as the performance incentive mechanism lasts. Stage 2 comprises three phases: i) the health care provider, who is aware of the rules of the game, produces his efforts and achieves a certain result; ii) it is then possible to calculate the performance bonus, and iii) the incentive provider, based on this calculation, must pay the health care provider. In stage 3, once the health care provider has received the funds from the incentive provider, he will use these. After the mechanism has been launched, there is a feedback loop between Stage 2 and Stage 3. Indeed, the funds used will constitute a motivation for the health care provider (himself directly and/or his staff) to produce even better results (first phase of Stage 2), and this will lead to a new cycle.

Quite logically, stage 1, i.e. the definition of the rules of the game, should take into account both stages 2 and 3. Yet, we can observe that in certain country-experiences there is rather more of a delay in the phase of distribution of the reward[14] than that of its use. For example, in certain pilot schemes in Rwanda, until quite recently, the phase of utilization of the reward was left entirely at the discretion of the health care provider, who used the reward solely for paying staff bonuses. Today, in Rwanda, the rules of the game have changed and have become more sophisticated: the bonus payment to staff cannot exceed 75% of the performance reward. Allowing the health care provider to freely use the funds received is in line with libertarian thinking. It is, therefore, assumed that it is the health care provider who knows best his needs and that he will know how to take the best decisions regarding the use of the funds for improving, in a second cycle, the production of results. In this case, the rules of the game do not need to cater for stage 3. On the contrary some will say that the incentive provider, under the rules of the game adopted, cannot lose interest in stage 3 concerning the use of funds. A first reason is the fact that it is generally public money and that the incentive provider is liable for its use. Another reason relates to the fact that the use of this money is in itself strategic, since it targets a better production of results in a second cycle. The incentive provider should therefore ensure that the health care provider will make best use of these funds. A final reason relates to the need to harmonize practices in the use of funds. Hence, it will perhaps not be in the interest of the incentive provider to allow everybody to do as he pleases and he might create guidelines for the use of performance funds.

In concrete terms, once the performance bonuses are calculated, the incentive provider makes the money available to the health care provider:

- If the use of this money is not conditioned or earmarked it means that the health care provider can use it as he judges best. This money is added to the budget of the health facility and therefore aggregated with other income. It is then spent on actions decided by the health care provider. For example, in Rwanda, it is stipulated that at least 25% of the performance bonuses should be used for non-salary recurrent expenditures. This 25% will, therefore, be added to other sources of income of the health care provider and used to finance operational activities, including investments needed to improve quality of care. Consequently, due to the pooling of funds, it becomes less visible what the exact attribution of this additional financing of quality improvements is;

- If this money is designated it can only be used for the intended purpose as per the prevalent rules of the game. For example, if it is stipulated that it should be used to pay staff bonuses, the health care provider cannot put it to other use. In some cases, the designation concerns a specific type of expenditure: hence, the money cannot be added to other incomes and should be used for specific purposes. In some cases, governments do not like performance bonuses to reach health staff, and stipulate that this money can be used for all possible expenditures, bar the payment of performance bonuses.

The use of regulation or contract will not necessarily be the same for the two phases above. Hence, in Rwanda, it is the regulation that takes precedence in the two phases at the level of the relationship between the incentive provider and the health institution. The contractual part concerns only the inclusion of the health institution in the performance bonus scheme. In other cases, the contract will concern the two phases. Still in other instances one may resort to regulation for phase 1 and the use of a contract for phase 2. In this case the distribution of rewards will be defined by a general rule valid for all health institutions, but phase 2 will be specific to each health institution and will be the subject of a contract based for example on a *"business plan"*.

Business Plans

The Dutch NGO CORDAID introduced the concept of Business Plans in its Performance-Based Financing (PBF) pilot schemes in Rwanda. These business plans are currently an integral part of its PBF schemes in Burundi and DRC. There were several reasons for this introduction.

First, It was observed that after an initial phase of rapid improvements in quantity but also quality of care, a ceiling was reached for most services. Rapid gains from economies of scale were made initially and the providers had become satisfied with increased revenues. Reaching the remotest individuals would have needed significant marginal efforts that were not in correlation any longer with the fixed unit fee reward that was offered for this service. For this reason, CORDAID constantly renegotiated the targets which were then put down in a "Business Plan": thus, the providers and the purchaser could negotiate on specific quantitative targets, and they could discuss and agree on the strategies and resources that would be needed for reaching these targets. Furthermore, the business plan allowed the purchaser to intercept moral hazard: some providers might focus on certain high-yielding services to the detriment of other services, but close monitoring of their production would enable the purchaser to adjust the volume of services purchased.

The Business Plan is an integral part of the purchase contract established between the provider and the purchaser and it is used as a "stick" that is additional to the incentive "carrot" (the "reward for services"). Conceptually, these Business Plans are similar to the "Action Plans" that have been used by most health facilities in the past. However, these Business Plans are more closely monitored by both parties (since there are financial consequences). Calling the action plan by a different name served also as a signal that things were not 'business as usual' any longer.

The second reason for introducing the Business plan concept was to get inside the "black

---

box" at the managerial level. In the first PBF pilot experiences the managers were thought and trusted to make good use of the resources and they were given large autonomy; it would of have been unnecessary and even inopportune to monitor too closely the use these resources. The Business Plan was designed to redefine this principle as it was deemed that the mangers did not always make use of the most suitable strategies for increasing their performance.

In the Rwandan national PBF scheme, the Business Plan was reintroduced in the beginning of 2008 in order to tackle the problem of stagnating performance after a rapid expansion of the quality and quantity of health services across the country.

Let us turn our attention to the performance bonuses. What are the criteria used by the incentive provider to determine the level of desired performance of the health care provider? There are, in reality two methods which are fairly distinct.

A first method is to consider that the benefit is entirely defined by the result.[15] For example we might propose that the health care provider will receive a certain sum per fully vaccinated child. There is therefore a direct relationship between the quantity or level of effort (which may be influenced by the quality if the purchaser decides to do so) of the services produced and the payment received by the health provider: *"working more and/or better to earn more"*. Libertarian medicine is in line with this logic. It is also practiced in Rwanda where health care providers are remunerated according to the activities they have carried out (taking into account both the quantitative and qualitative aspects). However, these types of schemes are a departure from pure market logic from various points of view. First, we see that the price fixed does not generally reflect the cost of production of this activity. If the level of the incentive would have been commensurate with the level of effort, then in that case a very low price for a service will not have an encouraging effect and a very high price will introduce a very strong incentive to produce more of this service. It is also necessary to underline that it is not a classical purchase act, since the incentive provider (the purchaser) knows the price of the activities, but is less certain about the quantity to purchase.[16] It is, thus, preferable to talk about purchase obligation, namely that the incentive provider will be obliged to buy at the price defined in the rules of the game all the quantities produced by the health care provider. This remark is important because, unless you have solid estimates on the quantities that will be produced by the providers the purchaser faces an unknown budget which may put him in difficulty. This also does not correspond to budgetary practices, notably those of the State. It presupposes that the purchaser can adapt his purchasing budget to the activity of the provider which is not always obvious when the purchaser is the State. As a countermeasure the State takes into account projected purchases and model these against budget available, in order to prevent budget blowouts. Finally, it may compel the provider to focus on certain high-yielding services only without the latter being always judicious all the more so since he knows that the buyer is solvent.

A second method consists of no longer associating results in terms of service provision but instead focusing on certain behaviours and practices. For example, in Mali hospitals, activities are funded from the operational budget defined according to classical input modalities. However, the Ministry of Health has established a special grant for improving performance. This grant makes it possible to pay a bonus to those who improved some of their practices (a bonus which is for example tied to the percentage of medical files correctly filled out). Hence, the processes are incentivized postulating that better processes of care will lead to better quality services and ultimately a better outcome. You act on contextual factors or processes which you believe will have an effect on the results. For example: a health care provider who reduces the waiting time of patients during consultation, will have an effect on patient perceptions, and possibly also on actual quality of care. The hypothesis here is that in order to improve results one cannot be interested only in the number of patients seen during a consultation but that it is important to open the 'black box' of the production processes.

We should of course always pursue the most efficient strategy. Advocates of results-based management will state that there is no need to enter the black box. The actors know what needs to be done and will put in place the production process that will yield desirable results. Others will claim that it is necessary to act on the production processes and that it is only by changing bad practices that one can influence (perhaps in a sustainable manner) the performance of health institutions and their health workers. We should note as is the case in Mali and in Rwanda, that it is possible to mix output indicators with process indicators for an effective performance framework.

How shall we determine the performance objectives? There are two slightly different methods to do so.

The first method consists in defining at the beginning of the incentive mechanism a result to be attained. Hence it will state, for example, the vaccine coverage rate to be attained by the end of a certain period of time. This target is, therefore, defined in the beginning of the mechanism (through a regulatory or contractual framework). For example, in Haiti, 95% of the negotiated budget is paid to NGOs in quarterly installments (output-based tied to certain deliverables), and 5% is put at risk. If the NGO reaches predefined performance targets, it can regain these 5% plus an additional 8% performance bonus.[17] The advantage of this technique is that the incentive provider and the health care provider agree on a target to attain, i.e. on what would be good to do. On the other hand, there is a risk that the health institution may not pursue its efforts beyond the target, as it has no interest in doing so.

The second method does not initially determine the target, but ensures that each additional effort made by the health institution is compensated. It is, therefore, in the interest of the health institution to pursue its efforts as long as the marginal benefit is higher than the marginal cost of an additional activity unit. Hence, if the incentive provider pays $1 per fully-vaccinated child, it is in the interest of the health institution to pursue its efforts as long as the additional child will not cost him more than $1.

Each of these two techniques has its advantages and disadvantages. The interesting aspect of "no target" is that no limit is placed on the effort of the health institution below the point where the incentive is higher than the cost of the marginal effort. However, it places the incentive provider at a greater risk for the quantities that will be produced and also gives no indication on the desired level of performance.

To sum up, to analyse the implementation of performance incentive mechanisms, five main elements may be retained:

1. Are the rules of the game defined in the sense of using regulation or using contracting?
2. Do the rules of the game concern Stage 2 (nearly) exclusively or simultaneously Stage 2 and Stage 3?
3. Does the appreciation of performance concern the outputs or also the production processes (behaviour change or process improvement in the implementation of activities)?
4. Is the objective of performance incentive to get the health care provider to attain a pre-defined target or to maximize his results?
5. Do performance bonuses represent a significant or a small share of the health care provider budget? are the rewards in cash or in kind and are they regular (e.g. monthly), or irregular (e.g. yearly)?

In order to see how its different elements are taken into account in the field, three experiences may be retained:

- The "Performance-Based Financing" (PBF) experience in Rwanda;
- The experience in hospitals in Mali;
- The experience of NGOs in Haiti;

The latter two country cases are presented in the annex.

	Rwanda Experience	Mali Experience	Haiti Experience On the award fee portion (5-10%)
1. Are the rules of the game defined in the sense of using regulation or using contracting?	The rules of the game are mainly defined by regulation, except the adherence of health care providers, which is the subject of a standard contract.	The rules of the game are mainly defined by regulation, except the adherence of hospital staff, which is the subject of a single contract signed by all participating hospitals.	The rules of the game are defined by a contract, whilst the award fee portion is regulated, with considerable constraints on how to use this award fee due to US government restrictions on the use of this money.
2. Do the rules of the game concern Stage 2 (nearly) exclusively or simultaneously Stage 2 and Stage 3?	The rule of the game concerns nearly exclusively Stage 2. A new rule related to the use of funds was introduced in 2006 during the national scale-up, and revised in 2008.	The rule of the game concerns explicitly Stage 2 and Stage 3.	The rule of the game concerns Stage 2 and cannot concern Stage 3, since the reward constitutes a part of the estimated operational budget; and the utilization follows the same modalities as for all the other funding streams outside the incentive scheme.
3. Does the appreciation of performance concern the outputs or also the production processes (behaviour change or process improvement in the implementation of activities)?	The performance assessment concerns the quantitative outputs attained by the health care provider and the process of care (quality aspect).	The performance assessment concerns some outputs but also processes (change of behaviours and practices in the activity production process).	The performance assessment concerns the public health results achieved by the health care provider, but also include certain process measures (quantitative and qualitative aspect).
4. Is the objective of performance incentive to get the health care provider to attain a pre-defined target or to maximize his results?	The objective of the incentive scheme is to get the health care provider to maximize its efforts and thereby its results. In addition since January 2008 the provider establishes in consultation with the administration a 'business plan' in which it will indicate the main population based targets that it will seek to attain for a more limited set of health indicators.	The objective of the incentive scheme is to get the health care provider to maximize his efforts and, thereby, his results.	The objective of the incentive scheme is to get the health care provider to attain pre-defined population based targets which have been defined at the beginning of the performance incentive cycle.

	Rwanda Experience	Mali Experience	Haiti Experience On the award fee portion (5-10%)
5. Do the performance bonuses represent a significant share of the budget of the health care provider or a small share; are the rewards in cash or in kind and are they regular for instance monthly, or irregular for instance once per year?	The performance bonuses represent a significant share of the budget of a health centre: about 30% of their overall recurrent budget. The staff gets paid performance incentives up to about an estimated 100% of its net base salary, which depends on the overall health facility performance, the staff is paid its performance bonus regularly once per month (after the health facility earns its performance bonus quarterly and distributes earnings once per month to its health staff).	The performance bonuses represent a minor sum compared to the actual hospital budget and are conceived as a bonus which is not intended to increase the hospital budget. The bonus is paid once per year.	The award constitutes only a minor sum related to the overall budget of the managing NGO. Health facilities under the management of the NGO could receive some share of this award fee, for instance in the form of a 13th month salary if the performance bonus was received by the NGO. The most important incentive for the participating NGO is the 'output' budget which allows it a high degree of flexibility in the management of project funds as compared to the traditional 'advance and then cost-reimbursement against receipts' micromanagement. The focus on results, due to the 5% of the budget 'at risk' and the 5% or so 'award fee' will focus the managing NGO more on what it needs to achieve.

316

5. PERFORMANCE ASSESSMENT: INDICATORS

Every performance incentive scheme will need to use tools to assess the performance of a health care provider. Indeed, the distribution of the performance bonuses can only be done on the basis of accurate assessments. Yet, the assessment of the performance of a health care provider is complex; its role is multidimensional all the more so as you go up the health pyramid. It is necessary therefore to adopt a method to measure performance; defining the indicator and its data-collection tools and methods is an indispensable part of this approach.

In general, there is quite some confusion surrounding performance indicators. In principle, the appropriateness of the types of indicators is related to the performance framework. For instance, in Haiti or Afghanistan, the performance framework consists primarily of certain desired public health targets related to the catchment population (percentage of fully vaccinated children; percentage of women coming for their first antenatal care visit, percentage of women delivering in health facilities etc). In Afghanistan, once per year a balanced score card score composed of various elements such as the results from health facility surveys also impact on the intermediate bonus payments for the contracted non-governmental organizations. These performance frameworks function in a 'contracting-out' situation, in which non-governmental organizations are contracted to deliver a defined package of health services to a distinct population. Different performance measures exist in Rwanda. In Rwanda's health center Performance-Based Financing model a Fee-For-Service system for 23 services/indicators is impacted by a composite quality measure which consists of a checklist of 1,058 data elements from 111 composite indicators. In Rwanda's hospital Performance-Based Financing model, a balanced score card is used with 57 composite indicators, and over 350 data elements. In the Rwandan models provision of health care is through individual health facilities which are a mix of public and faith-based organization managed facilities and who are individually contracted by the Government and bilateral donors and their agents. Purchase of performance in Rwanda is through a 'contracting-in' arrangement and an 'internal market'.

The tools used in various Performance-Based Financing systems differ depending on the kind of approach and the monitoring and evaluation system pertaining to their idiosyncratic approach. However, and fundamentally, patient register books and individual patient cards form an important backbone of any PBF system. In fact it is very important in the design phase to avoid introducing indicators that are not commonly known by the providers and for which no registers exist. Also, indicators chosen would preferably need to be SMART,[18] should be collected by the HMIS, and be verifiable through community client surveys. This seems all logical, but practice shows a large misunderstanding of policy makers and technicians on the exact 'how to do's' in PBF systems. For instance, it is generally considered unwise to link an indicator to age or a socio-culturally stigmatizing condition. If you were to pay bonuses for all new malaria cases in children under five years of age, you will be unable to verify this result in the registers or the community and introduce perverse incentives for the provider to cheat (there will be many more children under five years of age than expected, and also many more malaria cases than expected). If you pay providers to find women with a vesico-vaginal fistula (a debilitating condition necessitating surgery), you might not find even one in a whole country over one year, although you offer a high premium for this (evidence: Rwanda). If you attempt to monitor and pay for improved quality of care through using documents, be aware that some tools are hard to use and easy to fake, for instance the partogram (a tool used to monitor the progress of women giving birth in a health facility).

5.1   Definition

It is useful to come back to the notion of an indicator. The definitions of an indicator are quite plentiful but the following may be retained: *an indicator is a statistic created in order to assess as objectively as possible certain activity dimensions of an actor.* Hence, an indicator helps to assess a state (today the health centre of such locality has two nurses) or a development (between year t and year t+1, the number of nurses will increase by 50%). It is also necessary to adopt a typology of the different indicators. Here too, the typologies are extremely many; the following will be retained:

Inputs	Process	Output	Outcome	Impact
Who is investing?	What has been done?	What has been provided?	Short and medium term results	Long term results
Human resources, Equipment, Supplies, Money	Training, Meetings, Workshops, Supervisory visits	Directives, Trained staff, Strategies implemented, Drugs distributed, number of service outputs	Know-how, Attitudes, Practices, Competencies, Behaviour, Politic	Social and economical well fare, Morbidity, Mortality
	Implementation		Results	
Input indicators	Process indicators	Output Indicators	Outcome Indicators	Impact Indicators

318

The input indicators: help to measure the resources at the disposal of the health care provider.

Example: the number of doctors in a certain health facility, the number of beds, the operational budget, etc.

These indicators are necessary to assess the efficiency of the actions carried out, for it is necessary to establish a link between the resources used and the results achieved. It could also be possible to design an incentive system that would incite the managers to make the best use of the resources at their disposal. A health insurer for example can incite a provider to lower its operational costs by resorting to outsourcing in order to diminish the reimbursement claim amounts.

The process indicators provide information on the professional practices applied during the different stages and tasks, as well as on the operational and coordination modalities of activities carried out.

Example: delay in obtaining an appointment, rate of completion of the medical file, number of days of stock-outs of essential drugs, etc.

If the incentive provider beliefs that these factors are prerequisites for obtaining good results he may attempt to reward health care providers that will make efforts to improve these indicators.

The output indicators help to assess the immediate and concrete consequences of the measures taken and the resources available.

Example: number of new family planning acceptors, number of new curative consultations, number of fully vaccinated children, etc.

These indicators reflect the level of productivity of the provider but they frequently fail to inform on the nature or quality of this production. These indicators are of particular interest to the incentive provider as he will attempt to incentivize these services as these are easier to measure and are mostly linked through a logical chain with outcomes and impact.

The outcome indicators: indicates the level of health outcomes for the patients.

Example: change in the health status of well being of the patients, the level of anaemia in children under five years of age, the level of stunting of children under five years of age, etc

These indicators are of particular interest to the incentive provider. This is what the incentive provider aims to achieve, however, these types of indicators cause measurement problems. For instance, these effects can only be measured through expensive surveys which are held at long intervals, in addition to leading to confidence intervals which needs interpretation; therefore the incentive provider cannot use these indicators if his purpose is to pay providers a regular performance incentive.

The impact indicators: assess the long-term effects on population health. It is obvious that these indicators are those that should primarily be of interest to the incentive provider. But these indicators are very difficult and expensive to assess. Moreover, it is not easy to disaggregate in population health status what is attributable to the financial incentive and what is attributable to other causes such as an improvement in the economy, or conversely poor harvests due to prolonged drought. Finally, impact is usually measured over long time periods; this is only weakly compatible with the short cycle of action and reward. For these reasons, the performance incentive mechanisms never retain impact indicators to distribute a reward to a health care provider.

Example: life expectancy, percentage of women suffering from breast cancer, maternal mortality rate, etc.

5.2   Quantity and quality indicators

In performance incentive mechanisms, we need to consider another characteristic of indicators, namely the difference between quantity and quality indicators. In some cases, the incentive provider may only be interested in getting the health care provider to always produce more. In this case, he will retain indicators that assess quantities. On the other hand, the incentive provider may also be interested in certain characteristics of the product (e.g. absence of nosocomial infections, relevance of the treatments given to patients, no complications after a surgical operation, etc.) or the production process (good conservation of vaccines, conditions of confidentiality during the post natal care visit, correct management according to the guidelines of the National Tuberculosis Control Programme, cleanliness of the pharmacy premises, etc.). For the incentive provider these elements may be considered essential since he assumes that these conjointly determine the quality of the care and services that will be provided. The incentive provider can then take that into account in determining the compensation to be given to the health care provider, and the latter will be encouraged to change his behaviours and practices. The objective therefore is not just producing more but also producing better.

Finally, the incentive provider may be interested in the satisfaction of patients and the population in general. For that, he will retain indicators assessing this satisfaction. The reward may then take into account these factors as well. For example if an indicator measures and pays the provider according to client perceptions on how he or she is treated, or how long he or she had to wait before being attended, the health care provider will most likely attempt to satisfy the client's perceptions.

5.3   Choice of indicators

In the face of a complex reality a single indicator or even a limited set of indicators will not make it possible to account for the results of a health care provider. In order to take into account the multiple facets of the action of this health care provider it is tempting to enlarge the number of indicators: indicators will be retained for vaccination, delivery, family planning, treatment of diseases, reception of emergencies, etc. The more the number of indicators is multiplied, the more the chances that each of the missions of the health care provider will be taken into account. It can then be affirmed that such care provider is efficient on such indicator, is less efficient on such other indicator and is not at all efficient on yet another indicator. The compensation provided by the incentive provider can take into account these performance differences. Finally, the approach, which is based on specific indicators helps to take into account a target to be attained: e.g., if we retain as indicator the number of assisted deliveries at the health centre, we can relate the number attained by a health care provider to the number that was expected to be attained.[19]

It is also useful to recall criteria used to define the quality of an indicator:

Quality criteria for a performance assessment

Attributes	Explanation
Comprehensible	• Clear (defined in a clear and uniform manner) • Placed in the context (explained) • Concrete (measurable) • Without ambiguity on the orientation
Pertinent	• In relation to the objectives • Significant and useful for users • Attributable to the activities
Comparable	• Possibility of comparison over time or comparison with other organizations, activities and standards

321

Attributes	Explanation
Weak	• Quite representative of what is measured (valid, not biased) • Of which the data required may be reproduced (verifiable) • Of which the data and analysis are devoid of error • Not susceptible for manipulation • Capable of balancing (completing) the other indicators
Practical	• Feasible at the financial level • Possibility of obtaining up-to-date and regular data

The multiplication of the number of indicators has several disadvantages. Apart from the fact that the collection of these indicators will be heavy and expensive, the multiplication of indicators of all sorts leads to a great difficulty of interpretation and especially prevents one from seeing the essential. Certainly, the latter disadvantage may be compensated by weighting the indicators, i.e. by assigning a significant difference to each of them, or balancing this weighting carefully. In a performance incentive mechanism, a concrete way of weighting indicators may consist in granting a lesser weight to the less important indicators or services and a more important weight to indicators or services deemed more essential.

On the other hand, it will not be possible to have a general idea of the performance of the health care provider, based on a juxtaposition of indicators of all sorts and of equal importance. One may, therefore, resort to a composite or synthetic indicator. A composite indicator is an indicator that aggregates different indicators into a single value. The interest of a composite indicator is obvious: with only one value, it is possible to compare the performance of various health care providers. The calculation of a composite indicator demands that particular attention should be paid to the following two points:

- Indicators which will be part of this composite indicator will obviously be valued in different units of measure. Example: percentage of medical files correctly filled out + number of assisted deliveries at the health centre + average number of laboratory tests conducted per person hospitalized. It is not possible to just add up these three indicators to come up with the average. One technique, therefore, consists in using a scoring system, i.e. a rating that helps to transform indicators with assessment units into addable scores.

- To take into account the unequal importance of the different indicators retained in the composite indicator, it is possible to use a weighting system. The latter are discretionary. In other words, it is up to the officials of the performance incentive mechanism to establish these weights. They will depend on the importance that these policy-makers attach to each of the indicators. Choosing indicators and weighing them is often difficult. Each stakeholder will have their favourite indicators and finding a consensus is time consuming and laborious. Nevertheless, there are some techniques and tools, such as the DELPHI method, that can make more efficient and transparent this decision making process.

Performance assessment becomes important when it is used for decision-making. The pupil will be attentive to his marks, since they condition his graduation to a higher class, the sportsman will attempt better scores in order to advance in his ranking, and the enterprise will look for better results in order to maximize profits. The search for performance is motivated by the benefits that one can derive from it and this is what will motivate individuals to make efforts to achieve the best performance. If there are no benefits attached to performance, individuals or organizations will just contend themselves with a minimal effort or decide to invest no effort at all. Consequently, in a performance incentive mechanism, the indicator becomes a stake. It is no longer as in classical planning an objective that one will try to achieve. It becomes the tool with which one can change the funding that will be made available to the health care provider. Hence, the latter will be attentive to the indicators that will be retained. It is not in the interest of the health care provider that the indicators retained are those where he knows he is not efficient. Hence, during the negotiation, and if the purchaser or incentive provider goes along with this, the provider will try to ensure that the indicators retained concern areas are those where he knows he is efficient.

We need to point out that these indicators should not be considered static elements. They need to be permanently redefined following the developments in each country. A scheme can include an indicator that is linked to an activity for which the results are very low (for example institutional deliveries); after a certain period this indicator can have witnessed a remarkable improvement and there might be reasons for dropping this indicator or change its weight in the total scoring system. On the other hand new indicators can be introduced: for example indicators that take into account activities related to Influenza H1N1, if the need arises.

It is difficult to imagine that we could establish a standard list of indicators valid in all the countries and applicable to all contexts. Nevertheless, it should be possible to come up with a list of essential indicators that could be a source of inspiration for schemes in a low income country context. This type of list could be established once a critical mass of empiric lessons learned is reached; this is not yet the case, although valuable experience has been gained with effective PBF indicators over the past ten years or so.

It should also be born in mind that the choice of indicators should be closely monitored by the incentive financier since wrong choices in indicators can produce perverse effects, conversely right indicators can lead to wrong choices made by providers; the box below gives some examples.

Examples of indicators

New curative consultations (new cases) reflect the utilization of health services by the catchment population whereas the re-attendances (old cases) can represent either a high level of follow up (which is positive) or an ineffectiveness of the treatment (which is negative); this indicator is vulnerable for falsifications or visits that are done as a favor; if the provider wants to exploit the situation, the patient can be asked to return as often as possible, even without a real need, or, the provider can re-classify a re-attendance visit, which is not paid under PBF schemes, under a 'new curative consultation' and make additional money.

Deliveries: in most developing countries the number of institutional deliveries is low. In order to decrease maternal and perinatal mortality, this indicator needs to be considered; nevertheless there is a risk that the provider will keep the future mother tightly in its grip in order to benefit from the incentive; to avoid this problem and to promote a better global follow up and care during pregnancy, the rewards can be distributed to the facility that receives the first visit but also to the facility that receives the pregnant women during a referral for more specialized care. The second risk in this particular case is that the first contact facility will become a simple gateway for referrals since it will get it reward for this.

Antenatal consultations: antenatal consultations (ANC) help to detect and prevent maternal and infantile health risk factors; using ANC visits as an indicator seems to be ideal for monitoring the follow up of pregnancies; however, women can make 3 ANC visits in three months, when it is recommended that there should be one visit every three months. In order to avoid confusion tetanus vaccination can be used as an incentivized indicator since it will be related to a certain interval between two ANC visits and to the regularity of services provided for the future mother; the incentive financier should cover these two activities - ANC visits and tetanus vaccination separately. Another solution would be to incentivize the pregnant women to make their first ANC visit during the first three months of pregnancy; indeed, the principal reason for failing to accomplish the recommended four ANC visits is that the mothers start their visits too late. Thus, incentivizing pregnant women to make their first ANC visit during the firs three months would be a way to sensitize them on the importance of accomplishing the four recommended visits.

---

6. HONOURING COMMITMENTS

Once a performance incentive mechanism using regulation or contracting or a combination of the two tools, has been put in place, it is necessary to consider the elements that will ensure that the two parties – the incentive provider (purchaser) and the incentive beneficiary (health care provider) – will comply with the mechanism. Indeed, it is important to recall the prerequisite that this mechanism cannot be imposed by the incentive provider. Hence, either the mechanism is completely established under a contract or it is established under a regulation, which should be accepted by the health care provider, and which will consequently be based on a contract. It is not possible to rely on command and control and its corollary the sanction to get the parties in presence to respect the new mechanism.

Honouring commitments is based on the credibility of the actors, reputation, confidence, and good faith. These contracts are 'self-enforcing'. In other words, it is in the interest of each party to respect the agreement if he wants to maintain his reputation and credibility. For example, if similar contracts are signed by all hospitals in the country, it is likely that some form of emulation will be instituted to promote the respect of commitments. Similarly on the side of the health administration the non-respect of commitments affects credibility. The administration will therefore witness a reduction of its influence due to the non-respect of the contract, for the memory of the latter will compel the health provider to protect itself rather than having confidence. This form of contract is particularly significant when the results of the contract are difficult to verify and when the parties to the agreement are in a predictable situation such as for example the donor and the health services or between the health insurer and the health care providers.

When the contract corresponds to a task to be carried out punctually, there is no reason for the contractual relationship to continue beyond that. It is therefore tempting for the contracting partner who should accomplish this task to adopt an unfavourable opportunistic attitude towards the other contracting partner. Only the threat of sanction may dissuade him. On the contrary some contracts are renewable unless particular events intervene. In this case the sanction will be imposed mainly at the end of the contract. It will be in the interest of the contracting partner who knows that his contract ought to be renewed to not to adopt opportunistic attitudes. This depends to some degree on whether he places himself in the perspective of an "automatic renewal" or rather a "renewal of the competition". Generally for contracts that are renewed it is in the interest of the contracting parties to comply with the terms of the contract and not adopt an attitude aimed at maximizing profit to the detriment of the other party. The theory of "relational signs" is in line with this logic: a partner will send to the other partner signs to show that he is worthy of his confidence and that consequently the contractual relationship may be pursued. The non-renewal of the commitment within the mechanism or even suspension of the contractual relationship amounts to sanction. It is not a sanction in the classical sense such as forcing commitments through a tribunal, but rather a suspension of the relationship between the incentive provider and the health care provider.

In reality commitments that are made in performance frameworks are generally of short duration. The results are appreciated over periods varying from one month to one year, but never beyond that. The commitment of the incentive provider and the health care provider alike is therefore limited to this duration. The incentive is therefore related to this short-term commitment and consequently should be repeated constantly. When the incentive is considered in relation to the direct achievements it is clear that there are no sustainable effects since the purchase act must be repeated all the time; the remuneration of time t+1 does not depend on remuneration at time t. The institution must therefore at each period renew its efforts in order to take advantage of the remuneration according to the activities carried out. On the other hand when the incentive is considered in relation to the production process, we can consider that once the behaviour change is attained the effect will be sustainable. For example, health personnel that have become habituated filling out medical files might continue doing this as a routine task. Yet studies show that, at best, behaviour change takes a lot more time before becoming sustainable and that quite often the disappearance of the incentive (the abolition of the bonus) will lead to a return to the status quo ante. This is because the incentive does not act on the underlying causes of non-performance. Hence, if the latter have not changed, we will find ourselves in a situation where the same causes produce the same effects. Behaviour change will only last for the period of the incentive, which mobilizes a particular effort with a "cost" for those who carry it out.

Moreover, so far we have been assuming that the health provider was an institution, and that all its composing elements would be sensitive to the same incentives. Yet, the interests of each of these elements are not the same. Let's assume a hospital: it is composed of three elements. First, there is the institution itself, then each of the units and, finally, each of the persons working in this institution. The hospital institution on the whole will be sensitive to any indicator that acts on its fame, whereas the staff of this institution will be less sensitive to that. The health institution will prefer incentives which are not tied to individuals, whereas the staff will be more interested in bonuses tied to individuals. The head of a unit will be interested in taking into account team work, whereas the staff will be much less interested in such. It is therefore important that the incentive provider pays particular attention to the elements to be encouraged. The choices to be made will have a major effect on the results obtained by the health institution. Indeed, if

326

the incentive provider decides that the benefits of the incentive be specifically reserved for staff bonuses, it is not meant for improving the situation of the staff but to ensure that the resulting motivation has an effect on the effort of the latter and, consequently, on the results that will be achieved.

7. ADVANTAGES AND DISADVANTAGES OF THE PERFORMANCE INCENTIVE STRATEGY

A strategy which uses incentives to enhance performance of health care providers in low income countries has many advantages, of which several have been mentioned above. The rare publications on this strategy often show highly favourable results, even if these studies are not exempted from bias. An important reason why publications are rare is that the approach is fairly new, less than ten years old, and therefore not much has yet been documented in the peer-reviewed literature. The objective here is not to question these results but rather to draw attention to the difficulties and risks that will surely appear when you want to implement this strategy.

7.1   Advantages

We will try to summarize below principal arguments in favour of using performance incentives:

1. **Provider enthusiasm**. In all supply-side PBF systems, the greatest proponents seem to be the providers themselves: whether the providers are the NGO managers, or the health facility managers. Both groups are positive about the increase in resources, and the freedom to determine where and how to use these increased resources. Whether to use it for improving the quality of services, for instance by purchasing missing equipment, or rehabilitating a building or an office, or to pay staff a bonus, or a mix of the two is up to the manager. Whereas policy makers, unacquainted or relatively unfamiliar with PBF systems, might strike a cautious note when one speaks with the end users who are the providers and practitioners in the field, one notes a high degree of engagement, and plenty of ideas and opinions on how to move forward with the current systems.

2. **Increased use of data throughout the system**. PBF systems provide a more limited set of data which are scrutinized much more carefully by all stakeholders than typically would be the case in non-PBF information systems. Data in PBF systems tend to be of a higher quality, more reliable, timely, and lead to managerial action, whilst being used at all levels in the system.

3. **More reliable data to work with.** Due to much enhanced data validation systems, which include rigorous data quality audits and surveys, data tend to be 100% complete, timely and reliable. This by itself is an enormous benefit of PBF information systems. Quite simply: if performance data are not available, there will be no payment.

4. **Focus on harmonizing and aligning HMIS systems.** PBF information systems tend to be innovative in the sense that these focus on limited data sets. In any given poor-country context, many parallel information systems exist, for project specific information needs and as a rule the national information system would be infamous for incomplete or unreliable data (which formed the impetus to create parallel information systems). Creating PBF data sets typically involve many stakeholders and always lead to intense discussions on what types of indicators to choose and how to monitor these. Such an intense discussion can form a fertile basis from which to contemplate existing information systems, and can lead to reforms attempting to harmonize systems (such as is the case with Rwanda).

5. **Improved Equity (certain projects).** PBF systems can improve equity in various ways. From an equitable financing point of view, PBF systems can take stock of other financial flows and correct certain imbalances if need be (by providing a higher budget to certain facilities, this is the case in for instance the Haiti RBF system). Second, in FFS style PBF systems, some providers have found that by decreasing the co-payment for a curative visit, they would get more curative consultations (for which PBF would pay a FFS), which would also lead to a higher number of preventive care services offered (for which PBF would pay FFS), as the port d'entrée in preventive care services frequently are the curative services. Small-scale household surveys done in Rwanda, DRC and Burundi show that such systems have the potential to lower the total household expenditure on health in catchment areas of PBF facilities (this would predominantly be achieved through health services of better quality, a higher uptake of preventive services, and an earlier consultation in case of a disease episode due to lowered out of pocket expenses combined with a higher quality of services offered). The incentive providers can also 'compensate' health providers by allocating a specific 'equity bonuses' over and on top of the PBF earnings, to provide these providers more money to improve their services faster.

6. **Community perceptions feedback**. Certain PBF systems such as in DRC, Burundi and Rwanda rely on community client surveys to (a) detract phantom patients and (b) to elicit feedback on the patient's perception of the level of quality of the services received. This feedback from the patients is communicated to the health center management and to the district/province

328

level. In CORDAID PBF systems, the community client survey results contribute to determining the level of bonus payments for the health facility (on top of the earnings from the FFS system).

7. **Focus on quality (various mechanisms).** PBF systems allow for including quality measures in the results/performance framework. Whereas most PBF systems have a singular focus on results expressed in increased coverage rates (typically increasing vaccination coverage of children less than five years of age, or women delivering in health facilities), quite a few PBF systems have sophisticated measures that attempt to measure various dimensions of quality. For instance in the Afghanistan PBF, a comprehensive balanced scorecard measures structural quality through a facility equipment list, among many other elements. In Rwanda, a quarterly checklist with 1,058 data elements checks a variety of quality dimensions in all health centers, leading to a quality score that impacts directly on the health center earnings (Quantity * % Quality = Earnings). In the Rwandan district hospital PBF model, a balanced scorecard focuses on processes, all attempting to measure and qualify, quality.

8. **Focus on innovative strategies (demand side interventions).** PBF systems are never static but are ever-evolving, based on lessons and insights learned during implementation. There is a push to 'do what it takes', to experiment and to find innovative solutions to barriers to access and to provide services. Quite a few PBF systems have started looking holistically at health systems, and have started adding demand-side interventions to complement the supply side interventions. For instance, demand side PBF which includes conditional cash transfer, or conditional in-kind transfer programs aim at attracting more beneficiaries to health services. It is thought to work by lowering the financial barriers to access services, by compensating beneficiaries partially for their costs to access services (these costs can be direct and indirect costs). Demand side interventions can also consist of health insurance schemes, such as in Rwanda, where health insurance has been made obligatory and over 90% of Rwandans can now access health services for a contribution of USD$ 2 per person per year. Health facility managers can decide to attract pregnant women to deliver in their facilities by for instance offering a 'welcome baby package' consisting of e.g. soap and baby clothes. Or managers can mobilize traditional birth attendants by paying them a fee for every woman that they bring to deliver in their health facility (they might pay $1 per woman, whilst they earn $5 per woman plus get kudos for achieving public health targets). In Rwanda, the MOH will investigate whether offering a large scale conditional in-kind transfer program would increase the coverage for certain essential mother and child health services.

7.2   Inconveniences

We will summarize below some of the major difficulties and risks related to the use of performance incentives:

1. **Assessment**: performance must be measured in order to qualify the difference between actual performance and the target, to know when corrective measures are necessary. The results of the assessment will generally be compared to the expectations expressed by a performance objective (which could be based on a better reference practice, a technical norm or some progress indicated in relation to a basic value). Performance assessments should, therefore, correspond to performance objectives and indicate how the organization meets its performance expectations. The complexity of performance assessment should not be under-estimated. This issue has already been tackled and will be further developed in the following paragraphs.

2. **Expected benefit**: performance assessment assumes all its importance when it is used to take decisions. The search for performance is guided by the expected benefits, and this is what will motivate institutions and the individuals working in these institutions to unleash efforts to achieve the best performance. If there are no benefits associated with performance, the actors might content themselves with minimum effort.[20] From the point of view of the incentive provider the benefit expected must be appreciated from the notion of net profit. Indeed, profits in terms of improvement of the performance of health care providers must be added to the costs incurred on establishment of the mechanism; costs for remunerating performance but also costs of surveillance of the mechanism. Yet, many studies have shown that these costs are often high and may call into question the overall appreciation of the mechanism and efficiency of the use of incentives. This analysis of net profit is not always conducted and we often content ourselves with the appreciation in terms of gross output. Certainly, in the context of developing countries these types of studies are difficult to conduct due to the lack of data. But the absence of these studies gives arguments to those who are reticent towards the strategy of performance incentives.

3. **Equity**: we should always consider that the health care provider is dealing with a population that does not need to be penalized for the poor performance of the care provider, especially when the latter has a de facto monopoly. It could even be said that the performance incentive mechanism may induce a double punishment: first of all, because of the poor performance of the care provider and secondly, since the latter has not been efficient, he will not have the necessary resources to improve his services. In this case, corrective measures

330

can be taken. Once the problem has been identified, conditional incentives can be used, these incentives would take into account the deficits (in equipments, in personnel) if the provider commits itself to make the necessary efforts for improving the performance.

4. **Context**: contextual factors are always difficult to take into account. Performance contracts are based on the principle that if a care provider has not been efficient it is because he did not make sufficient efforts. Although this effectively reflects the reality in many situations, there are also situations in which care providers have done their best, despite the constraints encountered: lack of necessary human resources, non-delivery of drugs, reduction in the income of the local population for economic or climatic reasons, etc. Rather than penalizing this care provider for not achieving the expected results, we should instead assist him to look for ways and means of correcting this contextual situation. Under these circumstances if performance agreements value the effort by taking into account the context, then these contextual factors may be mitigated. It is also true that incentive mechanisms can resolve problems that seemed to be unsolvable before. For example, in Rwanda before PBF was implemented, health centres sent their tuberculosis and malaria samples to the capital city for quality control, but they rarely if ever got the results back. When the PBF mechanism introduced an indicator related to the quality control of laboratory results the problem was solved. In fact, health providers took adequate measures to convince the national laboratory to execute their work and to ensure that the quality counter-verification results were sent back to their facilities. Also, it is always possible to integrate contextual factors into a performance incentive mechanism. For example, even if the indicators are the same for all of the providers nothing would forbid different values for the indicators. Some experiences have introduced coefficients for isolated facilities : for example if every new consultation is worth 1$, this could be increased to 1.2$ dollars for remote and isolated health facilities (this is currently the case in the Burundian PBF model);[21]

5. **Flexibility of the financing**: we need to ensure flexible financing arrangements. We cannot fully predict the level of budget execution (in effect, if the budget is consumed near 100% we have either done a brilliant job calculating and forecasting, or a lousy job because we have paid insufficient attention to financial risk forecasting but got it accidentally right). Hence, the financier will put in place mechanisms to ensure that he will be able to deal with the financial effects of an exceptional performance. On the other hand, in case of insufficient performance, the financier will be saddled with unused budgetary capacities, which may be reflected by a loss of opportunity, if the

financing is provided in the framework of the annual budgeting. Hence, to deal with this risk, it seems necessary to envisage compensation or reservation mechanisms that are excluded from the annual budgeting cycle. The techniques thus exist for responding to these situations; nevertheless, the decision makers need to keep in mind that they are not always easy to implement;

6. **Opportunistic behaviours**: performance incentives may lead to opportunistic behaviours in favour of the care provider but, not desired by the incentive provider:

    a.   One of the problems treated in the literature is "Gaming."[22] Since he knows that he is rewarded on his results, it is in the interest of the care provider to ensure that he will look good. The idea is not to cheat, i.e. make false declarations, but simply arrange, embellish the reality. The care provider may also, during the negotiation, insist that only indicators on which he is sure of getting good results are retained for the assessment. He may also negotiate for modest objectives, where he is sure of achieving results. Finally, he will concentrate his efforts only on activities that are assessed by indicators and neglect the other activities;

    b.   Another problem is "Dumping". It is in the interest of a care provider to get rid of clients with serious health problems and who, consequently, cost him a lot of money and, for whom it is (all things being equal) more difficult to achieve results. This health care provider is only interested in getting good clients, i.e. clients who are not expensive and through whom it is easy to achieve results: "cherry picking". Hence, the care provider will have a better performance and can earn a higher bonus;

    c.   The third problem is that of "multitasking". A health service provider is an entity that has several tasks which can be grouped in three categories: curative, preventive and promotional. When this entity allocates its resources between these tasks, it will often arbitrate between the costs of the tasks and the relative advantages. Same applies to the employees of this entity when it comes to their working time. If the implemented incentives pay for a certain task, the provider or its employee will be tented to shift their effort on this task on the expense of the other ones. This effect will produce more frequently when there is a task that is easily measured and by consequence rewarded and another one that is difficultly quantifiable and does not thus easily open to rewarding. This is why it is easier to reward quantitative aspects of an activity over its qualitative aspects.

The behaviours presented above, luckily, do not occur all the time. Those who wish to set up performance incentive mechanisms should however be aware of them; the objective of this document is to portray them so that they can be avoided. To avoid the effects mentioned above the incentive provider must ensure close monitoring of the contract. He must also assess the compliance of the behaviour shown by the care provider. Yet it is obvious that it is not easy to provide evidence and hence this surveillance will entail costs thereby reducing the profits from the contract for the incentive provider (purchaser). Besides this surveillance or monitoring is difficult to implement by the incentive provider, since there could be a conflict of interests (especially when working through a 'contracting-in' or 'internal market' mechanism). The function of surveillance should therefore be entrusted to a "neutral" body, on behalf of the contracting parties.

Finally, we should never lose sight of diminishing returns at the margin. Let's take the example of vaccinations in a health centre. It is obvious that not much effort need to be made to reach the first children to be vaccinated. Populations close to the centre might naturally come. On the other hand, it will be more difficult to reach certain children, particularly those living far away and those from the most disadvantaged families. The health centre should produce greater efforts to reach these children. It will have to put in place communication strategies, an advanced strategy, all of which require efforts and entail costs. Vaccinating all children under five years of age, demands increasingly greater effort.

In light of the above, a performance incentive mechanism should have a reward mechanism based on the logic of increased costs at the margin. Hence it is not really necessary to incentivize the provider to vaccinate the first children. They will be vaccinated without incentive anyway as they will present to the health centre. On the other hand, the incentive should be commensurate with the extra effort made to reach additional children, perhaps those in the last 20% or so that need to be vaccinated. Yet, all the performance incentive mechanisms currently put in place are functioning with constant monetary incentive. This approach assumes a constant cost at the margin which obviously does not reflect the reality. One consequence is that this constant incentive cost leads to an insufficient incentive in the real world. In any case, when it is less than the marginal cost, the health centre might quickly interrupt its efforts since the reward would be less than the cost of the effort. On the contrary, with a reward that increases with the effort the health centre might be encouraged to make a greater effort.

Let's take the case of vaccination of children under five years of age. The representation diagram is as follows:

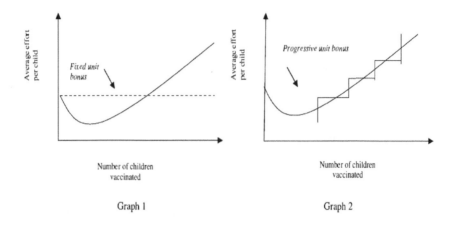

Graph 1   Graph 2

In Graph 1, the fixed unit bonus increases quite rapidly along the curve of the average effort; this means that quite rapidly the health care provider will have no interest in pursuing its efforts since the unit bonus is not sufficient compared to the additional effort that it should provide. On the contrary in Graph 2 the progressive unit bonus follows better the curve of the average effort and consequently it is in the interest of the health care provider to pursue its efforts. There are, however, some disadvantages in the progressive unit bonus approach. First of all, it can encourage the health care provider to cheat simply because its interest is higher than in the fixed unit bonus. Moreover, it can get the health care provider to overproduce. In the example given here – vaccination of children – this risk does not exist since the interest of the incentive provider is to ensure that all the children are vaccinated. On the other hand, if we take an indicator such as hospital inpatient days the hospital might not let the patients go, even if there is no real clinical need for hospitalization, in order to increase the number of total inpatient days.

Certainly, the establishment of a progressive rather than uniform compensation mechanism is not easy. First of all this progressiveness should no doubt be organized in stages. Moreover, it should be established through successive trial and error in order to test the adaptability of health care providers to this progressiveness. Such an approach is undoubtedly promising. With a constant budget, we should expect greater efficiency of the progressive reward mechanism, compared to a uniformed reward mechanism.

8. PERFORMANCE INCENTIVE MECHANISMS

The performance incentive mechanism is implemented within a particular institutional context. To understand its specificities it is important to review the development of the mechanisms observed during the past years. To simplify matters we should conceptualize that a health system performs three major functions: health care provision, health care financing and health administration. For a long time, in the public sector the State ensured these three functions. Health systems belonging to the State are deconcentrated services which receive their operational budget as defined by the central departments of the Ministry of Health. The 'Ministry of Budget' establishes the amount of the performance budget, the Ministry of Health is the fiscal officer, and the Ministry of Finance is the accountant of this expenditure. In the private sector, once their authorization to operate has been obtained from the health administration, health facilities operate with their resources (cost recovery, grants from donors and eventually a grant from the State).

A first series of reforms concern the notion of separating the provision of health services from other functions. Hence, we resort to autonomous health facilities and decentralization. Because of these reforms the Ministry of Health can no longer use conventional command and control in its relationships with public sector health facilities.[23] This separation of functions is never perfect especially due to the fact that, financially, public health facilities continue to depend largely on the Ministry of Health. Nevertheless, gradually the notion takes shape that the relationships between these health institutions, which still depend on the public sector but no longer directly on the health administration, must be based on a formalized agreement, i.e. a contract.

The establishment of the performance incentive mechanism opens a window of opportunity, which is based on two considerations:

- The financier, i.e. the incentive provider or purchaser, no longer produces virtually automatically his financing in favour of the health care provider. A mechanism is put in place to vary certain financing facilities depending on the efforts and, therefore, the results achieved by the health care provider. The incentive provider receives funding from either a development partner or the Ministry of Health. He will use these financing facilities as a means of exerting pressure to get health care providers to intensify their activities notably those he considers as priority activities.

- The incentive provider is not necessarily the Ministry of Health. PBF pilot projects are frequently initiated by development partners who establish the mechanisms. In other cases the lead is taken by the Ministry of Health with

335

support from development partners; this has been the case for example in Rwanda, Burundi, Ethiopia, Eritrea, Liberia and Afghanistan.

Consequently, the function of financing becomes a full-fledged function and should not be mistaken for the administration function. In reality, this new separation of functions is currently organized according to two models:

- Model 1: consists in putting in place complete separation between the two functions of purchasing and provision. To that end, a new distinct entity of the administration is created. This entity generally takes the form of a "Purchasing Agent";

- Model 2: the separation of the two functions results in the creation of two entities within the Ministry of Health: a unit in charge of health administration and a unit in charge of financing the provision of health services.

The creation of a central procurement agency raises a basic issue: who can play this role? A development partner may directly play this role. This is generally the case when a local experience is put in place. But to go on scale, the organization of health services must be formalized. We can then create a private law agency, a specific body grouping eventually development partners around the Ministry of Health. But it is generally a public law establishment created by the Ministry of Health to manage the funding intended for the provision of health services.

The entity or agency thus created may play a multi-purpose role. It may take on a general mission from conception to implementation of the mechanism or even that of verification (cf. above). But very often, the health administration reserves for itself, the conception of the mechanism and requests a specific entity to ensure the implementation.

Each of these two models has advantages and disadvantages, as summarized in the table below:

	Advantages	Disadvantages
Model 1: Purchasing Agent or private entity	- Separation of functions is clear - Independence, which facilitates greater efficiency in the implementation of the mechanism	- The public authorities lose their direct control over financing - The Ministry of Health is not usually well prepared for fulfilling the stewardship function - Implementation an administrative costs of this entity -The Ministry of Health does not want to part with this function

	Advantages	Disadvantages
Model 2: Service by the Ministry of Health 'contracting-in' approach	- No creation of a new external entity, hence possibly reduced costs - The health administration maintains considerable supervisory powers	- There is a risk that the separation of roles is only cosmetic,[24] since the health administration considers itself as the responsible authority

Besides, the introduction of performance incentives has created a new function in the organization of health services: that of certification. Indeed, performance incentives require that the output expected by the health care provider is verified, validated and certified. This can go through either one of the following methods, or a combination of these two:

- The care provider declares the results that he has achieved. He is paid according to the results he has claimed without further ado, and an external control is instituted (ex-post control, that is after payment for performance) to discourage fraud;

- Certification by an external controller of the results achieved before payment is done (ex-ante control). The care provider should, therefore, provide this controller with all the information he needs to accomplish his mission.

In all cases, it is in the interest of the care provider to give the impression that he has achieved high results: cheating[25]? Arranging the truth? The financial stakes are important for both parties. The health care provider expects the reward to finance certain actions (bonuses to staff, additional activities, etc.). The incentive provider wants to ensure that he does not disburse money (often public money for which he is liable) to finance imaginary or overestimated results.[26]

The agency theory *(cont'd)*

The agency problems are related to informational asymmetry. In other words, the agent has some information that the principal needs for remunerating at its just value the effort of his agent. But out of opportunism it is not in the interest of the latter to disclose all information fully.

Hence, the principal may be contended with the declaration of his agent, but he runs the risk that the latter does not reveal to him the correct information thereby compelling him to disburse more than necessary. This opportunistic behaviour of the agent may be penalized by the non-renewal of the contractual relationship, in case the principal discovers the fraud.

The behaviour of the agent will be determined by his risk aversion and the likelihood of detection of the fraud by the principal.

To avoid any opportunistic behaviour on the part of his agent, it is in the interest of the principal to put in place a mechanism for gathering sufficient information on the agent's performance. He will need to control the declarations of his agent or directly observe his behaviour. However, the agent, finding that the principal is both judge and defendant in this observation, may require that this control be made by an external entity.

The issue is identifying the entity that can perform this function. It could be conceivable that the incentive provider himself takes on this role. The advantage of this solution is that it might reduce considerably the costs of this function; however it is obvious that the incentive provider will then face a possible conflict of interest situation. This function may also be entrusted to the health administration. The latter has lesser conflict of interest, but is verification really its role? In playing this role, it interferes in the relationship between the incentive provider and the health care provider and can no longer play in all neutrality its main health administration role. On the other hand if this verification is coupled with the monitoring of activities then the involvement of the health administration may be justified. In this case the health administration takes advantage of the verification activity to initiate a real discussion with the health care provider on analysis of the causes of the outcome observed. This may result in an improvement of the situation.

The independence of the verifier is therefore absolutely essential. Who else could play this role?

- A foreign audit firm: it is the spirit of a scoring agency. This solution is no doubt the one that best guarantees (though not totally) independence. But this solution will obviously be very expensive and can be used only if the financial stakes are very important;[27]

- A national consultancy firm: the independence will be lesser and this solution is expensive;[28]

- A local NGO with which a contract is signed for this work. There is some experience[29] gained with this approach. It assumes that the NGO represents the voice of the population concerned by the activities of a given health care provider, and also assumes that the NGO is sufficiently impartial and that the results of its work will be credible. Nevertheless we may try to know whether this auditing and consequently policing role can be played by an NGO. Moreover, many NGOs are not channels for community voice since they are often organizations composed of a handful of individuals who can be easily influenced by external pressure;

338

- A "clients - patients" association: this solution is interesting for assessing client satisfaction and providing information to the incentive provider. But, they are not easy to put together and, in the poor-country contexts, they generally have several capacity constraints;

- A group of care providers from another region of the country: peer auditing has many advantages, notably the guarantee of having qualified persons to analyse the results produced by colleagues. But the disadvantage of this solution will be the relative independence of these persons. Indeed although coming from another region it is certain that they will know the persons whose performance they will have to verify. In fact it is never easy to challenge the performance of your colleagues (especially not when large sums of money depend on your assessment). Moreover, this certification may be vertical (conducted by peers of a higher level of the health pyramid) or horizontal (conducted by peers of comparable level in the health pyramid).

Furthermore, this issue of independence of the verifier becomes more acute when dealing with the financing of the verifier. In reality, this component is often entrusted to the incentive provider. This being the case it is clear that the independence of the auditor is not guaranteed. Undoubtedly, there is no perfect solution. The alternative solution is perhaps the one that consists in instituting a financing scheme that associates all the actors concerned by this mechanism: incentive provider, health care provider, health administration and development partner. In addition, it is extremely important that these mechanisms are operated transparently and that the results are known by all the stakeholders involved.

Certification is always an expensive function in the implementation of a performance incentive mechanism. The main actors of this mechanism, particularly the incentive provider, should be aware of that and ought to strive for a solution for achieving reliable results whilst balancing costs and risks. The balance is not easy and will depend a lot on the societal and cultural contexts. In any case, it will be necessary to compare the cost with the gross outcome of the performance incentive mechanism. The following equation may then be obtained:

Net profit = gross profit - (administrative costs of the mechanism + auditing costs)

Also, it may turn out that the health gains from a performance incentive intervention are only slightly positive, if not negative, once the costs induced by the implementation of the performance incentive mechanism are taken into account (although we do not have data on this yet).

The separation of functions in the organization of health services may be summarized in the diagram below:

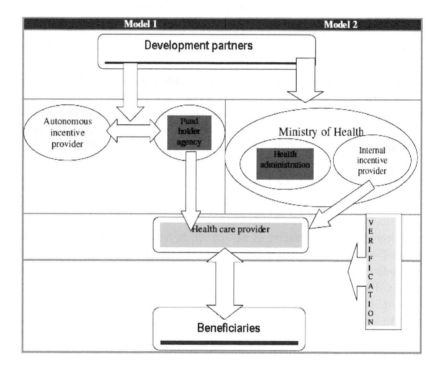

This figure indicates the different relationships that exist between the stakeholders in the context of a performance incentive scheme. The relationships represent agreements between the actors; these agreements are generally formalized in contracts. However, the nature of the contract will vary depending on the context:

- In some cases a classic contract will be used: an actor purchases services from another actor - both have their full legal autonomy : this is the case in model 1, where a purchasing agent belonging to the private sector through its statutes, "purchases" performance from a public or private health care provider. This type of arrangement is often referred to as "contracting out" situation or service delivery contract;

- In other cases the scheme will be based on internal contracting since the contract will be established between two institutions of a single legal entity. This is the case for model 2 where the contract is established between an internal incentive financier and a public health care provider that does not have legal autonomy. We can refer to this as a "contracting in" situation, and this concept is linked with the concept of an 'internal market' or 'quasi market';

- In some cases the contracting will be quasi-internal. This is the case when there are two separate public legal entities which are not fully independent. This type of situation is portrayed by the model 2 when the contract is between an internal incentive financier (an integral part of the Ministry of Health thus linked to the legal position of this Ministry) and a public health care provider that has a legal autonomy through its statutes (and thus has a separate legal position that is nevertheless linked with the public authorities (in different ways in different legal contexts)).

In reality the situation is often more complex and several types of relationships can cohabit.

9. A DIFFERENT VISION

In the preceding paragraphs we made the hypothesis that performance improvement depend mainly on incentives. The actors are not sensitive to the request for an increase in performance if this improvement of result does not lead to compensation, a compensation which is directly linked to the level of effort. Doing better because it is normal to always try and do better does not seem to reflect a normal behaviour. This focus on the link between result and financial encouragement is derived from an approach that places market mechanisms at the centre of the economic approach and which, consequently, seeks to please economic agents in a situation close to this logic within a paradigm built around value-utility and the theory that seeks to maximize its utility. Hence, the incentive is reduced to a form of purchase of an act/service produced by an economic agent. The impact of this incentive will be linked to the manner in which the agent expresses his preferences. Whilst sticking to this paradigm, we will attempt to look at non-financial factors whose importance is also acknowledged by economic actors.

What are institutions and their personnel prepared to do without hoping for an immediate and material reward? Several factors may help to achieve better results:

- Training: one can do better when one is better trained. Hence, better trained staff will be more efficient because they know better how to carry out their activities. Training enhances know-how. However, it is also observed that training is not always followed by improvement in productivity. Training is not always adequate and/or good quality, and therefore does not guarantee the improvement of know-how. In addition, know-how will only be reflected by a result when staff is capable of using and applying this know-how.

341

- Another method is based on performance assessment. The starting point is the analysis of the favourable factors and impediments to performance. Hence, performance assessment is used to identify the situation and the subsequent stages will be related to improving performance. This approach identifies strong points and weaknesses through an analysis of all variables that intervene in the production function. But what differentiates it here is the use of contracting. Two types of contracts could be imagined:

    - One consists in a situation whereby the two parties agree to provide solutions to the situation that has been analysed on the basis of the performance indicators retained. These two parties may, for example be a hospital and a health administration or the components of a hospital. The two parties both benefit from the agreement which is based on a strong dialogue on the means to improve the conditions for producing results;

    - The other consists in making a reward not only for the results achieved but also for the solutions that would have been proposed. Hence, if we retain an indicator like completing medical files, the reward does not only concern the number of well- completed files but also the measures taken for improving the completeness of the medical files.

In many performance-related approaches the incentives act directly on the outputs i.e. on the immediate performance but do not act on the causes that led to this outcome. Hence, just like the leaky barrels of Danaides, we might be forced to constantly provide incentives in order to maintain the best outcome. Changes are supported solely through the incentives and are artificial. If the incentive disappears the outcome will also disappear. To avoid that, this approach is often accompanied by funding modalities instituting the principle of service purchase. For health services, a large part of which is based on the logic of public good, this service purchase principle has some limits. It favours certain clearly identified services, the production process of which may be standardized, as for example vaccination. It is much less adapted to services like emergencies, which cannot be organized on a mere principle of pricing per activity. It is also much less adapted to complex medical care and support, which are developed with the ageing of the populations. [30] Finally, the analysis of the dynamics of organizations shows that the output is the result of the capacity to combine each of the variables that influences this output. This capacity is related to the management of organization methods and personal dynamics. In the above approach, the focus is on the fact that sustainable change requires that you act on the causes. Incentives are then mobilized on the one hand for identifying the causes and on the other, for implementing remedial actions. In such a strategy performance incentives are not used to obtain short-term outputs/outcomes but to analyse the causes of inadequate performance. Performance incentives will not be conceived as a mere reward mechanism leading to a mechanical response from the health staff, but as support for the change in practices. This type of approach needs to be based on trust between the contracting parties; this will build up progressively during the relationship and will consequently need time.

Is it possible today to steer away from a confrontation between the supporters (the champions) of incentives and those who, for some of the reasons discussed above, are fiercely (perhaps ideologically) against or are simply skeptical and are having some questions about it. One possible answer could be the following.[31]

An OECD study reminds us that while some studies show a positive effect of financial incentives on administration and civil servants, that others have pointed out that the effects on performance have been moderate or even negative. This conclusion is by no means a reason for abandoning performance incentive mechanisms. These mechanisms should not bee seen trough the simple mechanical effect of increasing individual remuneration based on the result. Implementing performance incentives always induce, more or less strongly (depending on the design), a change in the health system. A performance incentive mechanism will bring about a redefinition of the objectives of an institution, it will facilitate the dialogue between the different components of the institution and with the authorities, it will facilitate the evaluation of results by introducing explicitly defined indicators, it will stimulate the monitoring of the activities, etc. The reward that comes with performance incentives should be seen as a catalyst that will enable this transformational change, or reform of the health administration. The effect of the reward does not depend on the financial motivations of the staff; it affects the performance through the organizational and managerial changes that this strategy provokes.

These arguments could help to better understand the current situation in Rwanda. Indeed, the recent improvements in health service provider performance seem to be undeniable, even though there could be room for some discussion on the exact figures. On the other hand, it is also clear that there is no more room for the explication according to which all of the improvements were due to the implementation of "Performance-Based Financing"; we know that there were several other administrative reforms implemented simultaneously such as decentralization with performance contract written between the President and his Mayors; making health facilities more autonomous; decentralizing salary budgets of health staff) and the scaling up of community based health insurance. These reforms are factors which have contributed to the enabling environment in which PBF was scaled up as a national strategy. Nevertheless, this does not mean that PBF did not have its place in the performance improvements. Indeed, the introduction of PBF was also an opportunity for implementing important managerial and organizational changes. For example PBF has brought along profound modifications such as better definition of health service providers' objectives through the definition of indicators and their valuation, redefinition and redesign of supervision and monitoring functions for provider activities, and a revaluation and recognition of the health workers' effort and results (intrinsic motivation).[32]

The main question that should be asked is thus to know if similar results could have been obtained by focusing only on these reforms without using performance related pay (in the form of variable revenue bonuses).

CONCLUSION

The notion of performance opens new avenues for improving the practices of health care providers and consequently for getting them to contribute more to the health of the populations. But as shown in this chapter, the technical and methodological problems are important and far from being completely resolved. Beyond these difficulties, the main issue is certainly political acceptance which may be viewed at two levels:

At the content level: performance is related to the adoption of the market logic, which is not accepted by all. The vision, according to which the public service mission guides activities to be accomplished with the resources available, is still strong in countries where this notion is part of the values of the social pact. Yet such a vision is hard to reconcile with an approach that reduces the notion of performance to the sole achievement of specific objectives, and which depends on internal motivation only to produce results. Certainly there is a vast movement of reforms at the level of the administrations which largely adopt strategies such as "results-based management ". It is therefore necessary to go beyond health and see how these reforms are accepted on the whole by the State. The acceptance for other public good services such as justice, education, police or even the national defence;

At the strategy level: even if a Ministry of Health may be personally convinced about an approach using performance incentives, it may also fear the social consequences of such a reform. The change of social relationships is so profound that reluctances and resistances will be all the more intense since actors will have the feeling of losing part of their well-being (or perhaps their degrees of freedom). Undoubtedly, such a reform must be implemented by allowing sufficient time; time for discussion but also time for negotiation and experimentation before a nationwide scale-up is contemplated.

Despite the limitations and the doubts, there is an unavoidable movement towards implementing approaches that promote health service provider performance. It is too soon to judge how these approaches will fit in the spectrum of reforms that target health system performance improvement. However, the early results allow us to assert that the schemes need some refining and if there is an approach that becomes preeminent it is probable that it will not be the only one. Improving health service provider performance will need to be based on a combination of several approaches which all have their specificities but which seem complementary. The specificities of each country will determine the way the combination of approaches will be implemented. Indeed, the evolution of health systems will be guided by several concomitant reforms. In this scenario it is difficult to attribute the results to one of these reforms. It is also probable that certain combinations of reforms will yield better results than others. Thus one would think that performance incentives will be more effective if other actions are taken at the same time. For example, performance incentives will be more effective if at the same time the autonomy of the providers is reinforced or if there is an intervention improving drug supply.

This annex groups and describes three experiences of performance incentive.

Experience of Haiti

USAID, through Management Sciences for Health (MSH), has provided financial support for many years to local NGOs operating in the health sector in Haiti. These NGOs are owners of health facilities (notably Health Centres) which they manage. Until 1999 financial supports to these NGOs followed the classical logic: an amount was budgeted at the beginning of a period and the NGOs had to justify the expenditures they had incurred during the execution of their project. The objective was to finance the necessary inputs for carrying out health related activities.

In 1999, MSH introduced a new logic based on results. A pilot experience with three local NGOs, serving 534,000 people was launched. During this period, the mechanism was based on a contractual agreement between MSH and these three local NGOs. MSH agreed on a budget required for carrying out defined activities. This in fact was no more or less the historical budget (from the previous year). In the course of the fiscal year, MSH would pay by instalments 95% of this budget without asking for financial documentation of all minor expenses and allowing the implementing partner NGO to manage the various budget lines with fair degrees of freedom (it wrote an output based contract of a type called 'fixed price plus award fee schedule'). 5% of the historical budget was put 'at risk' that is, the implementing partner risked losing it when their performance would not reach pre-agreed basic performance results. Also 5% additional 'bonus' or 'award fee' was budgeted, which the implementing partner could gain if performance was exceptional. At the end of the year, and after evaluation MSH:

- would not pay the remaining 5% if the results were not sufficient;

- would pay the 5% if basic results were achieved;

- would pay 5% on top of these 5% if all performance results as stipulated in the contract would have been achieved.

The change of logic is therefore profound. MSH was not interested in how the implementing partner managed to achieve the objectives defined at the beginning of the period. It is up to the implementer to organize itself with the resources at its disposal to be the most efficient ...including by motivating its staff.

Two points of this mechanism must be underlined:

- objectives to be achieved are defined at the beginning of the contractual period: one-year contract;
- The performance bonuses are part of the ordinary budget and consequently the issue of use of the bonuses does not arise.

To determine the performance of NGOs, the following indicators are retained:

Indicators	Objective	% of the Bonus
1. Women using oral rehydration therapy to treat diarrhoea episode in children	15% increase	10%
2. Children aged 12 -23 months fully vaccinated	10% increase	20%
3. Pregnant women who have had at least 3 prenatal visits	10% increase	10%
4. Rate of abandon of injectable oral contraceptives	25% reduction	20%
5. HCs proposing at least 4 modern FP methods	100% of HCs	20%
6. Average waiting time for child consultation	50% reduction	10%
7. Participation in UCS and coordination with the Ministry of Health	Defined by the UCS	10%

The first 5 indicators concern the increase of the health services. Indicator 6 relates to the satisfaction of clients and indicator 7 to the level of community participation and coordination with others.

The results obtained by each of the NGOs were not declared by these NGOs but calculated by the *Institut haïtien de l'enfance* (IHE), through population-based surveys.

Since 2005 this experience has been scaled up to include 32 NGOs working for an estimated catchment population of about 2.8 million people. These NGOs were selected by MSH on the basis of their capacities to carry out the defined activities.

Factors taken into account include their organization, human resources, information system, financial management, management of drugs, etc.

Since 2005, the system has changed a bit. It may be summarized as follows:

Elements	% of the annual negotiated budget
On signing the contract	10%
Upon receipt of the annual action plan	15%
Upon receipt of the annual report	1/12 of 10% of approved budget each month
Request for quarterly payments	20% in March 20% in July 13 % in October 6% in November
80% of children under age 1 fully vaccinated (target for all NGOs)	1.5%
50% of pregnant women who paid at least 3 prenatal visits (target for all NGOs)	1.5%
Random choice of 1 indicator from the following list:	3%
– 50% of children under 5 were weighed	
– 63% deliveries were assisted by a trained staff	
– 44% of women who delivered received one home visit	
– 50% of pregnant women were tested for AIDS during a prenatal visit	
– 75% of new TB patients were also tested for AIDS	
– Timely submission of quarterly reports	
– Supervision system with defined criteria is in place	
Additional bonus if all above targets have been attained	6%
Maximum possible	106 % of the negotiated budget

Today, the mechanism is defined by the incentive provider -MoH- in consultation with the NGOs. We have therefore gradually moved from a system largely based on contracting to a system based on a rule defined by a development partner, as the contractual aspect is limited to a subscription contract established between the MoH and NGOs acknowledged as capable of being part of the mechanism.

This experience, apart from being among the first to have adopted the performance incentive mechanism, poses some problems. The approach based on targets to be attained has some consequences. Indeed, there is no incentive to maximize efforts but simply to maximize efforts to attain the targets set. For example, when we have attained the target "50% of children below 5 years have been weighed" it is in our interest to limit the efforts on this target and transfer these efforts to other targets.

What encourages NGOs to attain the targets set is not so much the financial bonus that can be derived from it but the non-renewal of the contract of the NGO, when the latter has not attained the targets defined. The sanction is, therefore, exclusion from the output based financing scheme rather than the non-payment of the bonus.

The budget of the health facility and the bonus received through MSH, which complement other sources of financing of health activities of these facilities, cover all activities of the health facility, whereas the indicators retained only concern certain activities. Consequently, such a system encourages implementers to adopt opportunistic behaviours, whereby they accord priority to efforts related to the indicators retained and do not make any effort on activities not related to an indicator of the mechanism.

Experience of Mali

In 2007, when Mali decided to institute a performance incentive mechanism in hospitals, the context was as follows:

- the country had 12 regional and national hospitals, mainly public hospitals (one hospital had the status of a private foundation, for historical reasons);
- since 2002, public hospitals have the status of "Public Hospital Establishment (PHE)", which gives them an autonomy in the legal sense, with, consequently, the possibility to sign contracts at their level;
- there is a National Hospital Evaluation Agency (ANEH), which, as a public institution, can conduct independent evaluations;
- the "project establishment" system is ongoing, enabling hospitals to have a vision of their future and strategies to be implemented;

-   the operational budget of these hospitals is prepared on the basis of an annual planning called "operational plans" (OPs).

Despite these reforms, the performance of hospitals is still inadequate. Because of an inadequately rigorous management, the following constraints are observed:

-   stock-outs of essential drugs are frequent
-   recovery of incomes is far from being total
-   medical files are not always completed
-   intra-hospital mortality remains high
-   hospital wastes are not always managed according to established standards
-   users are not always satisfied.

In the face of this situation, the Ministry of Health wished to institute, with the support of the World Bank, a performance incentive mechanism. The Ministry of Health entrusted to the ANEH the mission of developing a system in consultation with the hospitals. Several meetings were organized with the hospitals to discuss the mechanism to be put in place. Through targeted incentives, the Ministry of Health, as an incentive provider, wanted to encourage institutions to change their behaviours and practices. The Ministry of Health does not impose changes. It proposes to use incentives to make hospital institutions aware of the interest in changing their behaviours and improving their performance. No target is defined initially. Incentives are built in such a way that hospital institutions have every interest in maximizing their efforts in order to attain the highest level of performance with the resources at their disposal. The mechanism retained is based on the following approach:

-   the Ministry of Health, in agreement with the Ministry of Finance, adopts a budget line entitled *Special Grant for the Performance of Hospitals*. This line will be fully distributed to hospitals that will have accepted to participate in the mechanism. To mark their support, the hospitals should sign a contract entitled "*participation in the mechanism of award and use of a special grant to hospital establishments with the objective of improving upon their performance their performance, measured through a series of indicators*";

-   the share allocated to each hospital will depend on the results they will have achieved on a number of criteria, but also on the performance of the other hospitals. For better understanding, the situation can be illustrated with the picture of a cake. The size of the cake is defined at the beginning of the process, and, consequently, the size of the share a hospital will receive will depend on these efforts, but also the efforts of the other hospitals participating in the mechanism. To mark this interdependency, it was retained that only one contract should be signed between the Ministry of Health and hospitals that have agreed to participate in the mechanism;

- the originality of the approach retained by Mali relates to the fact that the contract signed between the Ministry of Health and the hospitals covers not only the distribution of the performance bonuses but also the utilization of the amounts received;

- the mechanism explicitly targets hospital institutions and not their staff. Hence, the mechanism stipulates that the amount received by the hospital cannot be used to pay bonuses to staff. It should also not form part of the operational budget of the hospital. The amount should be spent on collective actions, which are clearly an addition. For example, with this amount, the hospital can buy a television set for the room for staff on night duty or an equipment, which was not provided for in the operational plan.

Over time, the mechanism is as follows:

Contract

Previous Year	1st Year	2nd Year	Subsequent Year
Budget	Production of results	Allocation of the grant	Control
Subscription			
Signature	Collection and verification of results	Use of the grant	External evaluation

The contract between the Ministry of Health and hospitals that had agreed to participate in the mechanism was signed for two years. During the first year, the hospital produces its efforts and at the end of the year, the results achieved can be assessed. During the second year, the relevant grant is paid to the hospital and the latter has the rest of the year to use the grant according to the plan established at the beginning of the contractual period.

Before entering into the contractual period, certain prerequisites have to be met: inclusion of the item in the budget of the subsequent year, declaration of subscription to the mechanism from hospitals and signing of the contract.

During the year following the signing of the contract, certain controls must be carried out (e.g., the efficient use of the grant by the hospital) including, eventually, some external assessments of the mechanism put in place and the results achieved.

At cruising speed, there are always two projects ongoing, as shown in the table below:

	2007	2008	2009	2010	2011
Contract signed end 2006	1st Year	2nd Year			
Contract signed end 2007		1st Year	2nd Year		
Contract signed end 2008			1st Year	2nd Year	
Contract signed end 2009				1st Year	2nd Year

Indeed, it is not necessary to wait for the end of the second year of the contract to initiate a new contract. A hospital must constantly make efforts to improve its performance.

In this mechanism, the ANEH is in charge of collecting data, verifying their accuracy and calculating the grant to be paid to each of the hospitals that subscribed to the mechanism.

To assess performance, the mechanism retained 14 indicators, which are frequently produced in the framework of the monitoring of the planning and budgeting. Some of these indicators relate to the inputs and the production process: e.g., *"Rates of conformity of medical files"* or *"Number of days of stock-outs of essential and generic drugs"*. Other indicators concern the results achieved by the hospital: e.g., intra-hospital mortality rates (measures by the number of patients deceased at the hospital / total number total of patients admitted at the hospital) X 100).

The method for calculating the grant is described in detail in the *"Manual of procedures for implementation, under contract, of the mechanism for improving the performance of hospitals"*. All these 14 indicators are grouped under a synthetic indicator, which presents a general picture of the performance attained by each of the hospitals. It is this synthetic indicator that is then used to calculate the grant for the hospital.

It should suffice to mention that this performance mechanism was put in place. The contract of the first year was signed and the hospitals pledged to improve the indicators retained. Thereafter, the process was stopped. There is no point attempting to explain the reasons for this situation. However, it may be underlined that the establishment of such mechanisms requires a strong political commitment, which was lacking during the implementation of the performance mechanism in Mali.

Experience of Rwanda at the level of the health centres

Two main observations led some development partners to launch performance incentive experiences at the level of health centres:

- the activities of the health centres were inadequate and population was suffering from a lack of access to services, and poor quality services;

- The health staff were poorly paid, unmotivated, and therefore, inefficient and lesser effective. Notwithstanding significant salary 'top-up' payments by NGOs, there was no measurable result in population health.

Two experiences were launched in 2002:

- A pilot project was initiated in the Cyangugu province with the support of the international NGO, CORDAID. Two districts were concerned, with a total population of 620,000 inhabitants;

- A second pilot project was initiated in the Butare province with the support of the international NGO, HNI-TPO. Two districts were concerned, with a total population of 384,000 inhabitants.

By mid- 2005 a pilot project was initiated in the Kigali region with the support of the Belgian Technical Cooperation. It concerned five districts, with a total population of 1,402,000 inhabitants. Under this project, the Contractual Approach Support Unit (C.A.A.C.) was created.

From 2006 the Ministry of Health decided on the one hand, to gradually extend the performance incentive approach to the entire country and on the other hand, to harmonize the practices by adopting a single model.[33] The main elements of this model, called "Performance-based Financing (PBF)", are presented below.

The logic is the same as for the other incentive projects. It involves improving the performance of health centres using an incentive strategy. On the other hand, Rwanda's PBF experience is different from an implementation point of view.

The Ministry of Health, more specifically the Contractual Approach Support Unit developed with strong and consistent support of partners a national performance incentive mechanism. This mechanism recalls the principles and establishes in detail all the implementation modalities of the mechanism. The health centres are free to subscribe to this mechanism. The subscription is done through a standard contract in which the health centre indicates that it acknowledges and accepts the mechanism, and the Ministry of Health pledges to pay the amounts due. This contract is part of the tools defined in the mechanism. It is therefore only a contract on a subscription to the national performance mechanism; there is no possibility for negotiation.

The contract is presented as a purchase contract, namely that the incentive provider – the Ministry of Health – pledges to purchase the production of the health centres.[34] This production is defined according to a number of priority indicators focussing on mother and child health.[35] 14 indicators are currently retained:

- *number of new cases in curative consultations*
- *number of new antenatal care attendances*
- *number of pregnant women with 4 antenatal care visits*
- *number of pregnant women who have received the 2nd, 3rd, ... anti-tetanus vaccination*
- *number of pregnant women who have completed the 2nd dose of Sulfadoxine Pyrimethamine*
- *number of pregnant women referred before the 9th month*
- *number of children aged 12 – 59 months consulted at the health centre*
- *number of women newly registered for modern contraceptive methods*
- *number of users of modern contraceptive methods*
- *number of children fully vaccinated*
- *number of assisted deliveries at the health centre*
- *number of women referred for delivery*
- *number of children aged 0-59 months referred for severe malnutrition*
- *number of other referrals (other than for delivery, antenatal care and severe malnutrition)*

For each of these indicators, a price is defined in the mechanism. For example, the health centre knows that for each new case in curative consultation, it will receive FRW 100. It should however be noted that the prices do not necessarily refer to a notion of cost of the activity. It is rather an amount arbitrarily decided taking into account budgetary possibilities and as assessment what could be considered as adequately motivating. This assessment was done by a panel of experts, deliberating on the relative value of a health service in relation to public health targets.

There are therefore no targets to be attained. It is in the interest of the health centre to maximize its efforts in order to maximize profits.

354

The indicators therefore refer to quantities. However, the performance mechanism takes also into account the quality of services provided by the health centres. Hence, a composite index is calculated. It takes into account factors like *"existence of cleaning products"*, *"do the beds have mattresses with covers that are intact?"*, *"absence of dispersed wastes "*, etc, or about 1,085 such data elements, through 111 composite indicators covering 14 services, and yields one composite quality percentage.

The revenue that a health centre may obtain from performance is calculated as follows:

Revenue = $\sum$ (Quantity x Price) x % Quality [0-1]

From an operational point of view: controllers from the district health administration pass by the health centre each month to control at the source the monthly invoice. After control and validation, these controllers bring the validated invoices to the district. The Hospital separately applies the quality supervisory checklist once per quarter. Both data sets are entered into an internet-based management information system, a 'real time database'. Once per quarter, district PBF steering committees discuss and validate the 'quarterly consolidated PMA and HIV invoices' in the obligatory presence of civil society actors and purchasing agents. The validated paper invoices are compared with the printed invoices from the database, and eventual data entry errors are noted, documented, and corrected. After approval, the signed quarterly consolidated invoices ('consolidated' refers to the fact that the quantity has been consolidated/merged with the quality measure) together with the minutes of the meeting are sent to the CAAC, which does due diligence; it verifies whether processes have been followed as required through the procedures manual. After due diligence a national payment order is printed from the database, and sent to the Ministry of Finance for payment (payment goes directly to the bank accounts of the health facilities). Once per quarter, an independent third party carries out community client surveys following a national protocol. Its purpose is to (a) detract phantom patients and (b) to elicit feedback from the community. Results are communicated to the clients, the health centres, the district and the national level. After four such community client surveys, less than 5% of clients reported in the registers cannot be traced in the community, which is an encouraging finding. Also, important information related to the quality of care of certain health centres is obtained and action is being taken by district directors to correct eventual anomalies. In addition, once per six months, a national protocol to counter-verify the quality of care measured at health centres is carried out.

The performance mechanism details how performance incentives are allocated, but is almost silent on the use of these performance bonuses by the health centre.

The standard contract, which is signed stipulates simply: *Article 11: "The use of the revenues earned with the performance-based financing strategy is left to the discretion of the Management Committee of the health centre".* However, in Article 5, it is said: *"reserve at least 25% of the revenues of the PBF for the operational expenses of the health centre".* Consequently, up to 75% of the revenues may be used to pay bonuses to staff. Indeed, we should not lose sight of the fact that the logic of this mechanism is as follows: it is necessary to enhance the motivation of the staff working in health centres predominantly in the form of bonuses, in order to effectuate a performance enhancement by the health institution. There are few collective performance bonuses to be used by the institution for interventions other than performance bonuses (stipulated at about 25%). This approach somehow focuses unilaterally on the presumption that if we incentivize institutions directly, but indirectly its staff, that this will lead to an improved performance.

Presently, on the average, the revenues of the PBF represent between 25 and 30% of the budget of the health centre (50% come from the Ministry of Health for payment of salaries and 25-30% from cost recovery, notably through mutual health schemes). The monthly bonus supplement often represents between 50-100% of the salary of an employee (depending on the combined effects from various sources of income).

Experiences similar to those of Rwanda were initiated in 2006 in Burundi and the Democratic Republic of Congo. Moreover, development partners that are supporting these experiences are practically the same as those that initiated the first experiences in Rwanda.

Conclusion

It is interesting to observe that the three experiences presented above follow the same logic of using performance incentives to enhance the performance of health workers.

However, they use quite different methods to apply this logic.

Furthermore, the stability of the political context, in which they are implemented, is an important question. Contracting, in its "contracting out" form, is no doubt more appropriate in unstable countries (Haiti, but also Afghanistan, Liberia, Burundi, Democratic Republic of the Congo) than in the more stable countries (Rwanda, Mali) in which the Ministry of Health has the capacities to steer the performance incentive scheme.

Notes

[1] The below is translated from French. From the Merriam-Webster Online Dictionary: there are two definitions, one is 'the execution of an action', the second 'something accomplished'. The former is a 'deed', the latter a 'feat'.

[2] Some quantitative measures are excellent proxy performance measures; for instance the rate of nosocomial infections. However, the challenge is to translate such measures in actionable items through which to influence provider behavior. In poor-country settings where one aims to pay health providers regularly based on regularly and reliably measured performance results, measures such as the rate of nosocomial infections are simply not realistic.

[3] Effort = concentration of the physical, intellectual or moral forces with a view to achieving an aim.

[4] A distinction is made in the literature on intrinsic and extrinsic motivations: Intrinsic motivation is related to the fact that one exercises an activity for the pleasure and satisfaction that one gets from it. An intrinsically motivated individual carries out activities voluntarily driven by interest in the activity itself without expecting payment for it.
- extrinsic motivation is defined by the fact that the individual is working in order to obtain a consequence that is exterior to the activity itself; for example, receiving a reward or esteem are extrinsic motivations.

[5] This cost-benefit analysis is of course quite difficult to execute. Identifying the cost is not easy, and determining the benefits is even more complicated; unless using DALY type of instruments, it will be difficult to measure the benefits of a vaccination or of multiple preventive activities. Measuring the incremental health gains from much improved quality of services would also cause a challenge for health econonometrists.

[6] Also called 'inputism'

[7] We shall later in this document that the incentive provider's proposition can be more or less compelling, and, in some cases, it will be comparable to an imposed regulation that will leave the providers with little choice.

[8] In this case the implementation manual will be integrated in the contract and will be the same for all participating providers.

[9] In certain cases, the scaling up can be done by conserving the different modalities and functioning mechanisms in different geographical areas. This situation is in general transitory and it precedes the adopting of a general set of rules for the country. Moreover, in some cases a development partner sponsoring a specific intervention can accept the national rules but still implement a specific contract between itself and the providers in its intervention area: for example MSH and other US government financed purchasing agents in Rwanda, or Cordaid, HNI-TPO and the Swiss Agency for Development and Cooperation in Burundi.

[10] The administrative modalities of this type of arrangement will of course have to be specified.

[11] However, in the Rwanda scheme, the payment for performance for HIV services is linked to the level of quality of general services: the higher this quality the more will be reimbursed, the lower the quality, the lesser will be reimbursed.

[12] However, when the incentives are not financial, they are not meant as a provider payment method and have a different impact on provider behavior. This distinction is crucial.

[13] We assume here that the health care provider is the health care institution, for instance a health center or hospital. The 'health care provider' is then synonymous with the management of this institution.

[14] The reward has to be perceived as something that is directly linked to the performance incentive scheme.

[15] Terminology: **Inputs** are resources that you put at the disposal of your project for its direct implementation. They include time, money and premises. **Outputs** are the services offered. They comprise the number of services produced, training, the supervision, and the advanced strategies undertaken. Some of these are processes (such as the 'supervision' or 'training'), but can also be put under performance schemes. **Outcomes** are all the changes and effects induced by your work. **Impact** concerns a more enlarged and long-term horizon. It concerns your own objective. It may be very difficult to appreciate the long-term changes in a short-term project.

[16] In the Cordaid PBF pilot schemes, which cover distinct geographical areas such as a province or a district with a given population, the quantities to be purchased have been made overt through the business plans, and form part of the negotiated contract. This allows the purchaser to send out signals of what he wants to purchase, and presupposes a perfect knowledge from the purchaser side on the public health situation in the province or district. If such a system is scaled up to the national level, perfect information on baselines, and differing implementation modalities (through government instead of through an NGO) make such approaches more difficult or costly.

[17] The most powerful intervention in NGO financing here is not really the bonus...it is paying NGOs output-based budgets instead of input based ones...they do not have to stick to budget lines, and can freely move around money in their negotiated budgets, without having to ask the donor for permission every time they want to shift money from let us say salaries to other inputs such as trainings or so. This is also the case in Afghanistan's Performance Based Contracting. The performance bonus in these types of approaches is much hyped, but really, and in reality, it is the different way of financing providers that is of importance here. Conceptually, the difference between the PBC and the PBF approach is, the level of intervention: for PBF (Haiti and Afghanistan and Cambodia) it is the NGO, whereas in PBF, it is the health facility. NGOs in Haiti and Afghanistan still manage their health facilities through 'inputism', whilst they themselves are under a donor performance scheme. But in reality, these performance bonuses, awarded perhaps once per year, do rarely if ever reach the health workers on the frontlines. This is why for instance in

Afghanistan, the new phase of PBC involves stipulations that the much enlarged performance bonuses for at the least 50% need to reach the health workers.

[18] SMART: Specific; Measurable; Achievable; Realistic and Time-bound. In Performance-Based Financing there is a further departure and specification of the term 'SMART'; not all SMART indicators can be purchased...this is due to the peculiar fact that one attaches a financial incentive for each service, and as a consequence, the actual provision of such a service might become unreliable. The purchaser has to put into place mechanisms to verify performance using community client surveys. Some on the face of it 'SMART' indicators, might prove to be less SMART as the actual service might become hard to verify using community client survey techniques due to recall bias or ignorance of the client or surveyor on the exact elements of this service.

[19] For a basic package of health services, offered in health centers, about 15-20 services are purchased in PBF systems. The quality measures of these services, which impact on the payment for performance in various ways and degrees (either as a stick or a carrot), can consist of a multitude of these indicators, up to hundreds of indicators and composite elements, as these attempt to measure process of care (or 'quality of care').

[20] Although it is not "politically correct", we can consider that the principle of least effort guides behaviors. Making an effort "is expensive" and, consequently, we are prepared to make efforts if we derive some benefit from it as compensation. This benefit may vary feeling good by doing well; it may vary from attempting to get material gains, but also through the search for well-being to attain harmony. The actors are, therefore, guided by aspirations, values and the context.

[21] C.Bredenkamp "The puzzle of isolation bonuses for health workers", The World Bank, September 2009, www.rbfhealth.org

[22] Lu, M. 1999. *Separating the "True effect" from "Gaming" in Incentive-Based Contracts in Health Care. Journal of Economics and Management Strategy* 8, no. 3:383-432.

   - Shen, Y. 2003. *Selection Incentives in a Performance-Based Contracting System . Health care Research* 38, no. 2:535-552.

   - Commons M, T. G. McGuire, and M. H. Riordan. 1997. *Performance Contracting for Substance Abuse Treatment. Health care Research* 32, no. 5:631-650.

[23] Since the Ministry of Health is no longer responsibly of the health facilities it has no direct authority over them. Nevertheless, the Ministry of Health will keep its regulatory powers which in some cases can translate into a supervisory authority.

[24] It will all depend in the end on the organic framework. If the two units are attached to the same management, the risk of a purely artificial separation is high; on the contrary, if the two units are attached to different managements, the risk will be lower.

[25] The need for monitoring and verification is going to be even more important when contracts are incomplete, since incompleteness leaves room for opportunistic behaviour from the providers

[26] For an illustration of this problem, see Lim, S. S., D. B Stein, A. Charrow, and C. J. L. Murray. 2008. Tracking progress towards universal childhood immunization and the impact of global initiatives: a systematic analysis of three-dose diphtheria, tetanus, and pertussis immunization coverage. *The Lancet*:2031-2046.

[27] For example in Afghanistan, Johns Hopkins University in collaboration with the Indian Institute of Health Management Research, have taken up this role by managing the "Balanced Score Card" M&E tool.

[28] In Rwanda, the Ecole Supérieure Professionnelle de Kigali (ESP) did take up this role during the piloting phase.

[29] In Rwanda the NGO "Health, Development and Performance" (HDP), created from the former Cordaid Rwanda team, has this role

[30] Despite the sophistication of the homogeneous patient group systems (DRG), and the possibility of adding aggravating factors for establishing a mixed box, it is difficult to define the fair price of each service.

[31] The arguments of this answer are essentially inspired by the OECD study: " Performance-related Pay Policies for Government Employees ", 2005

[32] In econometrics, when performing a regression, we know that we can explain part of the variable explained by one explanatory variable that plays as a "proxy" for other variables.

[33] "Guide to the contractual approach for health centres – User's manual", Ministry of Health, May 2008: http://www.pbfrwanda.org.rw

[34] This is in reality a purchasing obligation contract. Indeed, unlike a classical contract, the Ministry of Health knows the price of what it is going to buy but not the quantity that it should mandatorily buy.

[35] A second category of indicators is defined around HIV. The mechanisms are quite similar but will not be presented here.

Part IV

Chapter 1

How to build and manage a contractual relation?

Jean Perrot

INTRODUCTION

This chapter aims to provide individuals in the field with a number of technical elements as food for thought and to guide their action. This is not really an operating manual in the prescriptive sense of the term, therefore, but rather a collection of elements that are useful for implementing a contractual relation.

Contractual relations can take very many forms and correspond to a wide variety of situations, and it would be very difficult to produce an operating manual encompassing this diversity. Nonetheless, some aspects of the implementation of a contractual relation are common to all situations; and this chapter aims to draw them together.

- The first stage aims to give actors in the field the tools they need to implement a contractual process;
- The second stage will identify the elements that need to be taken into account by the drafters of a contract.

1. THE CONTRACTUAL PROCESS

1.1   The prerequisites

Entering into a contractual process is not yet a habitual procedure, so its feasibility needs to be examined in advance. There is no use in a field worker being convinced of the validity of the procedure if the setting is unfavourable.

Political acceptance

Contractual relations concerning State matters are not yet a normal and habitual mode of operation. Nonetheless, this new culture is clearly starting to make inroads, particularly in developed countries and/or in domains other than health care. The "new public management" trend has developed very quickly over the last few years in sectors such as postal services, railways, telephone and television/radio, which in many countries have long been viewed as public services that should be operated directly by the State. This approach is even more recent in the health sector.

In developing countries, while reform of the State is generally proceeding under pressure from developed countries and international organizations, the health sector is still largely excluded from this trend, at least in terms of a common organizing principle. During discussions with a senior health official in a developing country, the author of this document mentioned the potential of contracting and received the following reply: "That's interesting, and I am convinced; but I'm not going to do anything about it!" Apart from a degree of provocation reflecting a friendly relationship, this reply can be explained as follows: the senior official in question was aware that this contractual approach was incompatible with the public sector culture of his country, and he knew that if he moved in this direction, without due caution, he risked being disowned at the highest level of State.

Political acceptance of an approach based on contractual relations is therefore essential if progress is to be made. Awareness-raising and advocacy are prerequisites for action and definitely cannot be neglected. Consequently, any party wishing to move towards a contractual relation must first make sure that all actions involved in this procedure are understood and accepted at the country's highest political level. If this is not the case, progress will need to be extremely cautious, and in some cases any action in this direction will need to be postponed.

As time goes by, this political acceptance will be facilitated by the international setting; and the fact that some neighbouring countries have already embarked on this path shows that it is not entirely new and revolutionary. This demonstration effect is reinforced by publications that are starting to appear describing experiments undertaken in individual countries, and also by inter-country meetings organized under various auspices, which allow new countries to take their place in this trend.

In May 2003, the Member States of the World Health Organization (WHO) adopted a resolution entitled "The role of contractual arrangements in improving health systems' performance." This resolution draws member States' attention to the opportunities of using contracting while inviting them to implement contractual policies that avoid the negative effects of ad hoc and uncoordinated contractual arrangements.

The technical capacities of the parties

As just noted, the contracting procedure is generally new in developing countries. Obviously, we all make contracts in our daily lives without realizing it: when you discuss with your partner whether to go out to see friends rather than staying at home, you are negotiating, and ultimately you reach a compromise and a contract. Nonetheless, in professional life, things are less simple; the issues are different, and more people are involved. Moreover, the negotiation often relates to events that will occur in the future. Thus, the technical skills that will need to be mobilized to implement contractual processes are a lot more demanding; and it is important to assess whether those skills are present, before entering into a contracting process.

Review of a large number of experiences in the field shows that contractual relations are often implemented in a very amateurish way, with the result that goodwill existing at the outset is often found wanting at the time of execution. For example, a district medical officer may be an excellent professional when undertaking health activities; but medical qualification does not necessarily make him/her likely to become a good negotiator. Contracting processes require specific skills for which health professionals are not generally trained. Negotiating with interlocutors or drafting a contract requires particular technical skills that goodwill cannot replace.

If there is no certainty that the parties possess the minimum level of technical skills needed, it is sometimes preferable to eschew a contractual relation. In fact contracting has no worse enemy than parties who lack technical skills; their lack of skills in the subject can discredit the whole process.

Nonetheless, one should not imagine that these technical shortcomings are the preserve of developing countries; developed countries face quite similar problems too.[1]

The appropriateness of contracting

Before entering into a contracting process, the parties should ask themselves whether this is the most appropriate strategy. In other words, when faced with a specific problem, an operator should always consider the steps needed to resolve it. Consider the example of a hospital in which the restaurant service is functioning badly. The hospital must investigate the reasons for this situation and analyse whether contracting is the best solution, or whether a different strategy — such as reorganization of the service within the hospital — would be better. Similarly, a Ministry of Health that owns and runs a hospital under direct management can consider whether it is worth improving its management, whether it is better to give the hospital autonomous status, whether management should be handed over as a concession to a non-profit or commercial organization, or lastly whether the hospital should be privatized. All of these alternatives should be analysed before entering into a contractual process.

2. THE PROCESS

Contracting is a lengthy process that takes its promoters from the stage of initial discussions to eventual renewal of the contract they signed. A contractual process is thus seen as a sequence of stages that need to be carried out properly if the contractual relation is to bear fruit. These stages can be presented in several ways. Some analysts distinguish between the pre-contractual phase and the contract implementation phase, the two phases being separated by contract signing which strictly speaking is a quasi-instantaneous act

In this document, the contractual process is presented in four successive phases:

1. Preparation for contracting
2. Formalization of the contractual relation
3. Implementation of the contract
4. The end of the contract

The four phases of the contracting process

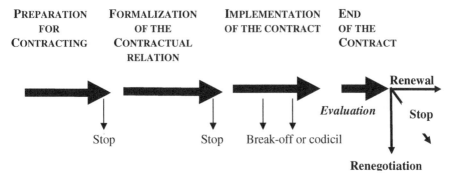

| PREPARATION FOR CONTRACTING | FORMALIZATION OF THE CONTRACTUAL RELATION | IMPLEMENTATION OF THE CONTRACT | END OF THE CONTRACT |

A contractual process that develops in full will pass through the stages or phases defined in the diagram above. These phases will assume a different dimension, however, depending on how the contractual relation is established. Thus, to simplify, a distinction will be made between "contracts based on open competition", and those based on "prior identification of the parties". As will be seen below, the two categories can be distinguished in several ways; but the fundamental point is that, at the outset, in contracts based on open competition many parties may try to obtain the contract award, whereas in those based on prior identification of stakeholders, the parties are predefined and known from the start of the process. Within these two categories, a number of distinctions can be made however: for example, in the first category, the competition can be more or less open. The category can also be changed during the course of the process: e.g. a largely competitive tendering process may be used to choose an interlocutor; but, once selected, the process becomes more of a negotiation.

2.1　　　　Phase I: Preparation for contracting

This phase starts when health sector stakeholders consider using contracting, and lasts until the moment when they actually formalize the contractual relation in question. The phase therefore involves the setting up of the process; it also has several stages:

- Identification of stakeholders and issues: the stakeholders are identified and apprised of the contracting process that could bring them together; they consider the issues involved, the advantages, the risks and the constraints of this contracting process. This is a stage of stakeholder engagement;
- The stakeholders put mechanisms in place to enable them to progress. This is an organization stage;
- Feasibility study of the putative contractual relation. This is a diagnostic phase.

At the end of this phase, the preparations are considered complete, and one can proceed to the next phase.

Naturally, at any time, it may be decided not to pursue further contacts. The parties involved then decide against entering into any formulation of a contractual relation. Phase I of preparation for contracting is crucially important because the entire unfolding of the contractual relation depends on its quality.

The initiative of a contractual relation

By definition, a contractual relation is not decreed. The initiative, i.e. entry into the contractual process, must come from the stakeholders themselves. Sometimes several stakeholders simultaneously perceive the need, in which case the preliminary contacts will be made easier. In most cases, however, the initiative consists of one stakeholder in particular recognizing the limits of its action, and realizing that it would definitely obtain better results by entering into a relationship with several other stakeholders. This starting point may take time: the self-analysis process is not easy and often involves reviewing actions undertaken thus far.

Thus, no contractual relation is possible without willingness on the part of at least one stakeholder. In some cases, this willingness exists; stakeholders are ready to enter into the relation. In other cases, willingness is not in evidence. Without wishing to create it artificially, there are means that can help generate it: for example, information on the potentialities of contracting or dissemination of the results of an experiment may lead certain actors to consider the process and decide to make use of it. This seeding role corresponds firstly to the Government and its representatives, who, when convinced of the potential of the approach, can take steps to promote it. The Government may be assisted in this role by outsiders, specifically international agencies providing technical support.

Why should one wish to enter into a contractual relation?

This question may seem simplistic; one might think that a stakeholder who decides to enter into a relation knows the reasons for doing so. However, in reality, the reasons are frequently vague, and parties ultimately are not very clear about the reasons why they decide to enter into a contractual relation. Nonetheless, it is very important that the stakeholders ask themselves this question at a very early stage.

For each of the potential parties in a contractual relation, this entails a self-analysis process that helps to clarify the situation. Each party must identify the benefits it expects to obtain from the contractual relation it wants to enter. The outcome of this will be very helpful in the negotiations to be undertaken with the interlocutor. These reasons clearly include some that are more worthy than others. For example, it is not hard for a Health Ministry to recognize that it wants to transfer the management of health centres to an NGO, because it does not have sufficient staff itself. It is harder for it to recognize that it wants to give up managing these health centres because the local population expresses great hostility towards it through its management committee.

But each stakeholder must also be able to identify the benefits its interlocutor expects to obtain from the contractual relationship. Thus, from the standpoint of the NGO, it is important to try to understand the Health Ministry's interests in outsourcing the management of its health centres under concession. Clearly, incorrect assessments can be made; so the stakeholder should also continuously check its assessment against reality and progressively fine-tune its judgment.

The situational analysis thus shows that the reasons that persuade two stakeholders to enter into a contractual relationship generally vary. Provided they are not fundamentally divergent, however, this will not handicap the negotiation and preparation of the contract. This might be the case in the above example if the NGO believes the Ministry of Health wants to impose family planning practices in its health care facilities, through this contractual relation. This analysis might also cause the NGO, for whom such an intention would be non-negotiable, to break off any further contact with the Health Ministry.

What is the object of the contractual relation?

In this contract preparation phase, defining the object of the contract is absolutely fundamental. A valid contract must have a certain purpose forming the subject of the undertaking. This may seem obvious, but an examination of numerous contracts shows that it is not at all obvious. The object of the contract is often found to be vague and liable to different interpretations by the different parties. Lack of precision in the object of the contract may be an undesired result; put simply, the parties have not been sufficiently aware of the need to clearly define its purpose. In other cases, it may reflect the deliberate desire of one of the parties to be in a position, cynically, to interpret the contract as best suits them. In all cases, the parties need to have a clear and identical understanding of the object of the contract, to ensure that its preparation and execution do not give rise to problems.

The "object" of the contract should not be confused with its "objective". The fact that the two terms are similar could lead to confusion. Moreover, while legal experts are familiar with the notion of "object", physicians are more familiar with the notion of "objectives", particularly since the development of activities planning. Thus, "Delegated management of the district X public hospital" is an appropriate title for the object of a contract; but "Improvement of the operation of the district X public hospital" is not an object but an objective. A great deal of attention must therefore be given to defining the object of the contract.

Who are the stakeholders in the contractual relation?

Simple contractual relations involve two parties that can be clearly identified: e.g. when the hospital contracts a private enterprise to maintain its premises, the parties are identified without any room for dispute. In contrast, in the case of a health district planning contract, the question of identity becomes relevant and can be addressed by asking the following complementary questions:

A- Do the identified parties have legal capacity?

Before parties embark upon a process that will lead them into a contract relation, it is important that their legal capacity be clarified, for processes have very often been initiated between parties who subsequently prove not to have the legal capacity to sign contracts.

In fact, there is often confusion between the status of a stakeholder and that of the health-care facility in question.

- Consider the situation in Mali, where "mutual assistance agreements" link the State to Community Health Associations (ASACO) and delegate the management of a public health centre to this association. In the event of termination of the agreement, or dissolution of ASACO, there may be questions as to the ownership of the health centre's assets. Should these devolve to the State or do they belong to ASACO?

368

- Now consider another case where the State associates a private NGO-run health centre with its geographical distribution of health services. The agreement will certainly allow the State to verify whether the activity carried out in the centre is in accordance with the commitments entered into. But, how will it then be possible to control the health centre's activity without controlling the NGO as a whole, since the NGO and the health centre are one and the same legal entity?

Although the solutions to these problems depend partly on the specific characteristics of national laws, they can be grouped in two categories:

- The first involves recognizing that it is possible to give one component of a given entity a degree of autonomy without thereby giving it separate legal status. This is the logic of deconcentration. Thus, this component (e.g. a hospital facility or a health centre) will be given a status that distinguishes it from the parent entity, characterized, for example, by an autonomous budget, specific norms applicable to the component in question, a specific internal organization and an internal regulation. But this component is not a separate legal entity and, therefore, cannot sign contracts in its own name. A specific contract can be entered into with this establishment, but it will have to be signed by the parent organization to be effective. This is usually the situation of public health establishments that do not have their own legal status. But it also corresponds to the situation of NGOs or associations that have multiple activities and various fields of action. Using this technique, health establishments can be individualized while preserving the pattern of the contractual relations of the establishments in question.

- The second solution involves attributing legal personality to the health-care facility itself. Examples are public hospitals that have autonomous status, in which the hospital board is the deliberative body that commits the hospital. This level of deliberation is therefore distinguished from the executive level represented by the hospital's chief physician, or director (as the case may be), who organizes activities on a day-to-day basis. This solution can also be adopted within large NGOs or associations, which, to clarify relations between the parent entity and the health care establishment, decide to give the latter full legal status. An example of this arrangement is provided by churches which separate mainly religious activities from those whose main objective is to improve people's health.

This separation does not mean independence, however; depending on the legal status used, the parent entity may retain de jure or de facto power in the new structure through the management board.

369

Each of these solutions has advantages and drawbacks which the personnel responsible must clearly identify. The partners of these entities must also be well informed of the status of each of entity so as to avoid any problem.

B - What is the status of the stakeholders identified (public or private)?

This distinction is important, because it affects the classification and execution of the contract. Public and private entities are not answerable to the same law. Public entities may have unilateral amendment rights in a contractual relation which a private person will not enjoy. Thus, a contract to provide a public service necessarily involves a public entity that will have amendment rights over the future contract that differs from those of the private party. This type of contract will not be subject to the same rules as a contract between a public and private entity to undertake a public health activity, for example, which is not in the realm of the general interest.

If there are no fixed criteria for distinguishing an administrative contract from a private contract, it needs to be decided whether the contract involves a public entity and/or an object that concerns a public service. To avoid misunderstandings at the time of contract execution, it is important for parties to be aware of the classification of the contract: either administrative (i.e. subject to administrative law) or private.

Within the public sector, however, a distinction needs to be made between the central State, autonomous entities, and decentralized authorities (common and other subnational entities that have contracting capacity).

Within the private sector, certain stakeholders classified in this sector nonetheless have quite vague charters. Churches often have charters that are quite difficult to understand. The same is true of certain NGOs, for which it is unclear whether the status concerns national or local representation, or else international.

C- Are the identified stakeholders recognized?

In a given country, health sector personnel are generally numerous, and the fact that their number is growing makes it is hard for any one of them to know all the others. In such conditions, how can a party be sure the counterpart with whom he wishes to deal is trustworthy and has the necessary competencies? Each party can make its own inquiry and obtain the necessary information, but this may take a long time and could prove costly in the end. The work can be done at the State and/or Health Ministry level through an accreditation system.

Accreditation is a procedure for identifying health sector stakeholders that are considered trustworthy, i.e. those with whom the population can deal safely. With a view to avoiding problems of conflict of interests, accreditation is generally entrusted to an independent organization, within which the diversity of health professionals and stakeholders is represented. This organization must evaluate each of the stakeholders participating in the health sector on the basis of pre-established criteria; and it will draw up a list of accredited stakeholders.

For an accredited stakeholder wishing to enter into a contractual relation, the fact that the identified partner is also accredited provides a guarantee and thus saves the stakeholder from having to make the evaluation itself.

D- What is the role of each stakeholder in the contractual relation?

In general, the role of each of these stakeholders in the contractual relation is simple: in a maintenance contract, for example, the enterprise must provide the service and the health-care facility must pay for it. But there are cases where the roles are much more complex, and a distinction needs to be made between the direct signatories of the contract and the stakeholders. The first category involves stakeholders that are directly committed with all associated duties and obligations. The second category encompasses actors who, without being directly involved in the contractual relation, are implicated; e.g. when a mutual insurance health company enters into an agreement with a private health centre, it is normal for the Ministry of Health, as guarantor of public health, to be involved. This involvement can take various forms:

- Information: it may be agreed that stakeholders will be informed by receiving a copy of the signed contract;
- Consultation: it may be useful for certain stakeholders to have been consulted during the contract preparation process, to obtain their opinion;
- Recognition - certification: in this case, the stakeholders give their opinion as to the soundness of the contract and its contents, before signing. This prerequisite may last up to the signing of the contract by these contracting parties, thus providing guarantees of its terms;
- Endorsement *(labellisation):* some stakeholders may go as far as authorizing signatories to inform their interlocutors that they have their endorsement. For example, the mutual health insurance company that signed a contract with a private health centre can state that the contract has received approval and encouragement from the Ministry of Health.

What types of commitments will be made?

From the outset, the future actors must identify the nature of the commitments they are going to enter into, i.e. the legal obligations that will be created. Two broad types of obligation are traditionally distinguished:

A- Obligations of means are traditionally illustrated by the contract between a doctor and his/her patient. The doctor promises to do everything possible to cure the patient's illness, without promising recovery. But the doctor undertakes to use all means available to him/her to cure the illness. The doctor's obligation therefore only relates to the means to be used.

B- Obligations of results involve a commitment by a contractor to strive for a specific result. For example an ambulance worker makes a commitment with a secondary hospital to transport a patient to a referral hospital. The secondary hospital has a guarantee of execution from the ambulance driver. If he fails to fulfil his commitment, the driver cannot evade responsibility by invoking force majeure or a fortuitous event. But ultimately, the means to be used by the ambulance driver are not very important.

It is often easier to identify means than results. It is also easy to list the people who will work within the contract framework, the payments to be made, the medications to be provided, etc. In contrast, while some results are easily identifiable and measurable, (e.g. the number of children immunized), others are very difficult (e.g. improving the quality of patient reception).

Over the last few years, the emphasis has been on "results-based management", which is a management strategy that targets stakeholders' efforts towards achieving precise results and direct effects, for which they have to be held to account, rather than towards undertaking certain activities. This approach means that the stakeholders are seen in terms of the aims of their action, identification of the results to be attained, and measurement of the results achieved through appropriate indicators. Under this approach, the administrators are accountable for the results of their actions: in return they have greater decision-making freedom (fungibility of funds). This new approach, which will be developed further, introduces another dimension of contracting.

On what bases will the contracting process be established?

This question needs to be addressed early on in this phase, since it affects the continuation of the process of preparing the contractual relation. Several characteristics can be used to define a contractual relation: we have considered two of them:

Competition-based relations. In this case there is a client who offers a contractual relation and actors who will respond to the offer: for example, in models based on a separation between financiers and service providers. Here, all potential providers must have the chance to compete to gain the market in question. Faith is thus placed in competition, to ensure that the optimal bid emerges. The actors do not develop any trust *a priori*, although they are not necessarily enemies. A process such as this clearly displays all the advantages of competition, specifically by allowing freedom to all potential actors to make their best offer according to their capacity; but it also contains several major disadvantages.

- The first of these concerns the potential for collusion between the various potential stakeholders. In any given region, the number of stakeholders is always small and generally they know each other quite well; this may provide a strong temptation for them to make an arrangement to divide up the market.

- The second disadvantage concerns the possible lack of competition in many areas of the country. In rural zones, the health services that actually operate, or could operate, are very few, or are even a monopoly. Very often, this situation is not the result of partners being driven from the market, but merely reflects the fact that population density is so low that there is no room for multiple partners. Thus, the institution already present enjoys a position advantage that is hard to overcome.

- The third disadvantage concerns the difficulty of evaluating the quality of services provided by a potential partner (cf. Agency theory, part III, chapter 1); But the service provider's experience could be taken into account by excluding providers who submit bids that are tempting but not backed by any experience. In practice, this problem can be eased by applying eligibility criteria that restrict access to the tender to bidders satisfying certain pre-requisites: a pre-qualification system in a tender.

- The fourth disadvantage involves "insider trading", specifically when public bodies participate in the tender. In this case, given their status, senior personnel may have access to information which partners in private entities find it harder to obtain.

- The fifth disadvantage relates to the consequence whereby, following the results of the tender, certain partners that are well established in the zone (e.g. NGOs) might be excluded from the market. This will pose a political problem that is even harder to resolve since those NGOs will be long established in the health zone in question, and will be undertaking activities there that are valued by the populations concerned.

- The sixth and perhaps greatest disadvantage stems from the scant room for negotiation available to future partners. The service provider proposes and the public authority disposes; i.e. the latter has to choose between the various bids submitted, using predefined selection criteria, but it will not really enter into negotiation with its future partner.

Cooperation-based relation. Stakeholders who want to enter into a contractual relation are not mutually dependent on each other, but partners who want to undertake something together and are ready to pool their efforts to achieve this. This relation is impossible without some degree of trust between the future partners - trust is the key for obtaining results from the relationship. For example, when the Ministry of Health knows the reputation of a given NGO, it considers negotiation is possible on the basis of mutual respect and trust. If this principle is established as a normal mode of relationship, it can even end up with each of the partners seeking to gain the trust of the other and adapting their behaviour accordingly, before entering into any relation. The relationship of trust must not lend itself to naivety, however; it is not a matter of blind trust, but a reasoned choice made by partners who are identified as trustworthy. For trust to be effective, it must be regularly validated. This trust can be viewed from several perspectives, such as trust in the partner's skills, or trust in the partner's honesty.

The contractual relation can be established either with no negotiation, or else with very lengthy and very open negotiations. In the first case, negotiation is not permitted; one party has prepared contractual conditions and a standard contract, and the parties who agree to enter this contractual relation will only have to sign the contract proposal. At the other extreme, nothing is predetermined and everything has to be negotiated; the parties jointly determine the terms of the contract without any *a priori*.

No single type of contractual relation is better than another; the choice must be made according to the setting. But it is important to remember that each type of relation involves different behaviour from the parties. Each party will adapt to the type of relation with which it is faced. For example, when negotiation plays a major role, it is not in the interest of individual parties to reveal their positions too early, so as to give themselves room for manoeuvre. In contrast, a bidder in a tendering process wants to make the fullest bid immediately and closest to its maximum capacities.

The dynamic of contract preparation

Once stakeholders have decided to enter into a process leading to a contractual relation, it is important that they implement mechanisms to start up the process rapidly. Otherwise, there is a risk that once the idea has been put forward, nothing will happen for some time.

A- Who will conduct the process?

A contracting process is generally implemented following an "initiative" by a given stakeholder. At the outset, this initiator probably needs to establish a certain number of objectives and the results expected for this phase, and inform the future partners of them. To some extent the initiator must act as leader to set the process in motion and propose a plan of activities, possibly proposing creation of a workgroup to which each of the potential parties appoints a member. This person will be responsible for conducting the process. This highly operational aspect may seem somewhat mundane, but it is crucial. Experience has often shown that the preparation of a contractual relation failed to develop simply because no one knew who was responsible for moving it forward. In fact, once agreement has been reached on the broad lines of the contractual relation (this is the role of the person in charge in the institution concerned), the practical methods of preparation must be entrusted to technicians. Each of the parties concerned must know which technicians have been appointed to conduct the process.

The parties in the contractual relation may also, by common agreement, decide to make use of a facilitator or "interface".

B- The communication space

From the outset of the process it is important for the initiator to introduce the notion of communication space among the future partners. This may emerge during meetings for training/information of stakeholders and then become the place of negotiation and preparation of the future contract. This communication space can also be created at the start of the process by putting certain elements of the process in writing: e.g. the objectives of the contractual relation, the type of contractual relation involved a timetable of progress in preparing the contractual relation, etc. This technique, known as *"Memorandum of understanding"* or *"Letter of intent"* makes it possible to enter into negotiation on the basis of sound foundations because care has been taken to make them explicit and thus avoid misunderstandings. A letter of this type, which is not a contractual document, can contain the following elements:

[1]   The object of the contractual relation;

[2]   Description of the parties, i.e. the stakeholders who will be contractual parties in the negotiations and will contribute to the successful implementation of the contract, and the specific reasons why they are essential in this implementation;

[3]   Identification of the negotiators who will conduct the negotiations/discussions. This approach clarifies, for all parties, the roles to be played by each one in establishing the contract;

[4]   The mandate given to negotiators and mechanisms for accountability to the decision-makers/signatories of the future contract;

[5]   A calendar with the stages to be completed and the deadlines to be met.

2.2 Phase II: Formalization of the contractual relation

This phase starts once the partners recognize that it is in their interest to establish a contractual relation; and it ends at the moment of contract signing. The phase may comprise the following stages:

- Negotiation: to establish all elements to be included in the contract. This makes it possible to forge understanding between the partners.
- Contract drafting: all of the above-mentioned elements need to be put in contractual form.
- Validity of the contract: once the contract has been established, and before signing, in some cases the co-contractors will need to obtain a prior approval; e.g. for some contracts an approval will need to be obtained from the health authority.
- Signature: This establishes the formalities for signing the contract. This stage lasts from the approval of the terms of the contract by the parties until the contract signing ceremony.
- Dissemination: Depending on the type of contract, once signed it will need to be (1) registered with the recognized authorities; and (2) disseminated, with the authentic copies specified in the contract.

The dynamic of contract preparation

As in the preparation phase, this stage of contract development may take time and also require a lot of energy from the parties. Several practical recommendations can be made to help attain the objective of this stage as quickly as possible:

A- The need for a leader: initiator or interface

This phase of contract development involves activities that the parties may not be used to performing. A leader is often needed to supervise this stage, which seems complex to persons who are not contracting professionals. The leader will have a mission to demystify the apparent difficulty of drafting a contract, and in particular for moving the negotiating process forward and technically supervising the contract drafting process. This person, as we have seen, may be the initiator of the partnership process or else a third party chosen by the parties to serve as interface.

B- The negotiation

Negotiation is an important stage wherever the contract is formed jointly by the parties. It is therefore necessary to be aware that the negotiation also involves techniques; a great deal of amateurism is too often displayed at this level. Persons in charge of this stage consider that everyone is, by default, capable of negotiating. Clearly everyone is continuously being faced with negotiations in their private and professional lives: with their partner, their parents, their children, their colleagues, etc. Nonetheless, the contractual negotiations being discussed here are of a different type: they are a lot more complex and, in particular, undertaken with partners with whom one is not used to negotiating.

Negotiating techniques have progressed considerably over the last few years. Knowledge of these techniques makes it possible to be a lot more effective and to reach more solid contractual arrangements, which, as a result, will have better chances of being implemented correctly. It is not our purpose here to discuss these techniques in detail, but simply to refer back to certain aspects to show how to deal professionally with a negotiation.

Preparing oneself for the negotiation

- Analyse the situation (divergences, issues, objectives): the feasibility analysis will provide numerous elements;
- Study the possible options: one should not enter a negotiation thinking that the other party is bound to accept one's own unbending position. It is also worth considering the different alternatives that one is willing to accept;
- Establish the strategy: this involves prioritizing options and defining the points on which compromise is unacceptable. It is also worth deciding on the negotiating style to be adopted: (1) A confrontational approach: in this case an attitude of domination will be projected, in which one party must win and the other lose; (2) A partnership approach: here the contractual relation must result in a situation where the parties involved all gain from participating in it.

Attitudes and rules of conduct during the negotiation

Several principles can be kept in mind at the time of negotiation:

- Accept differences: the other parties involved in the contract do not necessarily have the same interests as you, and this difference needs to be accepted; otherwise the negotiations will come to a halt;
- Respect the other party's point of view and try to understand the reasons underlying it. If one does not share this point of view, find ways to persuade the party to reconsider it;
- Arguments should be put forward calmly and without signs of subjectivity;
- Personal prejudices should not intrude in the arguments and they must not be allowed to colour the responses.

377

- Positions must be set out in full and backed by logical arguments;
- Unreasonable or arbitrary positions should be avoided;
- Ultimatums and other non-negotiable types of demand should also be avoided;
- Where appropriate, the validity of the other side's arguments and the legitimacy of their concerns should be admitted.

Contract signing

This stage involves knowing how the contract will be signed. It lasts from the approval of the terms of the contract by the parties involved, until the contract signing ceremony.

- Thus, once the negotiating team has finished its discussions, it needs to make the result known to decision-makers who will in turn give a ruling on the terms of the contract. There could thus be a lot of iteration before the negotiators and decision-makers agree upon the final version. It is therefore preferable for negotiators not to wait for the end of their discussions to inform decision-makers of consensus. This stage is often referred to as "validation" of the terms of the contract by the decision-makers. For example, the final version of the contract needs to be approved by the management board or by the Minister.
- The final version must bear the name of the signatory institutions but also the name of the individuals who, on their behalf, will sign the contractual document. A letter of mandate should accompany the individual signatories.
- The document must be reproduced, identically, as many times as originals are required.

To make this event more visible, it may be useful to organize a signing ceremony and invite all individuals and institutions that have helped prepare this contractual document and might later provide guarantees and support. The press can also be informed through this channel. Lastly, it is useful for representatives of the public to be invited.

Registration of the contract

The contract document must also indicate how the contract will be registered. It is not unusual to find that a contract is a secret document to which only the two parties have access. What rules are possible on this issue? In all cases, it is advisable that the Ministry of Health issues these rules for the contracting parties to refer to.

NB: This is not the place to consider the issue from the standpoint of a fiscal registration fee (e.g. in the form of a fiscal stamp).

- There are clearly cases where the contract does not need to be known by anyone other than the signatories: examples are contracts for non-medical subcontracting between private partners. Thus, if a private hospital wants to make a contract with a private firm for the maintenance of its premises, the contract does not need to be known by the Ministry of Health;

- There are cases where it would be appropriate for the contract to be registered at the local health administration level; contracts for local service provision by NGOs clearly do not need to be registered nationally. The health district and/or regional level will be appropriate for this type of registration;

- Nationwide contracts, however, must clearly be registered with the Ministry of Health at the central level. A ministry unit must therefore be made explicitly responsible for this task.

- But there are also cases where it is preferable for local contracts to be registered with the Ministry of Health at the central level; clear examples are all association contracts and contracts for delegated management of health care facilities. These are so important in terms of health coverage that they must be listed at the central level.

A contract between a health micro-insurance entity and a public or private health-care facility should definitely be registered at the local health administration level. In contrast, if this health micro-insurance entity uses a framework or standard agreement with several health care facilities, then any such agreements should be registered at a higher level of the health pyramid.

At the end of this phase, a contractual document that has been signed by all parties involved exists.

At any time it may be decided not to pursue further contacts, in which case the parties decide not to complete the formulation of the contractual relation they were envisaging.

2.3   Phase III: Implementation of the contract

Once the contract has been signed, the parties must execute it pursuant to its terms.

- Implementation of all contractual clauses: Obligations to make available all the resources envisaged in the contract, results monitoring, mechanisms for dialogue and settlement of disputes.

379

- Codicils [amendments]: As it is never possible to foresee everything, codicils to the initial contract could be introduced by the parties involved. These should be the subject of negotiation, irrespective of the methods used to establish the initial contract.

- Termination: The contract can be terminated at any time. Normally, the methods for doing this will have been provided for in the text of the contract itself.

- The State should also be in a position to ensure the good performance of the contract to safeguard the public interest.

Let's assume that the contract has been signed. The conditions under which it will be implemented will have been negotiated and appear in the contractual text. This does not require a rediscussion of implementation, but an analysis of what will happen during this stage after contract signing.

Information

One of the first questions to be raised is the extent to which the contract should be disseminated among stakeholders and the population at large.

It should never be forgotten that most contracts will be made known to the public, so the press may comment on the contracting process. Nonetheless, as this is a new subject, the press might interpret the information incorrectly and transmit false impressions.

An example of this is provided by the following article which appeared in the Senegalese press:

> *"Le soleil" Wednesday 5 March 2003: Article concerning the Dakar - Bamako railway line*
>
> *Title: Operation handed to a Canadian-French group*
>
> *Text: The Bamako - Dakar railway network is set to be transferred under concession in June 2003 to a consortium formed by the Canadian company Cnac and the French firm Getma, thereby completing a process of railway privatization in Mali and Senegal that began 10 years ago. Through this form of privatization, the enterprise ..."*

Clearly, the journalist is not entirely clear about the notion of delegated management and puts forward contradictory arguments that could be misleading to readers.

Who should have knowledge of the contract?

It is therefore very important that those who have signed a contract have considered how it will be made known to each person:

- It is also necessary to prevent the press form gaining information on the contract and misusing it simply through lack of knowledge. It may therefore be useful to produce a dossier containing all useful information to enable the press to understand the issues involved in the contract. This dossier could include elements such as the setting of the contract, arguments explaining why the contract has been entered into, making the object of the contract explicit, what is expected from it, and the participation of the various stakeholders. A press dossier of this type is not only defensive, however; it also aims to make sure that the press reports the contract and thus helps to disseminate it.

- The local authorities, who will not necessarily have been involved in all phases of the contract, should also be informed of its existence, depending on its importance and object.

- The population affected by the contract should also be informed: What steps should be taken to inform the public? Meetings, opinion leaders, press, ... are some possibilities that the signatories should consider. It is also necessary to bear in mind that providing good information to the population concerned will help implement the contract.

- This question may seem obvious, but generally it is not (only) those who have negotiated and signed a contract who will implement it on a day-to-day basis. It is often the case that those who have to take account of the provisions and clauses of the contract in their daily work are not informed of its existence or its contents. As a result, the contract fails to become the working tool it is intended to be.

- Contracts need to be available for consultation by anyone or any entity wishing to do so, especially by anyone involved in its implementation. This consultation must be possible not only for each of the contract signatories, but also for the health administration at both the national and decentralized levels.

How to make sure that the contract is used?

- The contract must become a daily working and reference tool for the persons responsible for implementing it:
    - The activities must be implemented in accordance with the terms of reference:
    - The resources (human and financial) must be mobilized according to

381

the clauses of the contract:

In a few cases, it will be necessary to provide for training for the staff who have to execute the contract.

- The signatories are responsible for implementing the contract; it is they who will be held accountable for its non-execution. Nonetheless, the signatory is not necessarily the person who actually implements the contract on a daily basis: For example, where a health-care facility is managed by an association, the contract will be signed by the president of the association; nonetheless, the daily implementation of the contract is more the responsibility of the director of the establishment. It is therefore important in this case that the president of the association explicitly delegates monitoring of the contract to the director of the establishment.

How to give due importance to implementation of the contract?

- Give the contract the place it deserves in daily work. Bear in mind that it is human nature to consider daily work as a relief from the humdrum, because "daily life is repetitive". Thus, the implementation of a contract may seem a lot less "noble" and exciting than its establishment and dissemination. It is therefore necessary to "value" its use and make it "visible" as a working tool.

What mechanisms are available for monitoring the contract?

- Establishment of a contract monitoring committee is recommended, and this will have been provided for in the clauses of the contract. It is now necessary to ensure its effective functioning.
- The monitoring committee is a mechanism of consensus between all parties to the contract and should be in a position to meet periodically. It is advisable for the minutes of these meetings to be made known to all contract signatories.
- Usually the contract provides for mid-term performance reports; but these actually need to be used and not remain as mere administrative items.
- Dispute settlement: mechanisms will have been provided for in the contract; but it will also be necessary to ensure they function properly. In particular, bear in mind that it will be easier to solve a dispute if it is addressed early. A dispute that has degenerated and become bitter is harder to deal with. Periodic meetings are mechanisms making it possible to identify potential disputes.

Contract and oversight

- The health administration is responsible for ensuring the provision of health services in accordance with the National Health Policy, particularly when it involves a public service. The health administration traditionally does this in the case of public health care facilities under direct management (hierarchical channel) and private health care facilities (while respecting the public health code and medical ethics). More recently, the health administration has learned to do this with the autonomous public health establishments (combining a degree of oversight with autonomy). Contracting changes the methods of oversight once again; this will also depend largely on the extent of the health administration's involvement in the contract. It is therefore advisable to avoid situations where the administration can find itself in a situation of conflict of interest (being at the same time a contracting party and an authority overseeing the contract).

- It is also recommended that the health administration, particularly at the central but also at the regional level, establish a structure (albeit lightweight) to monitor the main contractual arrangements, and which can also make evaluations for the purpose of reporting to the decision making authorities. The ongoing contracting process will cause changes in some of the procedures habitually followed by the central administration, which must take into account the legal and administrative implications induced by contracting, and implement the necessary acts that support this process.

- It is also recommended that, when networks of stakeholders exist, these should provide a mechanism for follow-up and regulation of the stakeholders they are responsible for: e.g. a federation of NGOs, a church, a medical association, or an association of paramedical staff. These entities will play different roles: prevention and settlement of disputes, evaluation ...

2.4   Phase IV: The End of the Contract

Any contract has a scheduled end as indicated in its terms. At the end of the contract, or sometimes slightly earlier, an evaluation will be made to draw up a balance sheet and draw lessons from the contracting experience. Three cases will now be presented:

- Renewal: The contract has given full satisfaction and the parties involved decide by common consent to renew it under the same terms as before (while amendments will often be foreseen, these respect the spirit of the previous contract). A new contract is then signed.

- Renegotiation: Although the parties consider it advisable to continue with a contractual relationship, they feel that the actual contract needs to be renegotiated. This renegotiation may be more or less comprehensive depending on the analysis of the previous contract as implemented. The process may be quite similar to that of the initial contract, although the identification of the partners is no longer an issue.

- Cancellation: The parties involved may decide not to renew their contractual relation, whether this has given satisfaction or whether it has ended in failure.

Contracting is therefore a lasting dynamic process. The length of each of the stages will depend on the circumstances; and it is important to clearly understand that time is needed, particularly at the start of the process. Too often stakeholders are swept along by enthusiasm and tend to precipitate things and move on to the next stage too quickly. It is thus useful, at the start of a contracting process, for the future partners to hold discussions to understand the normal duration of phases I and II. Poor understanding between actors can be damaging to the process.

3. THE STANDARD STRUCTURE OF A CONTRACT

Fieldworkers who enter a contracting process are always keen to use a model contract. Their rationale is always the same: why reinvent the wheel? If some part of a well drafted contract exists, then its example can be followed. This may nonetheless result in very different rationales:

- The rationale of the standard contract: This involves a standardized contract formula containing pre-established clauses, drafted by the "dominant" partner. If acceptable to the other party, it is sufficient for the latter to add its identity and signatures. This is sometimes referred to as "ready to sign". Affiliation contracts such as insurance agreements are examples of this.

- The logic of the standard contract structure: This involves a framework presenting the necessary and essential elements of a contract to enable it to respond to the key issues raised during the period of the partnership. The way they will be treated varies according to the parties and how the negotiation unfolds.

The standard contract formula is based on simple relations, in which the object of the contract may be clearly identified; for example, when a Health Ministry makes a contract with a private provider for it to monitor a specific type of disease (e.g. monitoring a TB patient using DOTS strategy) a standard contract may easily be established in conjunction with these private practitioners. In contrast, when the relation becomes more complex, the standard contract formula is no longer appropriate, since it leaves insufficient room for negotiation and adjustment to the specifics of the relation in question. The standard contract therefore cannot be generic because contractual situations differ widely, and it is inconceivable to envisage a standard contract that would fit all situations. In contrast, it is possible to develop standard contracts in well-defined situations; e.g., in the case of delegated management for a district public hospital.

Use of the standard contract formula also has the disadvantage of being unpedagogic; but the contractual process has the advantage of leading the parties to consider their activity, their behaviour, the objectives of their action, and the means to attain them. This aspect of the contractual relation is very important, and the standard contract formula approach breaks this dynamic which, in many cases, may be more important than the contract document itself.

Lastly, it is also very important to understand the purpose of the standard contract. Two approaches can be contrasted here. The first states that the standard contract that has been prepared stems from a model that is applicable to all, with no possibility of rejecting the model; this is then close to the idea of a ready-to-sign contract formula; the standard contract becomes mandatory for all parties. Alternatively, the standard contract may simply be seen as a guide, i.e. as a tool to assist the stakeholders in preparing the contract. The standard contract goes further than the standard structure for it proposes a contract formula, but it obeys the same rationale of helping stakeholders to formulate their contractual relations.

Joint preparation of the contractual relation and of the contract itself does not mean reinventing the wheel each time. The approach using a standard contract structure now becomes fully relevant. The way a contract is structured does not vary greatly, and it is useful to agree on this standard structure to guide firstly the negotiators and then the drafters of the contract. A standard contract structure should therefore be seen as a framework for gaining time and avoiding the omission of important points.

The contract preparation phase will lead into the drafting of the contract itself. The way this contract will be prepared depends greatly on the choices made in the previous stage, specifically on the foundations of the contractual relation:

- In the case of competitive processes, i.e. a tender, the contract will be drafted once the implementing agency has been selected. If a standard contract has been used, this phase will be very simple and consist merely of filling in the details of the parties involved. If negotiating opportunities are possible after selection, the standard contract will be adapted and the respective information will be obtained.

385

- When negotiation takes place, the negotiating team will establish the contract, based on situation and feasibility studies, as well as the outcome of discussions. Use of a standard contract is not recommended in this case.

Use of a standard contract therefore entails relying on a list of different elements that should be present in a contract: the prerequisites, the object of the contract, the role of each of the parties, the objectives to be attained (obligations of means or of results), the means to be implemented, the duration of the contract, performance indicators, monitoring and evaluation mechanisms, dispute settlement mechanisms, methods for disengagement ... then the signing of the contract and its registration. Elements of a model contract are discussed below. This is an operational tool that the drafters of the contract should use as a guide to ensure that no key element is missing from the specific contract they are drafting.

1. A clear reference to the National Health Policy and National Contracting Policy (if one exists). This initial point will also indicate the laws, decrees, and regulations governing the contracting to be referred to below.

   In addition, information on the parties to the contract will be repeated here: e.g. a historical memoir of the institutions involved.

   These different points are generally set out in a *preamble* to the contract, which contains elements relating to the contract's environment and setting. This information is intended for readers of the contract who are not the parties directly involved but who have an interest in the contract and must understand its context to appreciate the body of the text.

2. A contract is established between **the parties to the contract**: this involves the institutions that will have to implement the contract and fulfil its terms. There must be at least two parties, but there may be more. These are the institutions involved and not the name of the person who will sign the contract on behalf of each institution. The legal status of these parties to the contract must be indicated.

   The parties to the contract are directly responsible for implementing it. It is also possible for other entities to be involved: for example, in some cases funding for an NGO that is a party to the contract depends on an agreement with a development partner: in this case, it is advisable for this development partner to also be a signatory.

   It could also be useful to note here the institutions that guarantee the contract. These are not direct stakeholders in the contract, but institutions that certify its validity and justification. For example, in an association contract between a mutual health insurance company and a private hospital, the Ministry of Health may participate through its deconcentrated entity, thereby indicating its recognition of the contract between the parties that are responsible for implementing it.

3. **The object of the contract** should be precisely defined. Usually, a contract has a title reflecting its object. For example, Title: "Management concession contract for district X hospital"; Object: "The object of this contract is for the Ministry of Health to transfer the management of district X hospital to NGO Y under concession."

4. Specifically when the contract pertains to a public-sector service, it may invoke a number of **principles** that are not negotiable, such as:

    − the requirement to respect the rates set by the health administration;

    − the obligation to satisfy user demand in a non-discriminatory fashion;

    − the obligation not to engage in anti-competitive practices: e.g. to hold public tenders to select subcontractors;

    − the obligation to provide sufficient information to the health administration;

    − the obligation to respect a number of codes of good conduct: e.g. respect for patient confidentiality.

5. The **objectives to be attained** will also need to be defined precisely; the term "results to be achieved" is sometimes preferred to "objectives to be attained". These objectives are generally defined in a *schedule of conditions* which is attached to the contract (and forms an integral part of it). The objectives should be defined as clearly and precisely as possible They should also be realistic: there is no point in defining objectives that one knows to be unattainable. Thus, an objective specified as follows: "To improve accessibility to health care at hospital X" could be a necessary general objective, but it is insufficient. It is therefore advisable to indicate how this general objective translates in practice: opening hours, access to emergency services, dealing with severe poverty, etc.

The schedule of conditions (the *specifications*)

The schedule of conditions is the document (forming an integral part of the contract) that precisely defines the activities to be carried out under the contract by the parties.

Depending on the nature of the contract, but also on the ways the contractual relation was established (enforceable contract/relational contract), the schedule of conditions will be defined with greater or lesser precision. At the two extremes, there are:

- *Either:* A succinct schedule of conditions, allowing the parties broad scope for adaptation according to the reality in question;

- *Or else:* A schedule of conditions that attempts to foresee all scenarios, i.e. leaving the least possible freedom for adaptation. This runs the risk that the schedule of conditions may be difficult to establish and become extremely burdensome.

The schedule of conditions should however address the following points:

- Nature of the activities to be carried out under the contract: This involves precisely identifying the activities to be undertaken.

- Implementation methods: This not only means stating, for example, that one of the activities is the immunization of children under five years of age; but also indicating the strategy to be pursued: outreach strategy, vaccination campaign, etc.

- Objectives to be attained;

- Deadline for each of the activities;

- Role of each of the contracting parties;

- Collaboration with other stakeholders.

One also needs to be aware that a schedule of conditions is never entirely complete. This incompleteness may be greater or less but it always exists. It is therefore advisable for the schedule of conditions to name persons who will have power to interpret this incompleteness, as the case may be, and under what procedure will the interpretation be done.

6. **Duration of the contract**: The duration of the contract is a very important element, because it will determine the partners' behaviour. For example, after signing a management contract with the Health Ministry, the behaviour of the person in charge of the health centre will depend on the duration of the contract. If it is known that the management contract will last five years, for example, then it would be possible to implement a phase of awareness-raising among population groups, in the knowledge that the results are not immediate. This will not happen if the contract is only for two years. While there are no precise rules in this domain, classic contracts generally tend to be of short duration, whereas relational contracts tend to be long-term because they involve reaching an agreement to be further developed rather than a precise transaction. Each of the parties to the contract therefore needs carefully to analyse the advantages and disadvantages of different durations. It is also advisable to set the date on which the contract will enter into force, which could well be different from the signing date, especially when conditions must be fulfilled between that date and the project's entry into force. The contract must therefore precisely define the conditionalities that need to be fulfilled between these two dates.

7. The **resources** to be used for the contract should be defined in terms of the amounts of all inputs (human and material resources), also identifying the funding sources in terms of timeframe (linked to the duration of the contract). We shall note here that it will be essential for the success of the contracting process that all parties respect the commitments entered into. A contract always involves an obligation of means. For some contracts, an inventory of movable

and immovable property, as well as other contributions, should be made. It is advisable to specify, possibly in tabular form, the age of the assets, their condition, their residual value when the contract enters into force and, above all, who owns them and has to ensure their maintenance or replacement in the event of obsolescence or wearing out.

8. The **role of each of the parties must be** defined. It will be advisable to clearly distinguish the specific roles of each party in the contract and for each element in the process (signature, execution, monitoring, evaluation, resolution of problems and disputes), and to choose on the basis of valid criteria, such as the comparative advantages of each one.

9. **Results measurement.** It must be possible to say whether the objectives of the contract have been attained or not. For this purpose, the contract should indicate how the results are to be measured: this requires specifying the criteria or indicators to be used, and their measurement. These indicators should be relevant (measurement in line with the objectives), comprehensible (clear interpretation), reliable (no measurement problems), practical (easy and low-cost measurement) , and comparable (not affected by place or time). It will also be important to use indicators on the development of the contract: for example, it may be worthwhile measuring the difficulties encountered in implementing the contract, the disputes that have arisen, resistance by staff, the reaction of users, attitudes of stakeholders who are not directly contracting parties, etc. The indicators should refer to both *obligations of means* and the *results to be attained,* and they must be realistic and measurable. Their evaluation should make it possible to gauge the extent to which the activities have been fulfilled and the difficulties encountered overcome.

10. **Contract monitoring mechanisms** should be made explicit in the contract. A *monitoring committee* should be set up with representatives from all contracting parties. This committee will have the task of appraising the implementation of the contract on the basis of information to be transmitted to it by the different parties to the contract, and also of carrying out the investigations needed to be able to hold contract signatories to account. It will also have the task of making recommendations to resolve any problem arising in the implementation of the contract. This monitoring committee may also make it possible to make explicit, during implementation of the contract, certain aspects that would not have been anticipated at the time of its signing. Nonetheless, there again, the monitoring committee will not have decision-making power but a duty to put forward proposals; decision-making remains the prerogative of the signatories alone. The contract should identify the operational resources to be provided to the committee to ensure its viability. This

389

monitoring committee should consider the role of the population: should representatives of the population be included in the monitoring committee (with what roles and powers?), or should mechanisms be implemented to obtain their opinion? Sometimes it may also be useful to call in an outside agency to evaluate implementation of the contract and fulfilment of its performance criteria. For example, an audit institution may be hired to perform a survey of the population's satisfaction.

11. The evaluation mechanisms will **need to be defined.** It will be advisable to indicate the stages of this evaluation (evaluations during the contract, final evaluation), as well as the persons participating in these evaluations. It is worth distinguishing between the internal evaluation conducted by the parties in the contractual relation, which forms part of the routine health system monitoring-evaluation system, and the outside evaluation performed by external mechanisms that will need to be designated in the contract. In particular, it is important here to indicate the role of any NGO coordination mechanisms, when these exist. Funding for any external evaluations must be provided for in the clauses of the contract/project (the evaluation issues are discussed further).

12. The contract will need to indicate the **mechanisms for preventing and resolving problems and disputes**. The methods used should be progressive according to the seriousness of the dispute (amicable conciliation, arbitration, tribunals, etc.)

   - Inter-relational or collaboration difficulties, and minor management problems (such as small delays in the arrival of supplies or medication, staff illness) should be solved amicably either at the local level, or, failing that, at the intermediate or central level. If a contract monitoring committee has been implemented, it will endeavour to avert tensions and conflicts, and will also propose solutions.

   - In the case of problems relating to mismanagement or misappropriation of funds, the first step should make use of external mediators. Third parties should be appointed at the outset, who are not directly concerned in the implementation of the contract, such as federative religious associations or public bodies such as a provincial level health administration and/or the Ministry of Health. Only if these mediators are unable to obtain a result should the dispute be referred to the competent courts.

   Three successive stages are therefore proposed:

   1. Amicable settlement following a cooling-off period.

2. If, on expiry of the cooling-off period, the parties have not reached a settlement, the problem or dispute should be submitted to arbitration at the intermediate level; then if a solution still cannot be found, at the central level before the secretary general of the Ministry of Health and other partners whether or not affected by the contract in question.

3. When these two channels have been exhausted, the parties can refer the dispute to the local competent court.

Nonetheless, it is advisable for problems to be settled as early as possible using the initiative proposed under 1 and 2. The courts should really be the last resort.

13. It is also is worth remembering that the signed contract should be familiar to all parties and the personnel who will be responsible for implementing it in practice. It serves as a reference for all actions and becomes a working tool. In addition to registration methods (c.f. below), the contract should indicate methods for its publication.

14. Clauses concerning early termination of the contract. It is worth precisely specifying the methods and procedures whereby the parties can terminate the contract before its expiry date. As far as possible, the contract will foresee the consequences of early termination the contract.

15. Codicils to the contract. By common agreement, the parties should be able to change certain of the contractual terms during its implementation. As far as possible the contract will specify the elements of the contract that can be revised, and those that cannot, as well as methods for doing so. The procedures for revisions will be indicated precisely.

16. Methods for terminating and renewing the contract: When the contract reaches its expiry date, there should be an indication as to how it can be renewed (tacit renewal, renewal following an evaluation report, and the opinion of the commission), and the technique for doing this (e.g. by sending a letter). The contractual document should also indicate how it can be terminated in advance: methods and procedures, notice, etc. In all cases of contract termination, it is advisable to indicate the destination of the assets of the contract upon termination. Force majeure: This clause covers unforeseeable events that are independent of the wishes of the parties, which make it impossible to continue execution of the contract; e.g. war, coup d'état, natural catastrophe, interruption of funding.

17. Identification of the representatives of institutions that are signatories of the contract: The mandate given to the signatories will need to be witnessed; and the capacity of the signatories should be clearly indicated.

18. Registration of the contract. The contract should indicate how it is to be registered and how such registration can be accessed. Any contract that involves public issues is a tool that should be registered by the health administration. This involvement of public issues may in fact make the Ministry a contracting party or guarantor of the contract. In either case, the health administration must register the contract. It will therefore be important for the contract to identify the places in which the contract should be registered; and it should also identify which stakeholders can have knowledge of it, and methods for accessing this information.

With a view to avoiding disperse solutions, it is important that the health administration define rules to be adopted by all.

CONCLUSION

Implementation of a contractual relation requires skills that institutions do not always possess, even though they may wish to make use of contracting. Using contracting is never simple, and there are many examples to show that inadequate mastery leads to negative results. These elements will be important to consider when evaluating a contractual relation. Bad results may also arise from inappropriate use of the contractual tool, just as much as from inadequate mastery of that tool by the stakeholders concerned. In the first case, contracting should be blamed; in the second case, contracting as such is not at issue.

The conduct of a contractual relation is therefore not a matter of improvisation. The parties must learn to master this tool, which is not easy since it engages multiple subject areas, requiring legal, economic, managerial, administrative and organizational knowledge, as well as knowledge of public health issues. Any one individual would find it hard to embrace all these skills; so it is appropriate for the conduct of a contractual relation to be entrusted to a multidisciplinary team.

Notes

[1] This aspect is clearly highlighted in "Before you sign the dotted line...ensuring contracts can be managed" (1997). This document is available on the Internet: consulted on the website: Competitive Tendering and Contracting Branch (CTC) of the Department of Finance and Administration, Australia, on 2 October 2000: http://www.ctc.gov.au

Part V

Chapter 1

Tools for regulation

Jean Perrot

"The Fifty-sixth World Health Assembly,..... URGES Member States: ... 2) to frame contractual policies that maximize impact on the performance of health systems and harmonize the practices of all parties in a transparent way, in order to avoid adverse effects;" WHA56.25, 28 May 2003

Use of contracting by health systems is increasingly common in both developed and developing countries. However, at the same time, use of this tool has developed in the absence of any standards or coordination. Private actors use it as they see fit and Ministries of Health do not always have the technical capacity to use it judiciously.

If we want to avert the misuse and harmful consequences of contracting, the first thing to do is to ensure that all actors in the field of health have the technical skills needed to use the tool in a professional manner.

Use of contracting must be subject to systemic examination; the tool should be put into context. We need to examine the reasons why the tool is used: is the tool appropriate in comparison with other tools? What are the areas in which we want contracting to develop? How may we harmonize the contractual practices of all actors?

1. THE CONTEXT IN WHICH CONTRACTING HAS DEVELOPED

Increased use of contracting has been part of the evolution of health systems and of the relationships between actors in health systems. The position and role of the latter have evolved considerably, and the following changes may be identified:

The definition of the role of the State has been called into question: those analyses which concluded that privatization was the remedy for the State's inability to manage are increasingly giving way to a vision in which the State's role is to safeguard the public interest rather than to provide and finance services. The State should focus on its stewardship function and, as is suggested by the **World Health Report 2000,**[1]"row less and steer more". There is nothing new about this view of the State's stewardship function, which is defined as a "function of a government responsible for the welfare of the population, and concerned about the trust and legitimacy with which its activities are viewed by the citizenry" ; it was addressed by Jean-Jacques Rousseau in the 18th century, then by Max Weber at the beginning of the 20th century before being taken up by the public choice theory in the United States.

This vision reflects a substantial calling into question of the practices and techniques of public management. In the view of some analysts of government, we now stand at the watershed dividing two periods, that of the "commanding government", which is coming to an end and the dawn of the period of "government by partnership". The *commanding government,* which is constituted and acts by virtue of the impersonal and coercive general rule of law, seems to be increasingly less suited to the environment of modern societies, with the complexity that characterizes them. The current crisis of "governability" has revealed the inefficacy of the State and of its conventional legal regulatory mechanisms. No doubt laws, decrees and regulations and their application by an authoritarian bureaucratic organization were suited to a certain period. Nowadays, the results produced by this form of governance are less and less satisfactory. *Government by partnership* is characteristic of a State that no longer commands from the top down, but which negotiates with its societal environment. Consequently, modern law should assign an increasingly important place to "negotiated law" (flexible, reflexive and reactive), and no longer aspire to regulate everything but simply to provide frameworks for negotiation. The new style of government is that of government by delegation and through the coordination of interlinked networks. A contemporary administration thus becomes a cooperative one which generalizes the practice of negotiating as a day-to-day form of action. The Law increasingly resorts to contracts as a means of ensuring it is applied and less to an enabling, secondary, legislation, which imposes it unilaterally. We have seen instances in which a framework law, in addition to setting out the fields for negotiation, requires actors to conclude contractual arrangements by a fixed deadline. In France, Ordinance n°96-346 of 24 April 1996 requires hospitals to reach agreements with Regional Hospital Agencies.

In most health systems, **the private sector is developing**, becoming more diversified and already playing or aspiring to play a more and more important role. As regards provision of health services, private providers, both for-profit and non-profit, are sometimes more important than the public service. For example, the private sector provides one third or more of health services in most African countries. The sector has become diversified: private non-profit providers, who used to be mainly from religious orders, now include non-denominational organizations. The private for-profit sector, which used to be present mainly in towns and which essentially provided curative services for the well off, is now developing in more diverse locations and providing coverage for less privileged sectors of the population.

Working in isolation is no longer desirable; gradually, actors are beginning to understand the need to build relationships which they desire to be more and more formal. However, such relationships are still frequently based on ad hoc arrangements. As in the commercial sphere, the actors consider contracting as a tool that enables them to solve their problems, without regard for the public interest. We thus witness the existence side by side of specific contractual arrangements that suit everyone, including the health authorities, and this is all the more so since contracting remains limited and relatively unknown. However, there are drawbacks to such juxtaposition:

- Within the health sector, contracting is being used opportunistically, rather than as part of a strategy that has been clearly defined by the Ministry of Health. In Benin, the decision to delegate management of the Ménontin health centre is an isolated one (the relevant order was signed on 12 February 1992). Similarly, a study concerning ten countries in the eastern Mediterranean[2] which resort to subcontracting reveals considerable differences between them which cannot be accounted for by any explicit strategy.

- Occasionally, use of contracting entails excesses and abuses that are deemed unacceptable. For example, in Morocco, in some hospitals in which cleaning was subcontracted, the subcontractors were found to be paying their workers less than the minimum wage. Elsewhere, subcontracting has led to the dismissal of public employees and frequently the opposition of trade unions.

- There is too often a lack of professionalism in the decision to use contracting; some actors, captivated by a particular experience, take the plunge heedlessly, their amateurism often resulting in failure. Handling a contractual process and drafting a contract that sets out, in both text and spirit, the understanding reached between actors is far from being as easy as it seems. For example, in Senegal, the contracts signed between the Ministry of health and a number of NGOs as part of the Integrated Health Development Programme were badly worded, a fact which largely accounts for the poor results achieved.

- Juxtaposition of specific contractual arrangements will make coordination increasingly difficult: for example, the St Jean de Dieu hospital in Thiès, Senegal reports having signed agreements with some 20 mutual health insurance institutions in its catchment area. Each agreement is the outcome of ad hoc negotiations and is consequently different. This tangle makes it increasingly difficult to manage the hospital, which finds it ever harder to coordinate and justify these differences.

Such a juxtaposition of ad hoc contractual arrangements, each of which may possess its own rationale, does not necessarily result in a coherent health system. In some cases, contracting may even undermine a systemic approach. As an illustration, in a health district that is organized as a coherent local health system, contracting may introduce upheavals which jeopardize the system; for example, delegating the management of a public hospital to a private entity (even a non profit-making one) may, if it is poorly thought out, isolate the hospital from the other first level health facilities. We now know, however, that health services are only truly efficient if they are correctly incorporated within a coherent health system: this is the price of their performance in terms of better health for the populations.

When ill-used, contracting may also prove dangerous. For this reason, it is accused of being a vehicle for privatization or with signalling the withdrawal of the State, with as its corollary, a loss of concern for the public interest. The realization that contracting might be seen as a factor favouring the development of privatization and the withdrawal of the State has been one of the main arguments in favour of the development of a policy on contracting in Senegal and Chad. However, in Madagascar, the public-private partnership has been at the heart of concerns, although there has been some ambiguity over the word partnership, and this has not yet been fully dispelled.

2. REGULATORY TOOLS

In recent years, many countries have felt the need to introduce regulation of contractual practices. The need has been expressed by Ministries of Health, but also by other actors. Thus the NGO Medicus Mundi International wishes that a clearly defined framework would circumscribe the use of contracting between the state and NGOs in countries where it provides support to.

We need first of all to define the concept of regulation. We shall adopt a broad vision of regulation, encompassing both the texts and the tools used to control and supervise - the regulation in a narrow meaning - as well as the incentives, the orientations, the strategies and policies. The aim is at the same time to stimulate initiatives by all actors, to encourage them to contribute towards the health of populations, and to provide a framework for contracting so as to avert its potentially negative effects.

Definitions and concepts: régulation - réglementation

In French, the two terms -"*régulation*" et "*réglementation*"- are close but not synonymous. In English, "regulation" is synonymous with "réglementation" in French. For example, deregulation of air transport means the elimination of all regulations pertaining to fares, access rights and monopolies, etc. The idea is that the market will regulate itself by achieving a balance in the best interests of the consumer. In contrast, regulations are introduced by the State to channel the practices of the market.

Regulations thus consist of texts (laws and rules) that precisely define what can and what cannot be done. In one case, the regulations may be a regulatory text stating that management of a public hospital may not be delegated to a for-profit actor. There are those who consider that regulations provide an adequate framework for contracting. Advocates of the free market hold the view that such regulations should be kept to a minimum so as not to interfere with initiatives by the different actors. On the other hand, there are those who believe that regulations should be as comprehensive as possible, to ensure that actors comply with the provisions laid down in the texts.

Regulation - Régulation is a different concept. To take the example of two familiar expressions:

- *Régulation* of road traffic: *régulation* cannot be taken as synonymous with "regulations". There is a set of *régulations*, contained in the Highway Code. Their purpose, within the framework of the Highway Code is to ensure that traffic flows properly and smoothly: for example, the police may prohibit access to a motorway if there are already too many vehicles on it, until things return to normal;

- Birth control: in this case too, there are regulations (the right to abortion, methods of contraception, etc.). Here, in contrast, *régulation* involves making recommendations to individuals to help them plan births in their family.

Régulation in this sense may be seen as a contemporary form of State intervention in a sector of the economy, for the purpose of preserving the higher interests of the community and remedying the excesses that might upset the smooth and balanced operation of the market. By upholding a number of intangible principles that may not be called into question by the laws of the market, *régulation* nonetheless makes it possible to allow as much leeway as possible to professional actors. Developing *régulation* means instituting a framework within which it is possible gradually to get rid of regulations that are too restrictive. *Régulation* is not then just a matter of reducing traffic; in some cases it may make it possible to increase it. It's purpose is not solely to restrict use of contracting but also to encourage and facilitate its use.

Why is there any need for *régulation*? For the reasons evoked above: to avoid excesses and abuses by the market, to authorize healthy and honest competition, to allow initiatives to unfold, etc. However, it is obvious that where health is concerned, the purpose is to preserve the public interest. Health is not an ordinary good or service; the State is responsible for ensuring that actors operate within the framework of a public service mission (for example, equal treatment for the population) and that the services are sufficiently numerous and of satisfactory quality.

Regulation - *régulation* is thus less restrictive than regulations - *réglementation*. The latter impose, dictate and then penalize any departures from them; the former provides a framework within which there is room to adapt; moreover, the framework is not understood solely as laying down limits, it also provides encouragement. Finally, regulation - *régulation* is pragmatic: it is based on observation of what is happening at a particular moment.

Regulations are thus the first form of regulation, and there are those who are content with this: laws and rules are sufficient to prevent abuse and to smooth out the imperfections of the market. However, countries are increasingly introducing other methods of regulating contractual practices.

Many countries harmonize contractual documents by drawing up model or standard contracts: 1) the adoption, by health insurance organizations, of standard contracts governing their relations with their members; 2) in France, Act n° 99-477 of 9 June 1999, guaranteeing access to palliative care, stipulates that "those associations that organize voluntary work in public or private establishments, welfare and medical and welfare establishments must sign with the establishments concerned a standard agreement defined by a decree of the Council of State"; 3) in Canada (Quebec province), a standard contract has been drawn up to harmonize contracts between network clinics and Health and Social Services Centres (CSSS); the purpose of these contracts is to coordinate the services offered by the network clinics and the CSSS so as to offer clients access, via a clearly identified portal, to a continuous range of services required by their state of health, and 4) in Great Britain, the Department of Health has agreed the content of the General Medical Services Standard Contract with the general practitioners' committee (GPC) and the National Health Service (NHS) Confederation. Thus, by offering a formal framework for specific contractual relations, the standard contract technique makes it possible to harmonize practices even if it remains focused on well-defined aspects of contractual relations.

Certain countries use guidance documents relating to specific areas which resort to contracting. These include Canada (Quebec province), which has been inspired by Great Britain, and which is developing, through Act 61 of 2004, public - private partnerships to renovate public infrastructure and improve the quality of services provided to citizens. In France, the "Hospitals" ordinance of 4 September 2003 has authorized the use of "long-term *(emphyteutic) hospital leases" (BEH)*, a particular type of partnership contract, and established the National Mission to Support Investment in Hospitals (MAINH). This is a form of contractual arrangement covering the funding, design, construction, maintenance and operation of the building and in some cases the overall provision of services associated with it. These official documents precisely determine the use to be made of this type of contracting, albeit within a clearly determined area;

The use of framework agreements reflects different objectives:

- Certain framework agreements define contractual terms with which actors may or may not wish to comply. In France, this is the case of the agreement between health insurance funds and general practitioners' professional organizations: practitioners may simply send a letter stating that they wish to adhere to the general agreement regulating relations between the funds and general practitioners; this means that there is no specific contract binding a physician to a health insurance fund.

- Certain framework agreements are designed more as documents setting out the major contractual guidelines, leaving it for actors to define, within their framework, their specific contractual relations. For example, the major national NGOs and religious bodies that own and manage numerous health facilities in low-income countries are keen to have framework agreements drawn up, to which they may then refer in negotiating specific contractual agreements. For example, in Burundi and in Benin, churches find that specific contractual arrangements require often arduous case-by-case negotiations. Moreover, each contractual arrangement is considered an exception, as the contractual strategy is not part and parcel of the national health policy. In order to make up for these shortcomings, the churches have requested the introduction of a frame of reference for their negotiations in order to provide strength and credibility to any contractual arrangements into which they may subsequently enter.

In some cases, framework agreements take the form of a Memorandum of Understanding (MOU): for example, in order to implement the "Directly Observed Treatment Short-course - DOTS" strategy to treat tuberculosis, the WHO Stop TB department has recommended that Ministries of Health sign an MOU with private practitioners, setting out the terms of collaboration between the public and private sectors.[3] Private practitioners are then free to sign contracts to implement the DOTS strategy.

The choice of a particular vision actually depends on the notion of subsidiarity: what powers do mutual health insurance societies wish to transfer to a union or federation? Do they wish to vest in the latter extensive powers at the risk of losing many of their own prerogatives for negotiating with care providers or do they simply wish to hand give them a mandate to assure coordination and guidance while retaining negotiating rights at their level?

The benefits and limits of using framework agreements

There are numerous **benefits** to framework agreements:

A framework agreement makes it possible to harmonize practices among a group of actors operating in the field of health and who share the same goals. The framework agreement thus makes it possible *to define, for all the health facilities covered by the agreement, common terms for each of the specific contractual arrangements.*

Because it contains a number of elements that have been negotiated at this level, the framework agreement *facilitates and simplifies discussions in respect of each contractual arrangement.* There is no longer any need to discuss these elements as the specific contractual arrangement will refer to the clauses contained in the framework agreement. For example, in Ghana, for moral and ethical reasons some religious NGOs working in partnership with the Ministry of Health do not want their hospitals in the field to provide certain reproductive health services. To settle the matter, the "Memorandum of Understanding" (between the Ministry of Health and the Christian Health Association) allows the NGOs that so wish to opt out of certain reproductive health activities. Accordingly, when the specific contractual arrangement is drawn up, an NGO that so wishes may invoke the clause and state which activities it does not wish its hospital to perform.

By setting negotiations at a higher level, the framework agreement *involves those levels that possess greater negotiating capacity and are thus able to protect lower level health facilities* which do not always have sufficient capacity to engage in complex contractual negotiations. A framework agreement that has been signed with a federation of NGOs restores the power balance between a Ministry of Health and the NGOs which are able, thanks to the federations importance, to gain acceptance for their arguments;

The framework agreement may determine the stance to be adopted by each health facility controlled by the federation that signed the framework agreement. The framework agreement is thus *capable of encouraging or even of compelling health facilities controlled by the federation to develop contractual arrangements at the level of each health facility.* Likewise, a federation of NGOs that offers services outside a health facility is able to persuade the NGOs to develop specific contractual arrangements which are nevertheless to some extent harmonized;

The framework agreement *will determine the role to be played by the federation throughout the contractual process, and in particular as regards signature* (signature assuming responsibility or signature giving approval) but also as regards monitoring of specific contractual arrangements. This means that the federation can ensure that its members comply with those specific contractual arrangements they have drawn up. For example, a federation of physicians in private practice which has signed a framework agreement with the Ministry of Health will be able to ensure that all private practitioners belonging to the federation comply with the agreement: the federation plays an important role in monitoring.

However, as far as harmonizing contractual practices is concerned, it has its **limitations:**

- The framework agreement is a voluntary document drawn up by two willing actors. It thus applies only to those who have signed it, and does not make it possible to supervise those who have not signed.

- It concerns only part of the health system and certain contractual practices. There are no instances of a framework agreement that covers all forms of contracting.

If countries want the different actors to use contracting in a proper and professional manner that will guarantee success, it is important for the actors to receive every possible form of support to enable them to perform these tasks. Many of them will need help in order to properly conduct contractual relations. Such technical support may take a variety of forms: support-counselling for actors who require it, at each stage of the contractual process; prior advice to the signatories of a contract; preparation of guides and manuals on the use of contracting; training in contracting; evaluation of experiences; drafting regulatory instruments; etc. Several countries have set up specific entities responsible for each of these tasks. In this way, entities or cells providing technical support on contracting help to harmonize the contractual practices of actors in the field.

In order to guarantee the interests of the populations, it is important to rise barriers to counter harmful behavior. In the market sector contracting is controlled by the judiciary system; if an actor feels that another actor, with whom he is in a relation, has caused damaged, he can always appeal to a court of justice. In the health sector, the judiciary system can not act alone as the regulatory actor. It is also important that the State sets up regulatory bodies for contractual practices. These bodies should act on upstream of the judiciary system by preventing harmful behavior. They will also guarantee that the contractual relationships will function appropriately: they need to defend the interests of populations and, at the same time, defend the income of the private operators. Depending on the country, these bodies can be mandated to: 1) regulate the financial aspects (price, competition, etc.), 2) verify that the rules are obeyed to (for example, the labor legislation), 3) verify that the commitments are respected, 4) give an opinion on conflicts between the parties, 5) circulate information on contractual practices in the country. These bodies should be used as instruments for fighting against special interest groups, nepotism and corruption. Therefore there is a need to clearly define the powers of the body: investigation, recommendation or sanction powers.

The question of who should take control of these bodies is also important. As it is a matter of protecting the interest of populations, one would think that the Ministry of Health should take control of this body. However, the Ministry of Health is often a contractual partner, this will make it difficult for it to be at the same time involved, as an actor, in the contracting activities and regulating them. The solution often lies in the creation of an autonomous "agency" that would take over the mandates (this will subsequently pose the problem of the origins of the funding for the agency). This independence from the operators - the health service providers - as well as from the public authorities is important; however, in order to be effective, in other words credible, this agency should dispose of necessary technical capacities that allow it to fulfill its mandates; often, there are gaps in these capacities.

Finally, the question of the scope of this agency should be addressed: will it cover only some form of contracting (an agency for regulating the practices in outsourcing), the entire scope of contracting of the Ministry of Health or will it be established at the level of the general government with a general mandate over all the contracting activities of all the ministries?

The necessity to establish such agencies of regulation will be increasingly important when dealing with competition based contracting when there is a danger of opportunistic behavior of the actors. On the other hand, in a situation where the contracting is based on cooperative partnerships and on trust, such agency is less necessary. In this latter case the regulation mechanisms are already in the contract itself; it is in the actors' interest to implement auto-regulation if they desire to continue with a long term contractual relationship.

In developing countries, such agencies have already been set up in sectors like water, electricity, and telecommunication; there are no examples from the health sector. However, as the contractual practices develop, the necessity to set up these type of agencies will appear.

In comparison with laissez-faire, these tools provide a degree of control over contractual practices. From the practical angle, benchmarks and limits are laid down for certain types of contract, in respect of which the rules of the game need to be spelt out. However, this does not mean that contracting is part of a systemic approach, i.e. a framework within which it is considered to be a tool to improve health-system performance. If contracting is to be seen within the broader framework of health-sector reform, it is in countries' interest to integrate it within their health policy; to do so, they have two options:

- Numerous countries draw up "national health policy" documents, which address the evolution of the health sector together with the reforms required. Countries that wish to adopt contracting may define the terms and strategies for its implementation within this overall policy framework.

- Within national health policy, the potential role of contracting, which is but one tool, is modest and does not allow its use precisely to be determined. To offset this, a specific "contracting policy" document can be drawn up. This is recommended by the resolution adopted by the World Health Organization (WHO) on contracting,[4] which stipulates that "The Fifty-sixth World Health Assembly... URGES Member States:...2)to frame contractual policies that maximize impact on the performance of health systems and harmonize the practices of all parties in a transparent way, to avoid adverse effects;". The

403

purpose of a policy on contracting will thus be to define relations between actors; it will determine the place of the contract in relations between actors operating in the field, lay down the principles and objectives of contractual relations, determine priorities and which actions are subject to contract and lay down certain ground rules (such as requirements for registering contracts).

Few countries have actually formally drafted such "national contracting policy" documents: Burkina Faso, Burundi, Chad, Madagascar, Mali, Senegal and Togo.

Obviously, these two strategies are not mutually exclusive; ideally, they are complementary. Depending on when they are drafted, the latter will complete the former, or the former will incorporate the latter.

Of the tools described here, contracting policies are perhaps the most comprehensive and innovative; They lie at the policy-making level rather than the level of technical instruments. They make it possible to integrate contracting within a systemic approach, along the lines of policies adopted for other areas: drugs policy, human resources policy and health financing etc. Because in many cases it is a new tool which may occasionally give rise to criticism from certain actors, it is in the interest of the Ministry of Health carefully to define its orientations and strategy.

A systemic approach to contracting

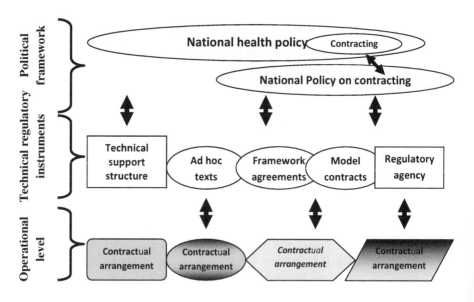

Thus, the majority of countries are currently in a **transition phase**, in other words, the recent period was characterized by the use of contracting as an exception, whereas the trend is now towards systematic use of it, the principles and strategies having been clearly defined by law. Nowadays, national policy documents on contracting are to be seen as the first drafts or as attempts to lay down the first elements of a comprehensive framework. Very frequently, examinations of the place assigned to contracting within the health system are only incipient, and national policy on contracting is taking a pause for reflection.

Notes

[1] WHO, The World Health Report 2000: Health Systems: Improving Performance, p.119.

[2] Siddiqi, S., T. I. Masud, and B. Sabri. Contracting but not without Caution: Analysis of Outsourcing of Health Services in Countries of the Eastern Mediterranean. 2006. World Health Organization, Division of Health System and Services Development, Eastern Mediterranean Regional Office (EMRO).

[3] WHO (2003) "Public-Private Mix for DOTS - Practical tools to help implementation", Stop TB Department, WHO/CDS/TB/2003.325

[4] World Health Organization (2003) "The role of contractual arrangements in improving health systems' performance", World Health Assembly Resolution 56.25, 28 May 2003

Part V

Chapter 2

The role of the government

Jean Perrot

INTRODUCTION

When one considers the role of government, what immediately springs to mind is the debate between "interventionism" and "laissez-faire". Interventionists will argue that the government is guarantor of the general interest and, as such, should intervene to make sure people have the best possible access to quality services — health care in particular. Nonetheless, agreement is needed on the modalities of such interventionism, and this is not that easy to achieve. The laissez-faire rationale, in contrast, relies on market mechanisms to ensure that contractual relations between stakeholders benefit the health system as a whole. Stakeholders know better than anyone what needs to be done, and their actions do not need restraints.

In the domain of contracting this debate is never far away. Without evading the issue, this document will try to avoid taking sides, but aim to show the various possible roles that the government can play.

1. LEADING BY EXAMPLE

This role is inevitable. The Ministry of Health will inevitably be a stakeholder of contracting through the contracts in which it is directly involved. Depending on the type of contracts it signs, it will provide impetus in one direction or another, and its action will never be neutral. By signing delegated management contracts with NGOs to run certain public hospitals, for example, the government indicates that it no longer wants to run its health institutions on a day-to-day basis, but it intends to retain ownership and thus preserve its influence. By choosing NGOs, it highlights the "non-profit" nature of its partners. Similarly, by signing partnership contracts with private health organizations, it shows its willingness to bring these actors into the public-service domain. Lastly, it signals its attitude even through the contracts it chooses not to sign; e.g. by not entering into delegated management contracts with private profit-making entities.

Moreover, without being a direct party in a contractual relation, the government acts as guarantor. Consider the example of a health insurance company that signs a contract with an NGO-owned health centre. While the government is not directly involved in this contractual relation, it cannot be indifferent. To publicly show that this contractual arrangement is consistent with the logic of its national health policy and is beneficial for the population concerned, the government can act as guarantor, by endorsing[1] the contractual relation. In this case the government will be a co-signatory, but will not have the same status as the parties themselves, and it will not interfere in the contractual relations between them. While it cannot be held responsible if the objectives are not achieved, it can intervene at any time by withdrawing its endorsement.

Health Ministry's actions thus send signals to other stakeholders in the health system, indicating the channels it prefers and those it wants to avoid. The attitude of the Health Ministry will always be interpreted by other actors in the health system; it can never claim to be neutral.

2. POLICIES ON CONTRACTING

The previous chapter demonstrated the importance and advisability of regulating contractual practices, and it highlighted a policy on contracting as a key tool of such regulation. While such policies must be designed in conjunction with the various players in the health sector, the Health Ministry plays a key role in steering their development. At each stage of this policy – preparation, elaboration, implementation and monitoring – the Ministry of Health has prime responsibility. Without it, nothing will be done, but without it nothing can be done. It thus plays an important role, but it must be aware that it is not just the policy of the Health Ministry itself, but the policy adopted by and for the country as a whole. Everyone must be a stakeholder of this policy and recognize themselves in it.

This procedure is clearly the best way to ensure that contracting policy will not put a straitjacket on the initiatives of the various agents. On the contrary, this framework should contribute to the coordinated development of contracting for the benefit of all the stakeholders, but especially for the population.

3. THE IMPORTANCE OF CONTRACTING TECHNIQUES

Agents often turn to contracting without the technical skills needed to implement a contractual process. The belief that contracting is a simple technique is still too prevalent. People sometimes think it is enough to find a good contract model and copy it, merely altering the names of the parties. Nonetheless, as Part IV of this book clearly showed, implementing a contractual process calls for substantial expertise from each of the parties involved.

It is up to the Health Ministry to ensure that agents wishing to engage in contracting have the necessary technical capacities. This is clearly not sufficient to ensure that a contractual relation will be beneficial, but it is almost certainly a necessary condition. Experience generally shows that a badly designed contractual relation never produces good results.

So what steps can the Health Ministry take to ensure that all health sector players (itself included) have the necessary technical skills?

- *Training*: As with all new tools, users need to acquire skills; and thorough mastery of the relevant tools is clearly a prerequisite for the success of any experiment. The Health Ministry must therefore ensure that all agents, itself included, have this mastery. Training in its various forms is the way to achieve this. While the Health Ministry is responsible for arranging this for the agents in question, it does not have to provide the training itself. The Health Ministry itself may organize training events on contracting, or it may help other agents to do so. For example, some NGOs nowadays offer training workshops on contracting for their members and also for other agents; the Health Ministry can then support these NGOs either through subsidies, by making expertise available, or providing various forms of documentation, etc. Moreover, with an eye to the future, the Ministry must also ensure that the topic of contracting is included in all initial training programs: in medical and paramedical studies, and in management and administration studies.

- *Development of technical tools:* Like other players in the health sector, the Health Ministry can produce materials of various types. It can also produce guidelines on contracting and brochures to inform and raise awareness among all stakeholders, including those who are not traditional health service agents, such as local authorities, elected officials, opinion leaders, etc. In some cases it may also draft model contracts (see previous chapter).

4. THE "STRATEGY" APPROACH

Many stakeholders, including Health Ministries themselves, see contracting as merely a simple tool to formalize a relation. One often hears comments such as: "Contracting is a health service tool", and as such it is neutral. Similarly, a hammer is a tool that can be used to build a good wall or to break down the door of a house to burglarize it. In this respect, the hammer is a neutral tool. One must not confuse contracting and contract. The contract itself is a tool and, as such, is neutral: anything can be put in a contract (subject to legal and regulatory restrictions). But contracting is not a tool: it is a strategy and is thus not neutral. Why engage in contracting? In any given situation, there are various strategies that agents can pursue, so they have to make choices. A detailed analysis of the situation might point to contracting as the most promising strategy (though the outcome is never certain). Only then can contracting be chosen and modalities defined. Contracting is thus neither good nor bad in itself. It is a strategy that will be more or less well adapted to the context in question ... but it will also depend on the technical skills of the people implementing it.

The rationale of *"Strategic contracting"* should guide the health Ministry's vision. Viewing contracting as a strategy changes the approach considerably. It is then up to the decision maker, in any given situation, to consider contracting as one of the strategies available to change the situation. Choosing contracting is never easy:

- other solutions need to be considered, and contracting can never be seen as the only alternative;
- the environment in which contracting will be used needs to be considered;
- do the technical skills needed for contracting exist?
- the risks must be taken into account; the success of contracting is never guaranteed;
- acceptance of this strategy by society at large needs to be considered, well beyond the health sector alone.

The Health Ministry must persuade all health sector stakeholders, itself included, to see contracting in strategic terms. It must coax stakeholders into adopting this approach.

The Health Ministry must set the example. Thus, every time it is decides to use contracting, it must demonstrate its capacity to visualize contracting as a strategy, i.e. as one possible alternative among the various available. Once again, this demonstration effect is important.

But it must also give leadership to other agents in this domain and here again the Ministry can call on training. Training in the strategic approach requires specific skills that have nothing to do with contractual techniques.

5. SUPPORT FOR CONTRACTING

Nowadays contracting is present in all health systems, although there are major differences in the types of contracting that different countries employ. Whether directly involved or not, the Ministry of Health cannot ignore this situation. The actions available to it may include the following:

- *A legal framework*: The government must ensure that the country's laws allow contracting. Beyond this, it must also take all steps to facilitate contractual relations. For example, it is not uncommon to find that health sector agents refuse to establish contractual relations because of difficulties encountered with a fastidious administration; in this case relations will remain informal even

411

though it would be beneficial for them to be formalized. The legal framework will define the "decision space"[,2,3] granted to each of the agents. Variations in the legal framework between countries will clearly be significant, depending on the institutional reforms that they have undertaken. For example, in Colombia, the law authorizes newly autonomous hospitals to make contracts with private health insurance systems, whereas there is no comparable law allowing this in Chile.

- *Accreditation:* From the initial stages of contractual relations, the government can help implement an accreditation system which, among other things, can facilitate contractual relations.

Accreditation

Accreditation is not:

- A planning procedure: this specifies the level of services to be provided in a given geographic space, and for a specific time period, based on health needs and existing facilities. The health map *(carte sanitaire)* is the tool of this planning procedure.
- A licensing procedure:[4] issued by the government, this licence allows a health institution to engage in an activity and specifies the minimum standards to be fulfilled. There are several types of licence:
  - Administrative: the government confirms that the activities undertaken by the entity in question are not harmful to the public; generally, this type of authorization is granted by the government agency responsible for the "interior"; with it -a health establishment can open its doors to the public; the authority gives entitlement to operate (some analysts call this process "habilitation" or "recognition" or "homologation");
  - Technical and/or financial: e.g. the procurement of heavy equipment may require prior authorization from the health administration;
  - Ethical: certain activities are prohibited: e.g., abortion after a specified number of weeks' gestation, human cloning, etc.
- A certification procedure: this recognizes quality system's conformity with ISO9000 norms; it is issued by a competent and independent agency by providing written assurance that a product, process or service satisfies specific requirements.[a]

Accreditation, sometimes also referred to in French as *"agrément"*, appeared first in the United States and has since spread to countries such as Canada, the United Kingdom, Australia, or France (after 1996). Despite a number of differences between countries, accreditation aims to:

- Obtain quality recognition for an establishment; i.e. formal recognition of the competency of a health care establishment to undertake quality activities – this is a regulatory function. In this sense, accreditation is very similar to certification
- Ensure continuous improvement of the quality and safety of health care actions – this is an incentivizing function. In this sense, accreditation can be seen as a tool for change.

To guarantee independence from the public supervisory authorities, health service funding agencies, and naturally the health establishment itself, the accreditation process is generally entrusted to a specific entity. Examples include the Joint Commission on Accreditation of Health

---

Organizations (JCAHO) in the United States, Agence Nationale d'Accréditation et d'Évaluation en Santé (ANAES) in France, the Australian Council on Health Care Standard (ACHS), the King's Fund Organisational Audit in England, Conseil Canadien d'Agrément des Services de Santé (CCASS) in Canada, and the Japan Council for Quality Health Care (JCQHC, 1995).

The accreditation procedure is external to a health establishment, and relates to its overall functioning and practices. Depending on the standards defined by each country, generally in conjunction with health system agents, the accreditation agency evaluates the following:

- The resources of the health care institution: upgrading of the facility (premises, equipment, etc.), mastery of production procedures and crosscutting processes (medications, blood, etc.);

- Procedures; professional practices (diagnostic and therapeutic procedures, organizational work, etc.);

- Outcomes: improved health status, patient satisfaction, etc.

But what really distinguishes it from certification is the fact that accreditation is seen as a driving force for continuous quality improvement within the health care establishment, and not only as a means of specific external evaluation. Recommendations issued by the accreditation organization thus provide guidelines for changes leading to higher quality.

What is at stake in health facility accreditation? The following situations can be distinguished:

- In the first case accreditation, for the healthcare establishment, is a matter of both internal management and external credibility, without necessarily having a formal influence with supervisory or financing agencies.

- The second case is the where accreditation is explicitly linked to obtaining a contract or funding, which are essential to the institution's existence. In the United States, to be accepted as an accredited provider of health care to Medicare patients (elderly people), a hospital must satisfy the quality standards set by the accreditation system. Globally there is a clear trend towards making an explicit link between accreditation and health facility financing procedures. Thus, accreditation becomes a condition for developing contractual relations – before entering into negotiation, the agents concerned need to have been accredited. It is thus possible that in future the capacity to develop contractual relations, either generally or in certain specific domains, will be included among the indicators on which accreditation is based.

- The third case is where accreditation does not formally contribute to planning or financing decisions, but forms part of the negotiations. In France, for example, the establishment's accreditation report is sent officially to the regional hospital board *l'Agence Régionale d'Hospitalisation* (ARH), which also negotiates contracts in terms of targets and resources between itself and the health care establishments. The accreditation report is not an official element in the contractual negotiation but forms part of the dialogue on which it is based. Accreditation can thus play a key role in contractual relations. As noted by C. Mathy,[5] accreditation provides an *ex ante* signal of the quality of the product or contracting entity. It thus reduces the risks for the other party, which now has assurance of the entity's "qualification", or competence, i.e. the efforts of its future partner. This makes it possible to reduce post-contractual controls and thus lower the cost of cooperation.

[a] *Definitions:*

   - Norm: A set of rules of conformity that are issued by a standardization organization.

   - Standard: A set of recommendations developed and advocated by a representative user group.

- *An information system*: It is the government's responsibility to implement an efficient system of information on contractual relations. This can include several elements: (i) registration of contracts: as the contracts relate to the specific product of health care, the government should at least have a copy of all contracts signed between the actors involved; (ii) analysis of the contracts; as with all information sources, the government should make a statistical analysis of the contracts (number of contracts signed in a country, stakeholders involved, financial value involved, contract type, etc). Ideally, this analysis should be entered into the national information system, but this seldom happens today.

- *Evaluation*: While evaluation is a specific feature of contracting at each stage, internal evaluation by the parties themselves is insufficient. It is also important to have external evaluations to assess the contractual process and its results and impacts. Only this type of evaluation can identify the bases for future actions, and persuade new stakeholders to make commitments on secure foundations. Here again, the government must guarantee this external and neutral evaluation.

- *Oversight*: The government can oversee contractual relations established between stakeholders. Without interfering in contract implementation, it can nonetheless make sure that they are implemented as intended and for the benefit of all parties, including the target populations. This contractual oversight function can be performed at the request of one of the parties involved or as a direct government decision. It can also be done through supervision mechanisms. Nonetheless, as the Health Ministry is more or less directly involved in many contracts, there is a risk that the health administration finds itself in a situation of conflict of interest.

To avoid this, the solution is to separate contractual oversight from the general administration function. One of the techniques used in this type of situation is to set up "autonomous agencies", which can be given mandates such as: (1) to regulate economic aspects (fees, competition, etc.); (2) to ensure regulations are complied with (e.g. labour legislation); (3) to check that commitments are fulfilled; (4) to make recommendations in disputes between the parties; (5) to disseminate information on the functioning of contractual practices in the country. These mechanisms will need to be able to combat cronyism and personalized relations, and prevent corruption of all types. The powers of these mechanisms therefore need to be clearly defined: e.g. enquiry, recommendation or sanctioning powers.

The agency's independence from the operators – the service providers and the public authorities - is important; nonetheless, to be effective, i.e. credible, it needs the technical skills to fulfil its mandates; but these skills or competencies are often lacking.

Lastly, a question arises as to the scope of the agency's prerogatives: will it cover just certain forms of contracting (e.g. regulation of practices involving subcontracting), or all Health Ministry contracting, or will it be established at the general government level and cover all forms of contracting by the various ministries?

Agencies of this type are even more necessary where contracting is based on competition, and opportunistic behaviour by agents can more easily occur. In contrast, they are less necessary when contracting is based on cooperative partnership and trust. Here, regulation mechanisms are built into the contract itself; stakeholders have an interest in self-regulation if they want the relation to last.

In developing countries, agencies of this type have been set up in sectors such as water, electricity and telecoms; but there are no examples in the health sector. Nonetheless, it will become necessary to put such agencies in place as contractual practices continue to develop.

6. COORDINATION WITH OTHER SECTORS

Contracting is obviously not the exclusive preserve of the health sector. All sectors, and consequently all ministries, have experiences that use contracting processes. The Health Ministry should therefore make contacts with other ministries to learn about their experiences and share their tools with them, for the purpose of updating synergies and harmonizing strategies.

In some cases, the government as a whole is also responsible for coordinating practices across sectors. All sectors make use of subcontracting, for example, so the government must harmonize procedures to prevent divergent (i.e. contradictory) practices from developing in the different sectors.

The Health Ministry needs to be mindful of the need for coordination and harmonization. It must always look "outside the box" to ensure that what it is implementing is consistent with what is being done elsewhere.

While this form of harmonization at the government level is still underdeveloped, the need for it will likely be felt as contracting develops in all sectors.

CONCLUSION

This regulation of contractual relations forms part of the government reforms that are unfolding in many countries. The role of the government is being reconsidered, and, particularly in the social sectors, the general direction, following many years based on privatization often advocated by certain international institutions, is now turning towards a stronger State but with functions that focus more on steering the general interest than acting as a provider and financier of services. The health sector, like education, is not immune from this general trend; the government, through the Health Ministry, must in particular strive to implement this general administration function (stewardship). As noted in *World Health Report 2000* "Health Systems: Improving Performance" (WHO), the government should be at the helm rather than rowing the boat. This reflection on the role of State stewardship is nothing new. As noted in R.B. Saltman and O. Ferroussier-Davis (2000),[6] the issue was addressed by J.J. Rousseau in the eighteenth century, then by M.Weber in the early twentieth century and, more recently by the public choice theory in the United States in the 1970s. We will use the definition they propose: stewardship is "a function of a government responsible for the welfare of the population and concerned about the trust and legitimacy with which its activities are viewed by the citizenry".[7]

Within this framework, the government must regulate contractual relations to ensure they contribute to the general interest and improve health system performance. Before reviewing the modalities through which it can implement this regulation, it is worth reflecting on the concept of regulation itself. Here we will draw on the definition given by L.Kumaranayake (1998) : *"Regulation occurs when government controls or deliberatively tries to influence the activities of individuals or actors through manipulation of target variables such as price, quantity and quality".*[8] We shall thus adopt this broad view of regulation that encompasses tools of oversight and surveillance along with incentives. [9] It is important to respect the spirit of regulation; it should always safeguard its objectives which are to ensure the performance of the health system, i.e. allow for effective supply of health care that is equitable and meets people's expectations. Regulation should therefore not be a handicap; some analysts will say that it should a simultaneously be a carrot and a stick, while others will describe it as an iron fist in a velvet glove.

While this seems to be a widely shared goal, regulation can be implemented in a number of ways. For some, it forms part of the logic of agency theory, i.e. the government – the principal – seeks ways to influence the agents – autonomous institutions, decentralized bodies, or private suppliers – to direct them towards attaining the goals it has set for health policy.[10] Others tend to see regulation more in the framework of cooperation, where stakeholders seek to pool efforts to attain jointly defined objectives.

This is an important issue; if the State is unable to play its stewardship role through its capacity to regulate contractual relations, there is good reason to think that contracting will rapidly prove ineffective, or even harmful, to the organization of health services. As a result, contracting may be discredited in the following ways:

- Higher transaction costs: To protect against malicious and opportunistic behaviour, stakeholders will be encouraged to develop all aspects of their contractual relations and to anticipate all possible scenarios, thus increasing the number of procedures involved in negotiating, drafting and monitoring contract implementation. The result will be higher transaction costs, which could cancel out the benefits expected from contracting.

- Corruption: Weakness in the government, and also among other stakeholders, opens the door to all forms of corruption. If stakeholders know that their contractual arrangements are not "supervised", they may be tempted into all sorts of corruption activities. Corruption at the negotiation phase, corruption at the time of drafting a contract (a skilled expert can easily find ambiguous formulations), corruption when signing the contract (the person with signing power is corruptible), corruption during implementation (withholding information, false evaluations, etc).

- New market for the distribution of financial resources; unless the government takes precautions, contracting could easily spawn a new market for obtaining funding. In some countries stakeholders have already realized that access to funding involves going through this new channel, whereas previously it was obtained administratively. If access to resources nowadays involves contracting, skilful agents will move quickly to offer services under a contractual form to take advantage of naive interlocutors.

The role played by the government is thus crucial for the future of this approach. Developing countries are clearly much less well equipped than developed countries, and it is urgent for them to develop skills in this area. The international community must play its part and help developing countries to meet these new challenges, by sharing resources and experiences. As the report by C. Ham (2000)[11] concludes: "Most countries are dealing with health-care reform as if each was on Mars. Few have tried to learn from others... This indifference to the international face of doctoring is a huge mistake... there are lessons to be learnt from looking at different ways of paying for and delivering the goods. Instead of each country trying out its own experiments, they should be studying each other's for ideas and pitfalls". These comments on the general problem of reforming health systems are particularly relevant to the field of contracting.

[1] Definition of an endorsement: recognition of the quality of the service provided by an agent or the quality of a contract between two agents; but the State will not step in should one of the agents fail.

[2] Th. Bossert (1999) *Decentralization of health systems: decision space, innovation and performance . LAC Health Sector Reform Initiative.* 17.

[3] Bossert, Th and J. C. Beauvais. 2002. *Decentralization of health systems in Ghana, Zambia, Uganda and the Philippines: a comparative analysis of decision space . Health Policy and Planning* 17, no. 1:14-31.

[4] Rooney, A. L. and P. R. van Ostenberg. *Licensure, Accreditation, and Certification: Approaches to health Services Quality.* 1999. USAID. *Quality Assurance Methodology Refinement Series.*

[5] Mathy, C. *La régulation hospitalière.* 2000. Paris, France., *Médica Éditions.*

[6] Salman, R. B. and O. Ferroussier-Davis. 2000. The concept of stewardship in health policy. *Bulletin of the World Health Organization* 78, no. 6.

[7] WHO. *World Health Report 2000 :Health Systems: Improving Performance.* 135. World Health Organization.

[8] Kumaranayake, L. Economic Aspects of Health Sector Regulation: Strategic Choices for Low and Middle Income Countries. *Departmental Publication N° 29,.* 1998. London, London School of Hygiene and Tropical Medicine.

[9] Some analysts distinguish an aspect of regulation consisting of government control from another involving incentives.

[10] Bossert, Th. 1999. *Decentralization of health systems: decision space, innovation and performance . LAC Health Sector Reform Initiative.* 17.

[11] Ham, Ch. *Health care reform: learning from international experience.* 2000. Buckingham, Philadelphia., Open University Press. *State of Health Series.*

Part V

Chapter 3

The role of other actors:
communities, labour unions, political parties, churches and private enterprises

Jean Perrot

INTRODUCTION

Part II considered the role of the key actors directly responsible for implementing contracting processes. While the previous chapter reviewed the specific role played by the government, i.e. the Health Ministry, this one will examine the role of various actors that are not actually parties in a contractual relation, but are nonetheless involved in several ways. We thus consider the specific role of population groups, unions, political parties and churches, as well as that of large private enterprises.

1. CONCEPTS

The terms "community" and "population" have very similar meanings; both can be defined as a group of people with something in common. The common factor in question might be:

- A group of people who share common interests or a common ideal; religion, culture, language, ethnic origin, profession ... The group is relatively homogeneous and people are aware about this membership of this group.
- A group of people living in a given geographic area. Unlike the previous case, membership of the group is automatic when a person inhabits the geographic zone in question. One cannot cease to be a member without moving;

Although the dictionary definitions of these two terms give both meanings, it can nonetheless be said that "community" relates more to the first meaning, while "population" tends more to the second. In this chapter we will mostly use the term "community" with the following meaning: "A community consists of people living together in some form of social organization and cohesion. Its members share in varying degrees political, economic, social and cultural characteristics, as well as by common interests and aspirations, including health. Communities vary widely in size and socioeconomic profile, ranging from clusters of isolated homesteads to more organized villages, towns and city districts."

One must not be naive however. Clearly, members of a given community are people who always share, albeit in different degrees, a common identity that distinguishes them from members of another community. Nonetheless, this definition considers the community as a relatively homogeneous group (as the adjective "communal" suggests), whereas a population is a heterogeneous group, even in a defined geographical area. This heterogeneity specifically implies the presence of divergent interests, conflicts, etc. Thus, the less group membership

420

stems from a voluntary act, the greater will be this heterogeneity and the harder it will be to maintain its cohesion. Harmony and cohesion are the exceptions rather than the rule.

"Community", in the sense of an individual's membership of a group, is a rich concept. But a problem of recognition immediately arises. Some communities enjoy recognition. In a society governed by the rule of law, this will be provided by a statute conferring legal status; in a traditional society it is provided by custom. In both cases, this community can act in its own name, and individuals can represent it. Otherwise, the community remains a group of individuals, unable to act as an entity; and, in particular, no individual can represent it since it is impossible to represent an entity that is not recognized (either legally or traditionally).

To overcome this situation, a community can give itself, or be given by law, a legal entity that enables it to act as such.

To have a legal identity, the community must be recognized in a specific organization. The latter acquires an identity that enables it to act on behalf of the community it represents. Individuals belonging to the community delegate to the organization the right to represent them and act on their behalf. This organization may take very different forms that can be divided into two broad categories:

Spontaneous organizations

Without any institutional obligation, the community organizes itself spontaneously very often following a process that is similar to self-promotion. This generally involves the stages of identification of a problem, chance to find a solution, preparation of solutions, design of operating rules for the organization, and control of its management. There are the following types:

- **Traditional organizations.** In modern societies, it is often forgotten that traditional societies continue to have an important place in the life of communities and that they have their own forms of organization. In some cases, this community organization is even recognized by modern States: traditional chiefs represent the community in the various mechanisms and specific tribunals that exist. Where there is no formal recognition by the modern State, this traditional structuring continues to permeate daily life, and ignoring this tradition can cause problems. The organization of this community does not depend on voluntary membership: the individual is conditioned by multiple criteria – ethnicity, caste, social rank, etc. – which are beyond his or her control. The organizational modes of this organization define its representatives – elders, nobles, etc. The legitimacy of this form of representation is enshrined in the customary rules of the organizations in question. Such communities form part of a social order.

- **Organizations based on voluntary membership:** This case covers all non-profit organizations encompassing people who have chosen to join the organization in question.[1] Firstly, there are "associations" defined as "groupings of people who join for a specific common purpose". Most national laws recognize the associative modality – clearly, the names will be different in each country, but they have the same foundations. The legal status conferred on them gives them full legal powers. Usually, the group of individuals that have joined the organization is quite homogeneous, which will make it easier to appoint representatives whose legitimacy will be unproblematic. Examples include a local mutual health insurance company for individuals in the same profession (health insurance for fishermen, merchants, cotton producers, etc). Similarly, an association of people living with HIV/AIDS is likely to be highly homogeneous because the frame of reference is broadly the same.

On the other hand, the representatives in question only represent the association as such, and not all the individuals living in a given geographic space. Nonetheless, the term "community association" is often used on the assumption that it represents the members of the community in a given geographic area. This is similar to the previous case, except that the organization is *de facto* rather than *de jure*. The law is no longer there to give legitimacy to the representatives of this community association; and the people living in a given geographic space do not have to be recognized through elected or appointed representatives.

Yet, despite being established on the basis of voluntary individual membership, some of these organizations do not have an explicit association charter, e.g. churches or religions. Their congregations are represented by the ecclesiastical authorities, but how these authorities are appointed is very different from the procedures followed by associations: in particular, they are not elected by their congregations.

Not all organizations pursue the same aim, and a typology is useful:

- Organizations that act as lobby [or advocacy] groups, aiming to promote specific ideas or defend particular interests. Their purpose is to gain acceptance for the interests of the group –e.g. political parties or labour unions, but also consumer or user associations. Such organizations want their points of view to be heard and taken into account. While they will generally act by positioning themselves outside the institutions they wish to influence, some of them will adopt a participatory strategy that leads them to act on the inside: e.g. by serving on the management board of a health institution.

- Organizations that exist to run health facilities: organizations of this type are sometimes created with this sole purpose: e.g. certain community associations (ASACO) in Mali exist exclusively to run grass-roots health centres. Although supposedly non-profit-making, in some cases these organizations are merely a regrouping of individuals for whom the organization is simply a way to obtain a remunerated activity.

- Organizations that manage health insurance contributions: these prepayment entities have no other purpose than to collect payments from their members and handle their health expenses;

- Ad hoc organizations: This category encompasses organizations that have generally been created at the request of the health authorities and often under strong recommendations by certain development partners, to provide an interlocutor that can give its opinion on the community's needs.

The reality is often less transparent. The purpose of these organizations is not clearly defined and the roles that they are supposed to play are vague.

Non-spontaneous or imposed organizations

Organizations of this type obtain their legitimacy from the law. The law accords legal status to a community defined as the group of people living in a given geographic space. Local authorities (region, municipality, etc.) are thus legally mandated to represent populations or communities. Membership of the community is automatic when a given individual starts to live in the area in question, although a nationality criterion is also generally added. This entity has its own legal identity which allows it to speak on behalf of the population and to commit it. Its representatives will be chosen by election, thus giving those elected legitimacy to represent the population. The community, which forms the basis of this organization, is not necessarily homogeneous; the election process makes it possible to identify a majority that will speak on behalf of everyone. These organizations have public mandates that generally are not rooted in the self-identification of a problem.

The two categories are not mutually exclusive; a given individual can be in both categories, and each of them is equally legitimate, in law, to represent communities. In the best of cases, these legitimacies may be mutually complementary; but they can also challenge each other.

2. POPULATIONS

In the 1970s, a joint WHO - UNICEF Committee on Health Policy declared: "Most systems of health service provision have failed to provide accessible and acceptable health care to those needing it ". Community participation is therefore proposed as specified in the Declaration of Alma Ata:

"Community participation is the process by which individuals and families assume responsibility for their own health and welfare and are motivated to solve their common problems. This enables them to become agents of their own development instead of passive beneficiaries of development aid. They therefore need to realize that they are not obliged to accept conventional solutions that are suitable but can improvise and innovate to find solutions that are suitable. They have to acquire the capacity to appraise a situation, weigh the various possibilities and estimate what their contribution can be."

"Primary Health Care"; A joint Report of The Director-General of the World Health Organization and The Executive Director the United Nations Children's Fund, International on Primary Health Care, para.44, International Conference on Primary Health Care Alma-Ata, USSR, 6-12 September 1978

There are two main reasons for community participation:

- No one knows better than the community itself what it needs are. It is not up to health workers to decide for people what services need to be put in place. The population must therefore be in a position to identify its needs and get them accepted. Furthermore, if the population is not involved, it will not feel responsible. This is true in the domain of cost recovery for example; unless the population accepts this, it will not make use of the corresponding health services. Public involvement is encouraged by awareness-raising; i.e. a population that is involved in implementing health services has become aware of the importance of health, and gives itself the tools to participate in decisions relating to the health of its members. These provide the foundations of the mechanism for matching supply and demand in providing the service.

- Many technical interventions in primary health care should be undertaken at the community level, and do not necessarily need medical personnel to be involved. The aims of primary health care are not confined to improving the cultural acceptance and use of medical services. They include improving the quality of water and local hygiene, and the preparation and consumption of food products, etc. – aims that depend on community participation.

Indisputably, participation of populations in health care services is now universally recognized. Without the involvement of community members, health standards are likely to remain low. Instead of being passive, populations needs to become actively involved.

Although everyone now shares this view, there are bound to be disagreements in translating this involvement into operational terms. The same joint UNICEF-WHO Committee also stated: *"There are many advantages in organizing health service provision in a way that services belong to those to whom they are directed. The ideal would be for health service provision to be put under the control and management of the community itself."*[2] Other people, in contrast, evoking the notion of counter-balance, will place community participation outside health care structures.

How can this community participation be assured? The role of communities has long been seen in terms of health services management. This whole line of action rests on this postulate and, according to its supporters, no alternative strategy is conceivable. The only divergences relate to how this type of community participation occurs in practice.

Naturally, a prerequisite is that community participation can only really occur if communities are organized through mechanisms that have the power to legally represent them, i.e. those with legal identity, either *de facto* or *de jure*. The Bamako Initiative has had many problems because it initially overlooked this dimension; in fact, the "representatives" of the community had no status at all. As soon as the community is given legal status, it can exert influence in various ways:

Participation through a self-owned health facility

In this situation, the community organization directly runs a health care institution of which it is the owner; e.g. a community association, a mutual health insurance society or municipality manages a health care facility that it has created or inherited (e.g. following an administrative decentralization programme). The community organization will thus have many powers. Legal arrangements may either be simple (the community organization directly manages the self-owned health facility), or more complex (the community organization sets up an autonomous but wholly-owned subsidiary). Unless it is to operate in total isolation however, this community organization will always need to interact with the Health Ministry and its deconcentrated agencies. To avoid the disadvantages of a vague situation, the community organization will want to obtain a contractual arrangement with the Health Ministry. One may also question whether it is appropriate for a community organization to manage such a technical institution itself when it does not necessarily have the technical skills to do so. Yet this is the approach advocated by the pioneers of community participation (see above).

Participation within the health care facility

In this case, community organization can have two strategies:

The first is where the organization aims to take over the management of a health care institution that does not belong to it, for which purpose it will sign a contract specifying how its management functions will be fulfilled. The rationale for this rests on the hypothesis that the community organization's impact on health service provision is greater when it can take its own decisions on the relevant issues. Rather than seeking to influence an external manager, it prefers to take responsibility and manage the health agency and its activities itself, as it sees fit, following the adage "if you want something done properly, do it yourself;"

The second case is where the community organization jointly manages all part of a health structure. This is consistent with the new forms of the Bamako Initiative. Specifically, the health structure will have a joint management committee or management board for the establishment in question, which consists of members of the health institution staff (the chief of post) and representatives of institutions representing the community: municipalities, associations ... A balance must be struck between the health administration, which has to make sure health institutions fulfil their public service mission, and the population, which, insofar as it participates significantly in the financing, must be able to give an opinion on and control the use made of its financial contribution. In practice, this joint management takes a variety of forms, however. Joint management can occur: (i) in daily management (e.g. shared management of the proceeds of cost recovery between members of the management committee and the director of the health centre); or (ii) in relation to the major orientations of the policy of the health care establishment (e.g. participation by the user association on a hospital management board). Joint management assumes the health institution has a status that takes account of this principle, and is run by a management board. In many cases this procedure is not in place, and a management committee runs a health care facility, which in fact is always legally under the entire responsibility of deconcentrated health services.

426

External community participation

This approach is based on the principle of separation of functions; the health institution is entirely responsible for supplying health services, but these must meet the needs of the community organizations involved. This is no longer a matter of acting within the health institution but outside it: this is the logic of partnership, which can take two forms:

Partnership based on consultation. Legally independent partners, with health service providers on one hand and community organizations on the other (associations, local collective institutions, mutual health insurance societies ...), enter into relations, but are not mutually obligated in the legal sense of the term. The relationship can therefore take various forms. Mutual recognition is the minimal form, and consists of recognizing that the other party is a valid interlocutor with which it can discuss and shares the main aims of action. This form of relation can also include information exchange, in which the partners keep each other mutually informed of their activities. Consultation between the parties is a supplementary stage. For example, a district management team (an offshoot of the Health Ministry) can consult the community organization's views when the district plan is being prepared, to seek to match supply and demand. It will then be said that this district plan has been prepared in conjunction with the communities, and they are therefore invited to take part in policy decisions relating to the evolution of health services in the district. At the national level, this partnership can be activated at the time of preparing a national health policy with these community representative mechanisms participating in a health sector roundtable.

It should simply be noted that consultation-based partnership of this type does not involve any legal commitment by the communities in question. Their voice may nonetheless be crucial for the district health authorities to take decisions based on the community's needs rather than merely fulfilling regulatory requirements defined by health professionals alone. In any event, the health authorities will not be required to follow the opinion of the communities; this is the basic principle of the consultation.

Partnership based on contractual relations. This differs from the case discussed above in terms of the commitment assumed by the communities. Partnership now entails an exchange of reciprocal commitments. Each partner undertakes to fulfil certain duties, in exchange for the benefits arising from the relationship. The relation now leads to a contract formalizing the rights and obligations of the partners.

427

These contractual relations give community organizations a powerful lever over health service provision:

- The community organization can now negotiate directly with the health institution; e.g. a mutual health insurance society can cause the health institution to change its behaviour, thanks to the purchasing power it obtains from its members' contributions. The negotiating process that will unfold between these two autonomous entities will allow the communities to express their own needs: they will negotiate fees, reception modalities, priority activities, etc. For example, in Burkina Faso, the FAARF mutual health insurance societies have decided to pay for children's medical expenses but not those involving syrups. The health institution for its part, has an interlocutor with which it can discuss the actions to be undertaken and can, for example, cause the insurer to raise awareness of preventive activities among its affiliates. Thus an insurer may decide to reimburse children's health expenses provided they are up-to-date with their immunization programmes. The same is true for a municipality (not a health institution manager) which, thanks to the subsidies it is able to provide to the health institution, can make sure its constituents' points of view are taken into account.

- The community organization can exert pressure on a contractual relation. For example, when the public service concession is awarded to a private supplier, the community organization (a user association) can negotiate to ensure that the contract signed between the two parties explicitly identifies mechanisms for coordinating with it. The community organization will thus make sure its points of view can be expressed and taken into consideration by the manager. There is in fact a risk that contracting, seen from the standpoint of subcontracting and delegation of responsibility, excludes communities from managing health services. It should be noted that communities had progressively succeeded in becoming involved in running health institutions, thus making sure their points of view are taken into account; management committees or participatory mechanisms are included in this framework. In the public sector, and also in the private sector although to a lesser extent, these participatory mechanisms have gained acceptance and recognition as partners. Contracting potentially puts these achievements in doubt, and community organizations can be excluded unless they are vigilant, as is clear in a health institution concession process.

3. LABOUR UNIONS

The union world is increasingly questioned on the issue of contracting. A few years ago, particularly in developing countries, where contracting was hardly known, it was not a cause for concern for unions. Today however, now that contracting has expanded into health systems, unions find themselves answering questions on which they are often inadequately informed.

Firstly, it should be noted that the union world concerned with health decisions is highly varied even within a single country. There are large unions that deal with the entire range of problems in defending their members in all sectors of economic life. Then there are specialized health sector unions which are generally built around a trade organization; unions of doctors (general practitioners and/or specialists), paramedics, other staff. Moreover, some unions may only concern personnel working in the public sector and/or undertaking civil service functions. The issues between the two categories are not the same, and can often be contradictory: e.g. a public sector union will defend the interests of the civil service charter, whereas a private sector union will argue that there should be no specific rules compared to another.

Unions are involved in contracting, in two ways:

- They are concerned with the contracts that their members' employers make with other partners, whose main objective does not directly relate to working conditions; e.g. an outsourcing contract for patient convalescence or delegated management of the public health institution. In this type of contract, unions normally act in two directions. The first consists of endeavouring to guarantee the quality of the service and promote the general interest. Here they will draw attention to the risks of privatization. The second direction consists of discussing the employment implications of these contracts: what will happen to the personnel who previously provided a contracted service; what will happen to the staff recruited by the public health institution? While unions cannot be the signatories of these contracts, they can be concerned in various ways.

- They are directly concerned because the object of the contract itself affects working conditions. They are also concerned for contracts that erode the benefits acquired by employees: particularly if the contract calls into question civil service charter, but also with all new approaches centred on the notion of performance. Merit pay, performance incentive systems, are among the changes that call into question the definition of a job based on the notion of "work correctly undertaken in relation to the means

429

available." Personnel are directly concerned in all these types of contract, even if they are not signatories.

Unions are therefore very often exercised by the contracts which employer institutions sign; yet they are very seldom involved in preparing such contracts. They therefore act either at the time of establishing a contract, by exerting pressure on negotiators through public opinion, or during the implementation phase "by dragging their feet."

The better organized are the unions, the more powerful they will be and more likely to represent factors that will cause the contract to fail. The power of unions in a contractual negotiation should therefore never be underestimated. They can be involved in three ways:

- Either through regular dissemination of information on the contract. Unions are kept informed of the contract at each stage in the contractual process.

- Or through more or less institutionalized consultation. At all points in the contractual process, the contracting parties can hold consultations with the unions. In some cases, this is institutionalized through commissions or groups in which unions participate as representatives.

- Or as contract signatories, or more likely co-signatories. For example, an outsourcing contract can require prior consultation with the unions, and signature of the contract can be on that basis.

Participation by unions in a contractual process is clearly a tricky issue to implement. They need to be involved, however, to prevent them blocking the process; but the protagonists of the contract must also not see their desire to reach agreement endangered.

4. THE CHURCHES

Churches have long played a major role in providing social services – education, and health in particular. They have traditionally provided these services "naturally". It goes without saying that the services they offered were useful to populations in question. They did not have to worry about public services, which often did not exist. Progressively, however, with the implementation of the State and its takeover of health services, the churches and their health organizations have had to take account of the existence of the State: In particular, they have had to gain accreditation and, for that purpose, prepare dossiers and submit them to the Health Ministry. The autonomous life of non-state health care institutions has nonetheless not been called into question by such accreditation. Once it has been obtained, church-based health institutions have continued to operate without taking account of the health system that was being set up around it. Only recently have these private health institutions come to realize that they could not continue to live on the fringes of the system.

"The public and private sectors must work together on public health". In fact there are no longer many grounds for arguing that the private sector should be excluded. Consequently, the public and private sectors are both present, albeit in different capacities, but they are present in practically all countries. It is also true that they must collaborate on public health issues. But what does that mean specifically? Collaborating may mean that each, in its own way, does its utmost to improve public health; in this context, the public and private sectors live in sealed compartments. But collaboration increasingly requires the public and private sectors to reach agreement and understanding on the response they provide to public health problems. Fine declarations of intent, by the public and private sectors alike, are not necessarily backed up by action. Lack of goodwill? No, often it is because the practical problems of implementation prevail over goodwill. Here we would like to make explicit some of the practical problems and suggest solutions to overcome them.

Firstly it is important to note that these health activities can be undertaken either by a health institution (health centre, dispensary, hospital, clinic, etc), or outside any health institution. This distinction may seem anodyne or trivial, but it is important as we shall see.

Suppose these health service providers and the Ministry of Health (or a local authority) [3] are seeking to agree upon the activities to be undertaken, i.e. the health services to be provided. This understanding will be formalized in an agreement, i.e. in a contract specifying the commitments of the two parties.

Where activities are undertaken outside a health institution (or more generally by any establishment) the situation is simple: the contract is made between the Ministry of Health and the institution that will carry out the activities specified in the contract. This institution may be an NGO, an association,[4] foundation, community group, church, health insurer, etc., provided the institution has a definite legal identity under the law of the country in question. It therefore involves a service contract in which the parties agree upon ways to implement the activities and each one's responsibilities.

When activities are channelled through a health institution, the situation becomes more complicated. There are now three actors: the Ministry of Health on the one hand, and an establishment and an institution of the other. The

431

establishment is the health care facility that is technically responsible for carrying out the activities specified in the contract; yet it seldom has a specific legal identity. The legal identity is to be found at the level of the institution that "owns" the establishment. This may be an NGO, an association, a foundation, a community group, a church, a health insurer, etc. This means there is an institution that has legal status but does not actually implement the activities, and an establishment, which carries out the activities but does not have its own legal identity. Clearly only the institution has the power to sign a contract with the Health Ministry. In a few cases, this situation may work without difficulty; but in other cases it can raise problems. The contract signatory (i.e. the institution) is not necessarily in a position to understand the issues involved in the contract with the Health Ministry; and the establishment, which does understand the issues of the contract, is not the signatory, so it cannot be held accountable. There are several ways to avoid these problems:

- Awareness raising activities can undertaken with senior staff to enable the managers of the institutions, which are not necessarily cognizant of the terms of the contract, to fulfil their responsibility and sign the contract in full knowledge of the facts. This is the approach adopted by Medicus Mundi International in the conferences of Kampala[5] and Cotonou;[6] the key objective of which was to raise awareness among bishops, who are the signatories of contracts committing establishments under their charge, on the issue of contracting.

- The second solution is to have the contract signed both by the representative of the institution and by the representative of the establishment. This makes it possible to ensure that the two parties that provide the service are involved. Needless to say, this solution does not solve all problems because, legally, only the institution is responsible; but the advantage is that the agency that will implement the contract on the ground to be involved in all phases of the contract.

- The third solution has two phases. The first involves setting up a management association for the health care establishment. This will likely be largely controlled by the "mother" institution in the sense that its affiliates will mainly be under its influence. Nonetheless, from the legal standpoint, this association has its own legal identity. There is therefore no longer any need for the mother institution to sign the contract with the Health Ministry. This separation of roles is clearly the best solution. The institution can ensure that its points of view are taken into account through its control of the institution, but it does not intervene in the day-to-day running of the facility. The latter fulfils its responsibilities through the

432

management association. This is how denominational education operates in France, for example: each school is directed by a management association, which signs the association contract with the government.

The object of the contractual relation between the Health Ministry and a heath care establishment must also be considered. Three situations can arise:

- The Health Ministry, as owner of a health structure, decides to entrust its management to a non-governmental institution. This type of delegated management corresponds to what is generally known as *"concession"* or *"affermage"* under French law, and "Build, Operate and Transfer (B.O.T.)" or "lease contract" under English law. The terms of the contract will define the roles of the two actors, but the non-governmental institution will generally act on behalf of the Health Ministry and be accountable for the activities undertaken vis-à-vis the Health Ministry. This does not imply disengagement by the Health Ministry, which retains ultimate responsibility, particularly in the eyes of the public.

- The institution, as owner of its health care facility, wants the best possible partnership with the Health Ministry, in particular to participate fully in the public service mission. Naturally, the institution already has accreditation, i.e. the establishment has been recognized by the Health Ministry. The two parties wish to deepen their relations through a contract. The Health Ministry wants to make sure that the private non-government establishment represents it in terms of the health card, and for that purpose it will grant certain advantages (subsidies, tax breaks, staff assignment, etc). For its part, the non-governmental organization undertakes to conduct all activities in the same way as a public establishment.

- The institution, as owner of the health care facility, signs a contract with the Health Ministry to perform specific activities only. The establishment therefore continues to operate as it did at the time of making the contract, which only relate to specific clearly defined activities.

These, at first sight, purely technical aspects often prove very important. In fact, the desire for collaboration, or more broadly, an understanding between the Health Ministry and non-governmental health service providers, is not always sufficient to produce a signed and clearly established contract. There are examples of negotiations that have started at the technical level between the Ministry of Health and the establishment, but which ultimately have not seen the light of day because at a certain moment it was found that the persons with power to sign were not involved in the negotiating phase.

The situation is further complicated when the institution owns several establishments, which happens quite often. If one applies the above approach, this means that the Health Ministry and the institution will sign as many contracts as there are establishments. Each contract will involve the same and specific parties to reflect the reality of each establishment. This solution is clearly cumbersome and it also fails to provide a separation between the strategic view at the institution level and the technical and managerial aspects specific to each establishment.

One possible solution, which has been adopted by the *Association des œuvres médicales privées confessionnelles et sociales – AMCES* (Private, Confessional. and Social Health Care Association) of Benin), consists of the following:

- Firstly, establish a framework agreement between the Health Ministry and the institution responsible for several establishments. This will contain the general guidelines of the agreement, general principles accepted by the two parties, and certain aspects that will be applied to all of the institution's establishments. This framework agreement will be signed by the institution, representing the group of establishments.

- Secondly, and based on this framework agreement, a specific contract will be signed for each establishment. As these contracts will define specific points for each establishment, there will be as many contracts as there are establishments wishing to have a contract with the Ministry of Health. One of the advantages of this approach is that there is no need to renegotiate the points that are negotiated in the framework agreement. The individual contracts will thus be signed at the establishment level either by delegation of signature by the mother institution, or by the management association if one exists.

This type of solution has the advantage of clearly separating the institution's policy orientation function from the technical and managerial function, which concerns the health services provider, i.e. the establishment.

On the basis of all the foregoing, the following prerequisites apply:

- The Health Ministry must first acknowledge that it cannot do everything, or should not do everything. The nuance is important. If the Health Ministry considers that it cannot do everything, this means that it will move towards contracting once it has identified its shortcomings. But it remains in the mindset that it should do something if it has the means. As it does not have the means, it accepts contracting. In contrast, if the Health Ministry

434

starts out from the principle that it should not do everything, then even if it had the means, it recognizes that is not necessarily its role to organize service provision, and that others can do this better. It will therefore not move toward privatization. By contracting, it keeps control over service provision; and its contractual action gives it a means of regulation.

- The private [non state] institution, on the other hand, must be aware that operating on the fringe of a health system is problematic. In fact, if it wishes to make use of contracting only to obtain certain advantages from the Health Ministry, then an ad hoc arrangement of this type could be of interest to the two parties. Nonetheless its influence on the functioning of the health system remains limited. In contrast, if the institution realizes that the interests of those for whom it is working, i.e. the public, require better integration into the health system, while safeguarding its specific nature, contracting is a strategy that makes it possible to obtain this objective.

These prerequisites are important. The contractual tool will be used for completely different objectives. In one case, it involves an ad hoc understanding that can regulate certain short-term problems in everyone's interest (institution, Health Ministry, and also the public). In another case, it involves a structural understanding that defines the role of each party in the health system; from purely technical, contracting now becomes a political issue in the "policy" sense.

If one now considers contracting as a strategy, it needs to be defined more explicitly. A framework needs to be laid down for regulating contractual practices and, more particularly here, to lay down a framework that will define forms of collaboration between the public and private sectors. This strategy can thus be defined:

- At the national health policy level; most countries adopt this type of document which must explicitly recognize the role of government organizations, but also define collaboration modalities;

- At the level of a national policy on contracting; when a country has this type of document, it is important that the principles of collaboration are specified in it, along with the specific modalities in each case.

Non-governmental organizations must also be involved at this level. By participating in the production of these documents, they can ensure that their points of view are taken into account. It should also be noted that this is the main reason why Medicus Mundi International (MMI) suggested that a WHO resolution be prepared and adopted, dealing largely with that issue; this was done in May 2003.[7]

MMI also considered that it was important that specific contractual arrangements be set in a framework that defined the roles of each party.

5. POLITICAL PARTIES

Whether it is the central government or local authorities, decision-making power does not belong to the management but to the political powers that are in place. It is they who ultimately decide the broad directions and strategies for health system development.

Several years ago, contracting was not in the politicians' lexicon, whatever their political persuasion or country. Contracting was regulated by the code of public tenders that set down rules for government procurement of goods and services. Contracting, seen as a strategy for organizing the health system, has only appeared recently. It has also appeared, albeit under slightly different forms, in domains such as education, water and sanitation, management of the major public utilities, etc. Political parties are thus confronted by the rise of a new strategy in which they have yet to master all the issues.

Many political parties still see contracting as a right-wing policy. It is viewed as a form of privatization, or disengagement of the State; and it belongs to neoliberal currents of opinion that advocate market forces for economic and social sector organization. The market must govern relations between the different economic and social actors. Of course the reality is different, as this book has demonstrated; but perceptions are often very persistent and we have to work with them

Clearly, there are parties claiming to be on the left that support the market economy; "Blairism", for example, did not reject all the reforms introduced during the time of "Thatcherism". Nonetheless, feelings on contracting still run strong. Here again, the aim is not to lobby on behalf of contracting. The message is more the following: as decision maker, if you want to use contracting, you must take account of political forces and the reticence of certain political parties, and in all cases take the political parties' understanding of contracting into account.

Ignoring the force of political parties can lead to serious problems, especially when understanding differs according to political persuasion. For example, the contract could become a political battleground if a health minister from a given political party intends to sign a contract with a hospital that has a public health establishment status, in a city whose mayor is from a different political party and is an influential member of the management board.

How can one then ensure that the political parties will adopt a conscious attitude towards contracting? Naturally, political parties represent different persuasions that exist among the population, and it would be foolish to think that there will be perfect agreement on contracting. Some will wait for equilibrium to be attained as a result of the forces at play. Thus, for example, a country might never use delegated management simply because the actors involved do not want it. But it is often preferable to reduce excessive divergences as soon as possible.

The first way is to improve understanding of contracting among political parties: in technical aspects first of all, but particularly with regard to the health system performance issues at stake. It is often surprising to still see a number of political parties or politicians from these parties adopt strong positions based on inadequate knowledge of this tool. The health sector, in conjunction with other sectors, must therefore provide political parties with information, training, visits to other countries, and exchanges of mutual experiences. Better understanding of the topic will progressively elicit a responsible attitude towards it.

The second channel involves the design of a contracting policy. This type of document should enable all actors, including political parties, to reach an understanding around a framework setting out broad rules on the use of contracting in the country. A policy document on contracting should represent consensus on the issue. This consensus is always out of date, however: it reflects the understanding that existed at the time and can always be questioned on the basis of current political forces ... making another policy document necessary.

6.   PRIVATE ENTERPRISES

For a long time now, enterprises, and particularly the largest among them, have shown concern for the health of their employees, providing health-related activities for them on topics such as workplace health, information on various risks, etc. These activities are undertaken within the enterprise and under its direct responsibility (even if it has to call upon specialists to carry out the activities themselves). In certain countries, such as the United States of America, some firms play an insurance broker role by affiliating their employees to service providers offering a predefined package of services.

Nowadays, corporate involvement also takes on another dimension with the development of the notion of "corporate social responsibility" (CSR). This is actually an old idea dating back to the 1950s, but it has mainly developed over the last 10 years.

> **A number of reference points:**
>
> - The ILO Declaration of 1998 defined four fundamental principles and rights at work: Freedom of association and representation, prohibition of forced labour, non-discrimination and abolition of child labour;
>
> - In 2000 the United Nations launched a "Global Compact" to which numerous firms have affiliated, which undertakes to respect 10 principles concerning human rights, the right to work, environmental protection and governance;
>
> - In 2001, the European Commission adopted a Green Paper entitled "Promoting a European Framework for Corporate Social Responsibility", which proposes the following definition: *"Corporate social responsibility: A concept whereby companies integrate social and environmental concerns in their business operations and in their interaction with stakeholders on a voluntary basis".*
>
> - In 2001, the French parliament passed a law requiring companies quoted on the stock market to publish certain information relating to the enterprise's social and environmental policy in their annual reports;
>
> - The French Development Agency (AFD) has developed eight CSR components, one of which is entitled: *"Improving the health of populations linked to the enterprise by promoting private hospital projects in the framework of public-private social partnerships and involving enterprises in the prevention of AIDS."*

From the enterprise standpoint, corporate social responsibility has two dimensions. The internal dimension concerns relations between the firm and its employees (continuous training, health and safety at the workplace, improvement of the work-family-leisure balance, application of the principle of equal pay and career prospects, profit-sharing and shareholding schemes).

The external dimension of CSR concerns relations between the enterprise and the outside world (protection of the environment, relations with suppliers, local residents and public authorities, application of codes of conduct covering work conditions, human rights, the funding of scientific, cultural and social actions).

Health is therefore an important component of CSR. Large firms also often have tools that enable them to signal their commitment:

- Certain firms prepare charters on health and/or the environment, specifying the rights of employees, and providing the means needed to guarantee them a safe and sound working environment, clearly defined work processes, freedom of opinion and expression, and open dialogue. A charter of this type is aimed at all of the company's employees, and reaches beyond to encompass suppliers and partners.

- Some firms set up foundations to help associations in their activities, signing contracts with the associations in question; they finance projects whose results are evaluated;

CSR also has another dimension with large firms operating in developing countries, which are encouraged to show concern for health:

They can do this when they first set up operations, i.e. "socially responsible investment". The enterprise can study the impact of its investment of the environment and also on the life of the inhabitants of the region. In Chad, for example, oil companies have joined forced with the World Bank to develop local health services for the entire local population.

Local health service systems are often so rundown that workers' health is impaired. From a strict profitability standpoint, the company is very interested in ensuring its employees find good health services for themselves and also for their families. An employee whose family has serious health problems cannot himself or herself be productive. Moreover, and particularly when the firm plays a major role in a given geographic area, it is in its interest to ensure that health systems operate properly. For that purpose, it can involve itself in the operations of the health facilities in question. It will seldom take direct charge of a health institution. But it may sign a contract with it. In return for sustainable financing, the institution provides better quality health services to the company's employees, as well as to their dependants and often also to the local population

---

The involvement of extractive and agricultural industries in health service provision in Papua New Guinea

According to the World Bank definition, Papua New Guinea (PNG) is considered a fragile state (2007). Yet, with a per capita GDP of nearly $ 2000 USD, it is classified as a middle income country. Concretely, these facts reveal the dual nature of this country where the private industry is active and producing wealth but where the wealth does not get redistributed, mainly because of the failure of the State to capture and use the resources for providing or financing services to the population.
In remote areas the government's presence is very limited, the public health facilities in rural areas are underfunded, understaffed or closed. It is in these type of contexts, often referred to as enclaves, that most of the big mining and oil industries operate. The insufficiency and lack of public health services has given rise to industry initiatives that have been implemented in order to establish a platform for health service delivery. The companies have in the first place focused on providing health services for their employers and their dependants. However, the companies have often later expanded their involvement in health; some of the companies have opened their clinics to the entire population in their impact zone, some others have started to finance the public or church run health facilities that are

situated in their operation area. The private corporations' involvement in health service delivery and financing in PNG is thus linked on one hand to a classic occupational health approach but also on the other hand to Social Responsibility actions.

The individual actions of the private companies have had considerable local impact on the health service supply in terms of quantity and quality. However, these actions often have a short or medium term objective since most of the mining and oil companies will be present only for some decades in a given extraction area. This sustainability problem has already materialized on the Island of Misima where a gold and silver mine was opened in 1990. The company running the mine built a high quality health clinic that offered services to the employees but also to the rest of the population. This clinic was never incorporated in the public health system or in any local level health service planning mechanisms; thus when the mine closed in 2004 there was no clear plan on how and with what resources would the activities in the clinic continue. Currently the clinic is underfunded and its activities have slowed down or ceased.

The Misima example demonstrates that the private industry involvement in health service delivery and financing can be a welcomed effort, however if this is done in an *ad hoc* manner without linking these activities into the general health system and planning framework they might pose problems later on.

The PNG National Department of Health (NDoH) has acknowledged these problems and it has already started to address them. A pilot project, that has created multi-stakeholder partnerships (local health authorities - Faith Based Organizations - corporations) has been established in a set of localities; these partnership arrangements have the objective to put in place a formalized system (through contractual agreements) that bring the different actors together. The next step for the NDoH is to strengthen its overall stewardship role by creating a general partnership framework that will bring the corporation based health financing and service delivery under a common health system planning and financing umbrella.

Firms may also make contracts with local NGOs/associations to help them to carry out actions in certain areas. For example, in Burkina Faso, the oil company Total signed a contract with an NGO to raise AIDS awareness among employees and their beneficiaries.

Involvement of Anglo Coal and Virgin Unite in the AIDS domain in South Africa

Anglo Coal and Virgin Unite (the charity arm of the Virgin Group) collaborated with a local community to build and open a health centre in rural Bushbuckridge. This centre provides free HIV treatment, TB and general services to around 70,000 people in the area (where around 20% of the population is estimated to be HIV+).

The attraction of this model for any MNC is the dual benefit of addressing' employees, and their families', needs as well as the community within a partnership structure.

From Overseas Development Institute London, U.K.), Briefing Paper 30, December 2007

Corporate involvement in the health of their workers and populations has nothing to do with altruism. It is in the firm's interest to have healthy workers. Moreover, the image of the firm is at stake both locally and internationally; and a firm recognized as socially responsible will see its share price rise.

CSR needs to be clearly distinguished from sponsorship. It is in the firm's interest to take account of the social and environmental aspects of its activity, but it will do so under its own criteria, i.e. as its action is voluntary, the money channelled into these activities will need to earn a return. CSR is an integral part of the firm's commercial strategy, and the firm expects to benefit from its commitments in these areas. This involves a process which is quite similar to corporate paternalism.

Notes

[1] Some people prefer the term "non-governmental organizations" (NGOs).

[2] Quoted in A.Goldsmith, B.Pillsbury, D.Nicholas (1986) "Organization communautaire", PRICOR, Monograph Series: Question, Brochure 3, Maryland, USA.

[3] For convenience we will refer to the Health Ministry hereinafter, but the argument applies equally to local authorities.

[4] An NGO is not a legal status but a label given to an association that fulfils certain clauses, even a foundation.

[5] Conference of English-speaking African bishops, Kampala, 22 - 24 March 2004.

[6] Conference for French-speaking African bishops, Cotonou, 31 May to 2 June 2005.

[7] *The role of contractual arrangements in improving health systems' performance*, World Health Assembly Resolution WHA56.25, of 28 May 2003.

Part V

Chapter 4

Elements for developing a national policy on contracting

Jean Perrot

1. THE PROCESS OF DEVELOPING A NATIONAL POLICY ON CONTRACTING

In order to draw up a national policy paper on contracting, it is advisable to follow the different stages of a process. There is nothing original about the one described below: it is more or less comparable to that followed in drawing up a document on national health policy or any other policy instrument.

Certain prerequisites need to be borne in mind:

- It takes time to draw up a policy paper on contracting; it is very difficult to do it in less than six months and in general it takes longer. For example, political validation is outside the control of technical specialists and may take a long time.

- Drafting a policy paper on contracting is the responsibility of the Ministry of Health, although not of the Ministry alone. The Ministry should involve other actors with an interest in health. If there is a desire for WHO to be involved, its role will clearly consist of assisting the Ministry of Health. It is imperative for this responsibility of the Ministry of Health to be made explicit: for this reason, it is recommended that consultants should not be given responsibility for drawing up the national policy paper on contracting, although they may be used to provide Ministry of Health officials with technical support. Ownership by the Ministry of Health is often delicate, as the Ministry frequently goes from one extreme to the other: either divesting itself of responsibility by calling on consultants or on the contrary jealously protecting its monopoly on drafting this document.

- Because contracting is a still unfamiliar tool, those who will bear responsibility for drafting the document are not necessarily acquainted with the approach. Moreover, globally, national policy papers on contracting are few and far between and finding inspiration elsewhere is not easy. This means that before setting to their task, those responsible for drafting the document must first of all perfect their skills, in other words acquire all the skills they need to perform their task.

444

The process may be conducted through the following stages.

STAGES

STAGE I : THE POLITICAL DECISION

Any process that leads to the drafting of a policy paper on contracting must begin with the development of political awareness of the need for such a document. This realization may spring from policy bodies - the Ministry of Health or occasionally the Government itself - which have understood its value. The document may also be requested by technical bodies, i.e. health executives. Awareness may also develop much further upstream from the implementation of contracting, as a sort of prerequisite for any development of contracting or, on the contrary, come in the wake of the multiplication of a range of experience of contracting, in this case out of a concern to harmonize contracting practices. Lastly, in some situations, there is no denying the involvement of development partners who, for a variety of reasons, want contracting to develop and need their actions to be based on a reference document.

The decision by the policy-making bodies within the Ministry of Health is based on the notion of public interest. In this instance, the Ministry of Health is not acting as a direct participant in order to define its policy for implementing contracting, but as the guardian of the public interest. The Ministry wishes to determine a policy on contracting that is valid for all actors involved in the field of health (including itself). Comparison with a national health policy paper is useful here. Such a policy paper does not set out the policy of the Ministry of Health as one of the actors in the sector, but rather determines the country's policy in the field of health for all actors working in the sector. Nevertheless, the Ministry of Health plays a vital role in this process; it is responsible for steering the drafting of the paper while of course ensuring that all the other actors participate in full. The same holds for a policy paper on contracting; the Ministry of Health must ensure coordination in the drafting of the document, while ensuring that all actors participate in and contribute to the process.

Political commitment should be clear and explicit; a note from the Ministry of Health or from the highest administrative authority indicating the onset of the process is valuable in vesting it with official status.

If the Ministry of Health wishes to receive support from WHO, it should make its request as early as possible in the process.

445

STAGE II : PREREQUISITES

The Ministry of Health must set up the entities that will direct the process. We recommend that a technical body be established to be responsible for drafting national policy on contracting.

Coordination of this "Technical committee" will be assured by an official from the Ministry of Health; The Committee, which will comprise at least 10 members, will be responsible 1) for directing the process and, 2) for drafting the policy paper on contracting. The members of the technical committee must be capable of devoting the necessary time to this task throughout the whole process. It should be borne in mind that the process will be very demanding on the members' time, even though they will not be entirely discharged of their regular tasks. This also means that their supervisors must be informed of the tasks assigned to their staff who have been assigned to the committee and that they must allow them properly to carry out their work.

The technical committee must be officially set up through the most appropriate channels in terms of the country's context: ministerial order, internal memorandum, etc.. This official document must both designate the members of the technical committee and define, as clearly as possible, its mandate. *If support from WHO is required, this must be explicitly mentioned.* It is advisable for the committee to be chaired by a senior official from the Ministry of Health so as to facilitate links with the Ministry's decision-making bodies. It must also include members from the Ministry of Health (from both the central and local levels, despite the difficulty of ensuring that the latter are able to make themselves available), together with external members (resource persons, private-sector representatives (in particular the non-profit private sector) and representatives of civil society, etc. Of course, it is important to take into account the ability of members to make themselves available.

STAGE III: LAUNCHING THE PROCESS

Stage III will be directed by the technical committee.

- It is quite probable that not all the members of the technical committee will be equally familiar with either contracting itself or the process of drafting national policy on contracting; some of them will have taken training in and some will have experience of contracting, others not. From the very outset, it is desirable for all the members of the technical committee to be brought up to the same level. This will require them to be given all the necessary information. the technical committee may also schedule training/information sessions for those who need them; the "training" may be provided by members who have already been trained or by resource persons (such as WHO staff, if any are involved in the process).

- Preparation of a detailed work plan, setting out everyone's responsibilities and the agenda for the processes. This work plan will observe the stages described here.

- Drawing up the detailed plan for the policy paper on contracting and assigning responsibility for drafting each part of it. For each part, an indicative number of pages will be set, to guide the authors in their work.

- Before beginning to examine national contracting policy, it is important for all member of the technical committee to have sound knowledge of contracting in the country. Ideally, whenever a policy paper on contracting is drawn up, it should be preceded by a study of the existing situation of contracting there. However, experience has shown that this requirement is rarely respected, and the study of the situation is in actual fact undertaken as part of stage IV below.

- Determining the main thrusts of national policy on contracting; it is important for the technical committee as quickly as possible to reach an understanding on what constitutes the core of national policy on contracting.

It is important for these elements to have been approved by the decision-making levels of the Ministry of Health; to this end, a " technical note " will be sent to the Ministry's decision-making authorities. This is a worthwhile precaution both for the technical committee (it is protected against any breakdown in communication with the decision-makers) and for the decision-makers themselves, who thus give their agreement to the conduct of the process and to the deadlines. Once it has been approved, this technical note will constitute the technical committee's "road map".

If WHO has been requested and has agreed to provide technical support, it is particularly important for it to be present at this stage.

STAGE IV : THE ACTUAL WORK

The technical committee will then have to carry out the following activities:

- Situation analysis: the policy paper on contracting will need to describe the situation regarding use of contracting in the country at the time the document is drafted. To do so, it may commission an ad-hoc study (or already have had it produced) or put together the necessary information itself. The aim is not to conduct an exhaustive survey of existing experience but rather to analyse the situation; in what spheres, who are the actors, what are the objects what are the factors of success and what difficulties were encountered, etc.? This snapshot of contracting at the time of drafting the policy on contracting will make it easier for the reader to understand the *raisons d'être* and the objectives of the proposed policy on contracting.

- Meetings between the members of the technical committee and the actors concerned: NGOs, health and management committees, religious orders, local authorities, trade unions and development partners etc. The purpose of these meetings is: 1) to develop a better understanding of the stance of each of them on contracting (i.e. the experience being garnered by each of them) but also to understand their point of view on contracting and its evolution within the health system, and 2) to provide these actors with information on the process of drafting the policy paper on contracting and the involvement expected from each of them. Specifically, it may involve working meetings with some of these actors, field visits in order better to grasp the actual situation and the difficulties, the exchange of information via notes or e-mail and the exchange of information documents, etc. These meetings will protect both the technical committee and the Ministry of Health from accusations that the national policy paper on contracting has been drawn up without consulting actors in the field.

- Each of those responsible for a part of the policy paper on contracting draws up a preliminary draft in accordance with the tasks assigned to them by the detailed plan. The drawback of this approach is the lack of internal harmonization of the document (although this will be corrected at the next stage), but it does offer the advantage of securing genuine commitment by each of the technical committee's members. Moreover, the determination in advance of the number of pages expected from each participant is a first step towards harmonization.

If WHO technical support has been obtained, at this stage it will be able to contribute by providing information from outside the country (such as documents from other countries), and commenting on the initial drafts, etc.

STAGE V : CONSOLIDATED DRAFTING OF THE POLICY PAPER ON CONTRACTING

When, and only when all the different elements have been put together, a consolidated and harmonized draft of the contracting policy paper is to be produced. One of the members of the technical committee must be assigned responsibility for this: it often proves to be a difficult task as those responsible are always late in submitting their work. In this connection, we recommend that the technical committee organize an outside retreat (of approximately on week) in order to finalize drafting of the policy document on contracting: it is important for all the members of the technical committee to be fully on hand at this crucial stage in the process. After the retreat, the technical committee will have a document that has been "harmonized" and which is complete. After this stage, a well-drafted and complete document which is no doubt quite close to the future final document should be available. All the members of the technical committee should be familiar with its entire contents and be capable, as a group and individually, of supporting it.

If technical support has been obtained from WHO, it should be particularly intensive during this stage.

STAGE VI : THE SEARCH FOR CONSENSUS

The technical committee must:

- Distribute the policy paper on contracting to those persons and/or institutions who are to be invited to the technical validation workshop. The document must be distributed at least two weeks before the workshop so as to give them time to read it (or to circulate it inside their institution) and to prepare for the workshop.

- Prepare and organize the technical workshop to validate the policy paper on contracting. This technical workshop (as a rule, one day is enough) will bring together all the persons or individuals who wish to contribute. This means that the purpose of the meeting is not to inform actors of the document's content (as they will already have received it), but to discuss its content, to say what they agree and disagree on and to make suggestions for improving the document. However, this is not a time for drafting: it is not advisable to form working groups to examine particular points. The objective is to adopt a position on the acceptability of the document as it stands. After the workshop, the following will have been achieved: 1) unreserved acceptance of the document (although this is no doubt rare), or alternatively 2) overall acceptance of the document, subject to certain amendments, or 3) rejection of the document: if this is the case, it will be necessary to resume the process further upstream, but the technical workshop will not be capable of solving the problem. If the document gives rise to substantial criticism, the Ministry of Health will no doubt indicate what steps it intends to take later.

- Appropriately revise the policy paper, i.e. on the basis of the recommendations clearly expressed and accepted during the workshop: this corresponds to situation 2) above. It will not take the technical committee long to incorporate these amendments.

STAGE VII : POLITICAL APPROVAL OF THE DOCUMENT

The document is now ready as far as the technical bodies are concerned. Before it is published, it will require political approval. It is a policy document which commits the Ministry of Health as the entity responsible for health.

Internal approval: here, the document requires the approval of the Ministry of

Health's policy-making bodies. Frequently, the Minister will ask for the views of his cabinet. The Minister of Health must give his official approval to the document, although he may also request certain improvements or amendments. However, these must not involve any substantive changes to the document, as this would require a return to the technical validation stage as the new text would no longer correspond to what was decided on at that stage. This could be confirmed by an internal memorandum. It might also be advisable for the Minister of Health to put his signature to a "foreword" or "preface" to the paper on national contracting policy;

External validation: the Minister of Health may also try to ensure the policy paper on contracting carries greater weight by seeking support from the Government. In practical terms, this involves presenting the paper to the Cabinet or persuading the Prime Minister or President to sign a foreword, etc.

The technical committee has but little control over the deadlines during this stage. In some cases, this stage may be a mere formality, while in others it may take a considerable time even if the process was set in motion by the Prime Minister himself. Of course, if the Minister of Health has changed during the process this might cause further delays.

Once the policy paper has been approved by the Minister of Health, it is ready for the next stage.

STAGE VIII : PUBLICATION AND LAUNCH

The document must now be printed. Some thought should be given to the number of copies required. If it is to serve as a basis for all those actors working in the country who wish to use contracting, it is important to ensure that enough copies are printed. In order to ensure it carries enough weight, its official nature should be made quite clear, for example by the presence of the national flag on the cover page.

It is also important for the policy paper on contracting to be accessible on-line on the Ministry of Health's internet site.

When the document has been printed, it must be distributed, and a distribution list should be drawn up for this.

It might also be a good idea to organize a campaign to raise awareness. The press, radio and television could be involved in this. This awareness campaign will make it possible for all actors, both those who were involved in the previous stages and those who were not, occasionally simply because they were remote, to acquaint themselves with the existence of the policy paper on contracting. A launch ceremony could be held.

The technical committee will need to ensure that the monitoring bodies, as defined in the policy paper on contracting, are set up. This is an important stage, because it is often the case that monitoring, despite being provided for in the document, is not actually carried out because no-one has actually been made responsible for it. For this reason, we recommend that the technical committee remain in place until the monitoring bodies have been established. Once this has been done, the technical committee may be dissolved.

It is quite possible that most of the members of the technical committee will be appointed to the bodies responsible for monitoring national contracting policy, thereby ensuring the continuity of the process.

2. THE CONTENT OF THE NATIONAL CONTRACTING POLICY PAPER

We may now consider the content of a policy paper on contracting. There is nothing compulsory about the elements suggested; they are simply suggestions on which the authors of the national policy on contracting may draw in order to draft the document, which must mirror national cultural sensitivity.

Title and size of the document

We suggest that the document bear the title: "National policy on contracting in the health sector in *(name of country)*". A policy paper on contracting need not be very long: some 40 pages are often sufficient. However, in all likelihood it will be necessary to complete the document with operational documents, regulations and operational manuals etc. when it is actually implemented.

Some people believe that 40 pages is too long for such a document; they explain this by referring to the notion of "policy statement" a document of just a few pages which simply sets forth the main lines of the policy in question. They consider that a document of this length is not a policy paper but rather a "strategy" paper. On the other hand, a strategy paper needs to be more precise and no doubt more operational than the vision set out here. Clearly, there is no hard and fast rule; it is up to those concerned to choose the most suitable formulation. For this reason, it has been suggested that the document should be entitled: "National policy and strategy on contracting in the health sector in …".

The national policy paper on contracting will be an "official" document. It sets out the country's position on contracting: it sets the desired orientations and (sometimes implicitly) indicates those to be avoided. In order to ensure it enjoys due official status we recommend:

- That it be published under the name of the Ministry of Health and display the national flag; this will give the document the status it deserves. It is not simply a document that sets out a point of view but one that expresses the will of the nation in respect of contracting.

- That a "foreword" or "preface be written setting out the intention of the Ministry of Health's decision-making bodies to institute a national policy on contracting. If this foreword or preface is signed by the Minister of Health it will lend even greater weight to the document.

3. TECHNICAL NOTE ON THE PROCESS OF DRAWING UP A NATIONAL POLICY ON CONTRACTING

The policy paper on national contracting policy might first of all recall the background to the decision to prepare it. It is worthwhile knowing the reasons for the decision as they allow the document to be placed in its country context.

The document might also provide a reminder of the drafting process adopted: this is a summary description of the main lines of the approach described in the previous paragraph.

This information is not an integral part of the policy paper on contracting; consequently, we suggest that it be set out in a technical note. This will indicate to readers that the note contains information on the manner in which the document has been prepared, but no details of the contracting policy *per se*.

3.1. The context

A document on national contracting policy cannot be isolated from its context:

- National health policy: it is important to recall how contracting fits into national health policy. If there is a national health policy document, it is worthwhile recalling what the document says about contracting. Alternatively, an indication could be provided of how the policy paper on contracting complements national health policy.

- Government policy: the objective is to demonstrate that contracting is not necessarily a tool that is specific to the Ministry of Health, but that other sectors resort to it or plan to do so. It may also represent a general policy orientation, i.e. one decided by the Prime Minister or the President. If there are any landmark documents on this, attention should be drawn to them here.

- Similarly, it might be valuable to draw attention to the experience of neighbouring countries.

Contracting is part of the institutional environment of the health system. Reference should be made to the main features of the system necessary to understand the context of contracting; for example:

- Do health facilities possess a specific legal status, and if so what is it?

- Who manages private health facilities?

- What is the status of the populations when they are associated in the management of health facilities?

- What are the mechanisms for accrediting NGOs? Is there a special status for them?

- Are there any federations or unions of either health-service providers or of funding bodies (mutual health insurance societies)?

- What is the status of the local health administrations?

- Within administrative decentralization, what is the role of the local authorities within the health sector?

Clearly, the legal status of the different actors is important in contracting, because it determines their capacity to sign contracts. This part should include only those elements considered essential to an understanding of the context into which contracting is being introduced.

3.2 The situation as it stands

Different forms of contracting are always present in countries. When drawing up the national policy on contracting, it is worthwhile to get an idea of the existing situation in respect of contracting. Obviously, national policy on contracting should base itself on existing practice in order to envisage the potential and desirable trends. If there is already a more or less comprehensive document setting out the existing situation in regard to use of contracting in the country, the job will be made easier as the document may provide a form of summary.

453

This is not intended to describe each and every experience, but to provide an overview of the situation and to draw the main lessons from it, in order to indicate, via an analytical approach, those areas in which contracting is used and the type of contractual relations that exist in them. It might be worthwhile to recall the main results and difficulties of previous or ongoing experiences and the actors mainly responsible for developing experience of contracting.

This is a snapshot, taken at the time of drafting the national policy on contracting, whose purpose is to demonstrate that the national policy is intended to provide a framework for the overall experience being developed and to set future orientations with reference to what exists: will it be designed so as to reinforce what exists or rather to develop new fields for contracting?

3.3   The *raisons d'être* for a national policy on contracting

The national policy paper on contracting must set forth the reasons why decision-makers have decided to draw up a national policy on contracting. Caution is to be exercised in this respect: it is not a question of justifying the use of contracting, but of explaining why it has become important to draw up a national policy on contracting. For example, a country may favour contracting without feeling the need to draw up a national policy in that respect. This means that it is necessary to account for the need to draw up a national policy on contracting at this particular moment.

The reasons put forward may depend on the level of development of contracting in the country. For example, a country that has developed broad experience of contracting in recent years will place greater emphasis on the need to harmonize contracting practices. On the other hand, a country with scant experience of contracting will place greater stress on national policy on contracting as a tool to facilitate and stimulate the development of experience.

Some countries may see the national policy paper on contracting as a prerequisite for the development of contracting in the health sector, while others may prefer to wait until they have acquired sufficient experience before consolidating it in a national policy paper.

For example, the national policy paper on contracting in Chad states that *"The purpose of contracting policy in the health sector in Chad is to ensure that contractual arrangements between actors in the health sector help to improve the performance of the health system in compliance with the national health policy and its principles of equity"*. While it is important to set forth this ultimate objective, other objectives may also be mentioned, such as:

454

- The desire to better associate the private sector in the implementation of the national health policy. This is what is generally meant by expressions such as "Public Private Partnership". This desire may take different forms:

  - Entrusting the private sector with the management of public health facilities: management by delegation;

  - persuading private health facilities better to integrate their activities into national health policy and the public service mission: association with the public service;

  - encouraging private actors, and in particular NGOs, to carry out activities with an impact on the health of populations, at the explicit request or proposal of the Ministry of Health;

- The desire to base the forms of technical and/or financial support on contractual relations that define the roles of the lead and supporting actors.

- The desire to persuade the different parts of the public sector to consider their relations in contractual terms: for example, contractual relations between autonomous entitities (hospitals) and the central authority and the central and regional administration.

- The need to define the principles of a contractual process.

- The need to harmonize the drafting of contractual documents by defining a standard model which actors must comply with.

3.4   The fundamental principles of national policy on contracting

It is important for the national policy paper on contracting to recall the main fundamental principles underlying the country's national policy on contracting. A number of these are set out below:

- The State is the guarantor of the general interest: consequently, the Ministry of Health, out of a concern to ensure the population as a whole has access to high-quality health services, must be able to ensure that all contractual arrangements observe this objective of national health policy.

- Contractual policy in the health sector asserts that contracting is a tool that makes it possible to establish sustainable and sound relations between actors working in the sphere of health and in no way signifies a withdrawal by the State nor any desire to privatise health services.

455

- Given the novel nature of this tool within the health sector, existing policy on contracting is a first stage. On the basis of the assessment of experience, and drawing on experience in similar countries, contracting policy in the health sector will have to be gradually revised and improved.

- The policy on contracting offers a reminder that contracting concerns all the actors working in the field of health: the State and its various branches, populations, financing institutions, civil society organizations, the for-profit and non-profit private sectors and development partners. It is the duty of the State to ensure observance of this principle. In this way, the actors must all feel concerned by this policy and the State must help them to do so.

- By defining a framework that favours and encourages contracting, the policy on contracting is intended to help all actors in the health sector, and in particular the private sector and civil society, to develop their competencies. However, pursuit of the public service mission remains a fundamental element of contracting.

- The policy on contracting asserts that contracting must be based on mutual respect between actors, whoever they may be, in their contractual relations. This means that even in situations that resort to rivalry and competition to provide health services, it is important for the actors as far as possible to avoid conflict and to give preference to negotiated solutions. Likewise, although the State is undeniably a singular partner on account of its status, it must always try to ensure that its partners provide the population with the best possible service, while taking into consideration that partner's possibilities.

- The policy on contracting asserts that contracting must safeguard the interests of populations and their involvement in the running of health services. This means that the mechanisms that have gradually been put in place to allow the populations to participate must not be called into question by contracting.

- The policy on contracting affirms the freedom of actors to enter into contracts. Nevertheless, because it is health, and more particularly public health that is concerned, the State must ensure that this contractual freedom does not work to the detriment of the population's interest.

- The policy on contracting provides a reminder that contractual relations must be developed between actors who possess the legal capacity to sign contracts. Nevertheless, forms of internal contracting may be developed provided it is clearly established that they are of an ad hoc nature.

- In order to harmonize practice in respect of contracting, it is recommended that a standard model contract serve as a reference.

These fundamental principles will undoubtedly be quite similar from one country to the next. It is nevertheless important for countries to bear them in mind. At a later stage, during an evaluation, the country will be able to ascertain whether the country's experience has observed these fundamental principles or whether it has departed from or even undermined them. These fundamental principles thus constitute reference points to guide the use of contracting.

3.5 The strategic thrusts of contracting

This is the very heart of the national policy paper on contracting because it addresses the strategic thrusts of contracting in the health sector. The paper describes the desired types of contracting. For each of them, the document must set out the reasons which led to the adoption of a given line of action: how this particular type of contracting will make it possible to resolve certain problems and what are the benefits of resorting to contracting rather than other tools. Similarly, for each of them the document will need to indicate what barriers are in place to avert the negative effects of using contracting.

It is important for the national policy paper on contracting to indicate whether contracting may apply to every possible type of contractual relationship between actors, or whether it applies only to certain forms of contractual relationships. For example:

- The national policy on contracting may declare that while on the one hand, management by delegation in order to run public health facilities is generally acceptable, it may not be used for health centres, and on the other that only NGOs of a certain size (and which have been awarded a form of approval) are eligible.

- The national policy on contracting may state that the twinning of a public hospital is possible only with a public hospital in a developed country and not with a private hospital.

- The national policy on contracting may stipulate that management by delegation may be used to manage public health facilities but not for the administrative functions of health districts or regions.

How may the strategic lines of action of contracting be presented? Once again, there is no hard and fast rule, and each country will need to choose the manner best suited to it. One attractive approach is to use the objectives of the different forms of contracting as a starting point, in other words to use the problems that each form of contracting is intended to solve. For example:

Ensuring that health service providers fulfil their public service mission as well as possible

For many years, health services were provided by establishments operated by the Ministry via their decentralized services. Nowadays, the Ministry wishes to address its responsibility in different terms: authorizing management by delegation of its health facilities, improving the links between autonomous establishments and the entity responsible for oversight, associating private health facilities in the public service mission and facilitating the introduction of decentralization, etc.

Ensuring that health activities are carried out by securing the commitment of all actors

This category includes contracts with NGOs and associations to carry out activities from their health facilities or outside any health facilities. These are service contracts which the Ministry of Health may sign with NGOs to help them carry out certain activities manifestly connected with health.

Improving actors' productivity

This category includes contracts for out-sourcing or subcontracting, contracts with suppliers (improving the skills of actors, and especially newcomers), contracts of employment, especially in the civil service (contractual employees, performance contracts for civil servants, etc.). This area concerns health facilities (especially hospitals) but also the Ministry of Health's central and decentralized administration. Those areas in which subcontracting may be used without posing any difficulties should be indicated, as well as those in which it is best avoided. The necessary safeguards to avoid harmful effects should also be put in place and attention drawn to the importance of the environment (i. e the presence of firms capable of working as subcontractors), consideration of the time factor (i.e. spreading subcontracting over time), and of the importance of the notions of "lowest bid" and of "best bid", with reference to the code applicable to public contracts.

Improving relations between financing institutions (mutual health insurance societies, health insurance companies) and service providers

Specific contractual arrangements: the importance, for both of these actors, of using contracting to establish relations between them, should be recalled, together with the elements that the contract may cover (rates, terms of admittance...). The text should refer to the evolution of the code applicable to mutual insurance societies. It

458

should also show the limits of too "specific" an approach and the need to develop framework agreements, by drawing attention to their advantages.

Facilitating inter-institutional cooperation

This concerns all those contracts whose explicit purpose is cooperation between actors: twinning contracts, cooperation contracts with the "North" (States, communes, regions), contracts with training institutions (Universities and schools), and networks.

It should be emphasized that such contracts are broadly inspired by the notion of cooperation and by the idea of working together; it should also be mentioned that on account of the nature of these contracts, the notion of their legal enforceability should no doubt be replaced by the importance of mutual trust, with as its corollary the possibility for one of the actors to end the relationship without the other resorting to the courts.

Improving the performance of health actors

The objective here is to introduce the notion of performance contract. This category of contract has a multitude of forms. It may involve introducing the notion of performance into the purchase of health services from public or private providers. It may also introduce performance incentive mechanisms, in which case it concerns both service providers and the health administration. The purpose is clearly to demonstrate the innovative nature of this type of contractual relationship and at the same time to show that it is a continuation of the notion of strategic planning. The notion of "results-based management" which is new to the administrative environment, should also be recalled.

To permit the use of advanced technology

The Ministry of Health needs to use advanced technology to perform certain tasks:

- Delegated contracting authority (DCO) for construction: this is an area in which technical factors are of a complexity that is beyond the technical and financial means of the Ministry of Health itself. However, it should also be explained that DCO should not result in the Ministry giving up its responsibility.

- Medicines: a central drug procurement office exercises a form of delegation: programme contract. Here the technical aspect is complemented by the desire for independence on account of the important financial elements.

- Health insurance: delegation to an agency.

- Relations with development partners: the relationship between the Ministry of Health and a development partner always involves a contract; however, generally speaking, this is an understanding between these two actors regarding the support provided by the development partner. Moreover, this understanding evolves into a contract setting out the commitments made by both actors and results indicators for their relationship. Besides, the application of contracts is an increasingly common requisite for the initial understanding.

Better defining the role of institutions in terms of technical or financial support

Institutions providing technical or financial support for national institutions (health service providers or central or local administration) are recommended to define in a contract their respective roles and mutual expectations. These institutions, as well as certain international NGOs, may be development partners. Budgetary support is a form of contracting, and it would be worthwhile recalling the issues involved.

3.6   The ways in which contractual relations are established

The policy paper on contracting will need to address the question of how contractual relations are established and indicate the country's preferences. For example, the way in which contractual relations are established is important. The country has no wish to impose a particular procedure and it is up to the actors concerned to choose the most suitable path. However, it draws the attention of the actors on stage to the need to define, at the outset of the contractual process, how these relations will be established:

- Encouraging rivalry and competition between potential actors: in this case, an actor proposes a contractual relationship and will choose its partner using conventional tendering techniques or by mutual consent. Such contracts are subject to enforcement by the law.

- Relational contracts correspond to situations in which the actors negotiate their relationship without one of them being in the position of calling for tenders or the other of submitting a tender. Such contracts are based on joint development of the contractual relationship."

The adoption of one of these contractual forms must first of all depend on the situation; however, the national context is also important; some countries will prefer to use legally enforceable, i.e. legally binding contracts, while others will naturally prefer relational contracts.

Lastly, it should always be borne in mind that there are a number of instruments that the Ministry of Health has to comply with: the Code applicable to public contracts - where certain forms of contracts are concerned, the civil service Code - where anything affecting civil servants is concerned and the Code of Commerce where other forms of contract are concerned. The Ministry's action is circumscribed by these instruments and it may not deviate from them, except to negotiate with the competent entities. For example, management by delegation is as a rule defined in texts that then apply to all sectors of activity. However, by virtue of its specific nature, the Ministry of Health may supplement these general texts: for example, it may indicate that one of the eligibility criteria for institutions is non-profit status.

3.7   The role of the Ministry of Health

The role of the State, in other words of the Ministry of Health, is crucial: it appreciates the risks inherent in uncontrolled development of ad hoc contractual arrangements, and must be the guarantor of a systemic approach, which alone is capable of bringing about a lasting improvement in health system performance.

The State as an actor in a contractual relationship

Although the State does not wish to be the only actor on stage, at the same time it has no wish to exit the stage. Contracting is a means of allowing it to reconcile these two positions. In   this case, the State becomes the signatory of a contract into which it enters with other actors.

The State as regulator of contractual relations

The role of the State in respect of contracting is not limited to its direct involvement in a specific contractual relationship. The State appreciates the limits of its direct involvement and measures the importance of the action of all the other actors, be they from the public sector or from the different private sectors, as well as that of the populations themselves.

It is more and more common for these different actors to interact, occasionally with the participation of the State, but more and more often without it. This diversification of actors and the concomitant separation of roles necessarily leads to the emergence of multiple interactions between the actors, who will try to formalize them by means of contractual arrangements so as to protect themselves with regard to their commitments. Can or should the State simply let things be? Because health is a good which concerns the public interest, it cannot and should not. If it simply lets things be, the result may be contractual relations that are harmful for the populations: unscrupulous health actors may reach understandings that are detrimental to the population. Regulation of contractual relations is part and parcel of reform of the State; the ways in which this regulatory function may be exercised vary considerably:

A- Accompanying contractual relations

- *Advocacy on behalf of contracting:* by putting the case for contracting to actors and other ministries concerned and by continuing discussions with external partners. The senior echelons of the Ministry of Health are responsible for organizing and carrying out this advocacy.

- *A legal framework*: The State must ensure that the country's legislation permits partnership based on contractual relations. However, beyond this, it must also adopt all the measures needed to facilitate such contractual relations. This legal framework will determine the leeway for decision-making allowed to each of the actors.

- The State must encourage a constructive dialogue among all the actors present in the sphere of health to urge them to develop the synergies capable of improving the system's performance.

- *An information system*: the State is responsible for setting up an effective information system on contractual relations. The information system may comprise several elements: i) contract registration; ii) analysis of contracts: as with any information system, the State must conduct a statistical analysis of contracts (number of contracts signed in the country, actors involved, volume of funds involved, type of contracts, etc.)

- *Control*: The State exercises control over contractual relations in the following manner:

    - E*nsuring contractual arrangements are in conformity* with the national policy on contracting on which they depend. Such control is exercised «a posteriori» by an entity with responsibility for monitoring contracting.

    - Without involving itself in the implementation of contracts, the State may nevertheless ensure that they are applied as planned and for the benefit of all the parties, including the populations concerned. Monitoring of the contract may be done at the request of one of the parties concerned or by direct decision of the State.

- *Evaluation of contractual arrangements.* The entity responsible for monitoring contracting must also be capable of evaluating practice in this respect.

- *Training*: as with any new tool, those who use it need to learn how to do so. Contracting calls on numerous notions drawn from different disciplines (law, economics, public health, science political and administrative science, etc.). A sound understanding of these tools is certainly a prerequisite for a successful contractual arrangement. Consequently, the State must ensure that each actor, including itself, has this understanding. Training, in all its forms, is the means of achieving it.

- *Mediation in case of disputes*: disputes are inherent to contractual relations. For their part, the actors must do everything possible to resolve conflicts. In the last resort, they may set the matter before the courts. However, between these two extremes, they may call on the State to mediate. The State must be capable of performing this often delicate role.

- *Registration:* The national policy on contracting must also prescribe how contracts are to be registered. It is not uncommon for a contract to be a confidential document to which only the two parties have access. What rules are possible in this respect? In all cases, it is recommended that the Ministry of Health determine these rules;

- *Evaluation of the national policy on contracting.* This evaluation must be conducted under the aegis of the highest authorities of the Ministry of Health. It will make it possible to assess the policy's impact on the performance of the health system and to draw lessons for improving action

B- Incentives

The State may influence contractual relations via incentives. On the basis of the above definition of a contractual relation, the State may, by means of appropriate incentives, influence actors' decisions by persuading them to consider their interest in subscribing to a contract. For example, the Ministry of Health may decide to award a bonus, subsidy or tax exemption when contractual arrangements are signed.

Incentives will be particularly relevant to all national contracting policies whose purpose is to persuade the public sector to work in coordination with the public sector.

The incentives that a Ministry of Health may offer are essentially financial. However, it may also make use of other incentives, such as labelling, which involve the Ministry of Health giving recognition to a contract between actors.

3.8 The legal environment

The policy paper on national contracting policy must indicate whether it is feasible under the country's prevailing legal environment. It is not enough simply to assert that this is the case; it is necessary to put forward evidence of its legal feasibility. For example, the document may indicate if and how public hospitals may outsource certain activities.

However, in all likelihood, implementation of the national contracting policy will require the amendment of certain legal texts. The policy paper on contracting will thus need to indicate how this policy will affect laws and regulations, in other words what adjustments will have to be made in order to permit the policy's implementation. For example, the document might indicate what regulatory framework will be needed to permit delegation to sign contracts to the local health authorities.

3.9 Responsibilities for implementing the national policy on contracting

The paper on national contracting policy will need to recall that the preparation and implementation of a contractual relationship is a matter for the contractual parties. This means that the Ministry of Health is directly implicated, via its different entities and services, in contractual relations when it is one of the signatories; in this capacity, it is bears responsibility at all stages of the contractual relationship.

We cannot over-emphasize this principle. There is frequently a tendency among organizations, when a new problem or a new field appears, to set up a new entity to take responsibility for it. For example, this was often the case with cost recovery or fields such as primary health care in the wake of Alma Ata or with community health; when faced with new tasks, Ministries of Health have set up units specifically responsible for them within the Ministry. While this approach has the merit of providing specific resources, it has the major drawback of isolating the topic within a "ghetto". For this reason, we do not recommend establishing a unit responsible for managing each stage in the establishment of a contractual relationship: identification, negotiation, drafting the contract document, implementation of the contract and evaluation. Of course, this also holds for the other health actors. If an NGO wishes to sign a contract with the Ministry of Health, it will draw up the contract itself.

However, on the one hand contracting is a recent practice within health systems and on the other it is never as simple as it seems. In order to manage a contractual relationship, those responsible require skills they do not always possess. Consequently, if the different health actors are to resort to contracting in a duly professional manner that will ensure its success, it is important that they receive all the support they need to help them perform these tasks.

In order to address these problems, it might be advisable to set up a *"technical support structure for contracting"*. This structure would assist health actors who feel the need for help, whether they are actors who belong to the public sector or private actors. It is not advisable for such assistance to be reserved for the Ministry of Health; it is important for private actors, should they express the need, also to be able to benefit from this support, which may take two forms:

- Support-counselling at each stage in the contractual process. Here are a few examples. The Director of Hospital may turn to this entity to request the texts in force in the country in respect of management by delegation. The director of an autonomous hospital may ask it for information on the provisions of the Code applicable to public contracts concerning sub-contracting of caretaking services. The chief regional medical officer may enquire of it whether he is authorized to negotiate payment on a capitation basis with a micro health insurance scheme or ask for advice on the signing of a contract.

- Prior opinion to the signatories to a contract; the entity may give its opinion on a contract that has been drawn up but not yet signed. This is the case within the Ministry of Health: before signing, the future signatory may ask the unit whether the contractual document it intends to sign has been properly drawn up. Likewise, a micro health insurance scheme may ask the unit for its opinion. These examples illustrate the need for the unit to be utterly impartial. The opinions it gives must not be influenced by anyone. Consequently, its position within the institutional structure must be carefully chosen.

However, the unit's mandate is not restricted to the two tasks described above. In order to properly perform its tasks, it will also need to:

- Coordinate the preparation of guides to the use of contracting in the main areas defined.

- Coordinate training in contracting for all actors, in particular at the peripheral level.

- Undertake an evaluation of the different contractual relations and their impact and publicize the findings of the evaluation.

- Ensure that the necessary regulatory texts to permit the use of contracting in all the selected fields are drafted.

Thanks to these activities, the entity ensures that the actors will have the means of improving their skills and qualifications in order to manage their contractual relations. These different tools will enable the actors to develop more satisfactory contractual relations.

It should be stressed that this "technical support structure for contracting" may be set up regardless of whether there is a national policy on contracting. It should be clearly stated that the entity's mandate is technical and not political. It should not express an opinion as to the wisdom of using a particular form of contracting: its role is restricted to the following: 1)"This is, or is not possible, 2)"If you want to do it, here's how to go about it, and 3)the contract document you submitted to us for our opinion is good or bad".

Moreover, it should be emphasized that this entity should possess the means of fulfilling its mandates: sufficient staff and appropriate operating resources. These operational considerations are important; there is no point in setting up such an entity if it is not given the means to carry out its task. Ideally, since it is at the service of all actors, it is conceivable for its means also to be provided by these other actors: for example, it is possible to imagine a federation of micro health insurances seconding one of its executives to the entity.

When a national policy on contracting has been drawn up in the country; provision must have been made in the policy for the means of monitoring the policy. Thus, once the Ministry of Health has drawn up its policy on contracting, it must ensure that it is implemented and that all the actors in the health sector comply with it. In order to perform this task, it is desirable that a *"Implementation monitoring committee"* be set up. The committee, which would be headed by a Coordinator/Chairman from the Ministry of Health, has the following main responsibilities:

- Developing advocacy actions directed at the political and administrative authorities and at civil society bodies, concerning the national policy paper on contracting.

- Informing and permanently raising awareness of the different health actors about the orientations and principles of the national policy on contracting and of the main areas concerned by it.

- Ensuring that the Ministry of Health takes all the steps required to enable it to perform its regulatory role over contracting.

- Issuing opinions on the orientations and priorities of the Ministry of Health in respect of contracting. The opinions may concern the new fields of application of contracting, the specific involvement of partners or the strategy for implementation in a given area.

466

- Organizing exchanges with countries that have drawn up their national policy on contracting.

- Initiating and providing support for the organization of periodic evaluations of the policy on contracting and proposing revisions of the policy paper.

A committee will no doubt have been established to draw up the national policy on contracting. The committee's task will have been completed once the Policy has been made official and distributed and the monitoring body set up. Moreover, it is possible that some of its members will be on the monitoring committee, thereby ensuring a degree of continuity.

Contrary to the entity described above, whose mandate is technical, the monitoring committee's mandate is political. Its task is to inform and provide guidance for policy makers concerning the implementation of the national policy on contracting adopted by them. Inasmuch as the policy in question will have been adopted by consensus among the different actors in the health system and, frequently with the support of the development partners, it might be advisable for the monitoring committee also to consist of representatives of these organizations. It is important for the monitoring committee to be under the direct responsibility of the Ministry of Health so that it is directly accountable to it. This means that it is not an operational and decision-making entity, but one that proposes actions to the decision-making authorities in order to ensure that the national policy on contracting is introduced as planned.

Accordingly, the monitoring committee will consist of individuals who will continue to perform their usual activities (contrary to those belonging to the technical support structure); nevertheless, if the committee is fully to play its part, it must possess a permanent secretariat to ensure that it carries out its activities in accordance with its mandates. It is a lightweight structure; however, the permanent secretariat is essential for it to operate smoothly.

Naturally, both these structures are independent from one another, despite occasionally sharing common interests. For example, the technical support structure must help to provide training in contracting: this does not mean that it does so alone, but it must help to set up the training. In turn, the monitoring committee will ascertain that the training actually takes place, as provided for in the national policy paper on contracting. If the training does take place, it will have to ensure that it has achieved the expected results; if it has not taken place, it will have to find out why and suggest solutions.

It is important therefore that the technical structure be under the responsibility of the Ministry of Health's senior technical body (the Secretariat-general) while the political structure (the monitoring committee) will be under the responsibility of the highest political authority (the Minister of Health).

CONCLUSION

By way of conclusion, the national policy paper on contracting may emphasize the following two elements:

- Contracting policy is a new process that will need to be carefully implemented and closely monitored.
- It is a dynamic process, requiring revisions that depend on the changes that may occur in its legal and institutional environment and the results achieved.

Significant use of contracting within a health system almost necessarily leads to forms of regulation. While perhaps regulation is not necessary as long as contracting is used only exceptionally, it will become indispensable when contracting is used by a variety of actors in varied settings. The need to lay down a framework is self-evident, and the need for it is frequently felt and expressed by the actors themselves. However, it may prove to be a perilous exercise, as the framework should not be too restrictive, so as not to sap the inherent vitality of the contractual approach. Regardless of its nature, a regulatory instrument has little chance of achieving satisfactory results if it is imposed by those who have drafted it, and this is all the more true in the case of contracting; coercion is a poor partner for the spirit of contracting, which relies on mutual understanding between actors. In Benin, the Ministry of Health realized that some trade unions were bitterly opposed to certain forms of contracting (management by delegation of certain public hospitals and certain types of subcontracting). Rather than imposing its point of view in the national policy paper on contracting which it plans to prepare, the Ministry has preferred first of all to persuade the unions to discuss the strategy.

The development of national policies on contracting will make it possible to address all the facets of contracting and to define sound orientations and strategies that will be adopted by health actors. However, it is impossible first to develop and then to implement a national policy on contracting without firm commitment by the policy-making bodies of the Ministry of Health, or, even better, the Government. An understanding of the need to determine a framework for contractual practices may come about simply for technical reasons; however, without political commitment the technical arguments are likely to fall short. Besides, the different actors will show all the more respect for a policy on contracting if politicians are genuinely committed to it.

EVALUATION OF A CONTRACTING POLICY

Part VI, which follows, will focus on the evaluation of contracting experiments. However, at the level of a national policy on contracting, the issue of evaluation also needs to be considered. Even where it is clearly indicated that a national contracting policy is a policy paper, it is nonetheless important, following its adoption, to reflect on whether the chosen policies have been implemented as desired. If this is not the case, the evaluation will prompt the policy-maker to consider revising the previously-adopted national contracting policy.

Suppose that a country wishes to monitor the implementation of contractual arrangements and to this end develops a contracting policy that provides a framework for all contractual arrangements. Let us suppose, for example, that the country has developed this contracting policy at the health-district level to enable stakeholders to collaborate in implementing district-level priorities and ensure better management of health facilities. Once this contracting policy is in place, all the contractual arrangements that it covers should make reference to it and be consistent with it.

The evaluation of contracting policies is part of a dynamic process. As we have stated on a previous occasion, contracting policies are the result of successive layers of experience. The evaluation must be seen primarily as a stage in the development of contracting policies; in this sense, evaluation is not a goal but a means to an end.

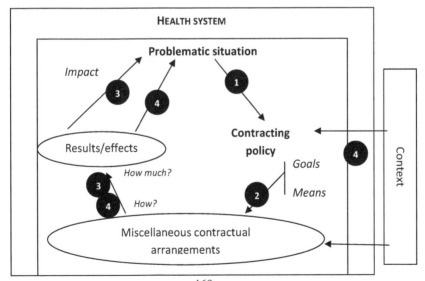

Before discussing the evaluation process in greater depth, we must agree on the rationale for the policy constituting the subject of the evaluation.

The rationale for the policy is as follows:

a. A specific issue arises in a given health system. For example, insufficient use is made of the various health stakeholders at the health district level.

b. To resolve this problem it is decided to develop a contracting policy. This policy establishes a frame of reference covering all the contractual arrangements that will be put in place in this area. Both the objectives of the contracting policy and its means of implementation (legal regulations, financial incentives) are thus specified.

c. Various contractual arrangements exist.

d. The effects of these various contractual arrangements will directly impact the problematic situation and, more generally, the performance of the health system

e. Additionally, this contracting policy exists within a given, specific context and will inevitably influence the development and implementation of the policy.

The evaluation will therefore be part of this process and will focus on various elements within it:

 Analysis of suitability

The first stage of the evaluation will question the suitability of the chosen contracting policy for resolving the identified problems. This is a two-pronged issue. Upstream, we should ask why contractual arrangements were preferred to other solutions to the identified problems. We should also seek to understand why a contracting policy was imposed instead of allowing contractual arrangements to develop naturally.

 Analysis of consistency

The consistency between the contracting policy and the various contractual arrangements implemented within the framework of the policy should be analysed. The contracting policy will have defined the objectives of the contracting arrangements: Are the implemented contractual arrangements clearly consistent with the objectives of the contracting policy? The contracting policy will also have defined the means of implementation (texts, regulations, financial incentives, etc.). To what extent has the contracting policy contributed to the emergence of contractual

470

arrangements? The analysis may reveal divergences whose causes should be identified. This analysis of the consistency between contractual arrangements and the contracting policy should lead to proposals for harmonization without aiming for standardization of practice.

 Analysis of results

The contracting policy will have facilitated the establishment of contractual arrangements. Evaluation at this stage consists of analysing the aggregated results of all the contracts, not just one single contract.

The results could be viewed as follows:

- First, we must fully understand the status of contracting in the area under consideration, for example by counting the number of contracts drawn up, the financial turnover they represent, the number of people affected by them, etc. These tracking indicators should be adapted for each contracting policy. In any given situation, it will no doubt be rare for all health services to be contracted out. It is therefore useful to understand the relative status of contracting with a view to gauging whether it is the exception rather than the norm. Let us consider the example of a contracting policy for the management of State-run health clinics by private operators. How prevalent are these private managers? We could also inventory the number of State-run health centres managed by private operators and ascertain how many are still directly administered by the Ministry of Health. In another scenario, we could, for example, calculate the amount of money handled under contractual arrangements to gain an idea of their importance. All contractual arrangements should be analysed to ascertain how many work well, how many are encountering problems, and how many are dysfunctional. Naturally, the reasons for this should also be determined.

- Harmonization of contractual practices: one of the prime objectives of a contracting policy is to try to harmonize the contractual practices of health stakeholders. Through the framework it offers, a contracting policy seeks to prevent disparate or contradictory contractual arrangements from arising. Evaluating the contracting policy therefore consists in determining whether the contractual arrangements conform to the contracting policy. In addition, the contracting policy may have included conditions or recommendations for evaluating each contractual arrangement. For example, the contracting policy may have specified a

471

certain number of indicators that must be present in each contractual arrangement, thus making comparison between arrangements easier. The contracting policy could, for example, recommend the same financial reporting cycle for all contracts, or a standard financial reporting format, or even that all contracts for health facilities must include standard attendance indicators such as the number of children immunized or the number of consultations, etc.

- The analysis of the results obtained in turn prompts an assessment of whether these results have provided a satisfactory solution to the problematic situation which led to the contractual arrangements. The changes brought about by contracting should be investigated. To the extent possible, changes directly attributable to the contracting policy should be distinguished from those that could have been brought about without a contracting policy. Organizational changes are of particular interest, but the benefits gained also need to be weighed against the costs incurred as a result of the contracting option. The cost of overseeing the implementation of a contracting policy and monitoring existing contracts are sometimes quite high, as a number of studies have shown, and can negate the benefits. Oversight should not only be carefully costed but also assessed in terms of deliverables.

- Analysis of health system performance: has the response to the identified problematic situation had an impact on the performance of the health system? Taken together, have the contracting policy and the contractual arrangements led to an improvement in public health and enabled the health system to better meet patient expectations and achieve more equitable results in terms of health financing?

 Analysis of integration

The integration of a contracting policy is how well it fits into a given organizational context. It is more about "how" than "how much". Analysis of integration focuses on two elements:

Analysis of the process

The evaluation should not only focus on the results of the contracting policy. It should also focus on how the contracting policy functions and how this process leads to high-quality results. This type of evaluation should be recorded in a "black box" so that the conditions under which a contracting policy works well and the conditions required for positive results can be identified. The methods for developing and implementing the contracting policy should be examined, as well as the linkage between the contracting policy and the operation of the various contractual arrangements. For example, the following points could be analysed:

- The genesis of the contracting policy could be described: did the policy predate the formation of contracts, or was it the result of existing arrangements, i.e. the desire to situate previous action in a coherent framework? But causes and developments over time should also be studied. This analysis is important because it facilitates an assessment of the results of the contracting policy. Because contracting arrangements are often innovative, no one expects the first few versions of a contracting policy to be perfect. Improvements are made gradually.

- Responsibilities within the Ministry of Health: it is useful to examine the division of responsibilities in the process of developing a contracting policy. What was the role of the Minister of Health, his closest advisers, or the highest echelon in the administrative hierarchy (the office of the permanent under-secretary at the Ministry of Health), technical departments, the legal counsellor, etc.? This analysis will be useful for subsequent understanding of the various difficulties encountered in the course of implementation.

- Stakeholder involvement: how were the relevant stakeholders involved in the development and implementation of the contracting policy? Were they merely consulted or was there real collaboration? Did the contracting policy result from strong pressure exerted by one or more development partners, or was it the result of a process of discussion and negotiation among the stakeholders? For example, if when private practitioners implemented the DOTS strategy, only young health professionals agreed to enter into contractual arrangements with the Ministry of Health, this is a crucial piece of information that might prompt us to reconsider the contracting policy in this area;

- The problems encountered: the analysis should highlight the main problems encountered during the development of the contracting policy and identify their causes;

- Change over time: with the benefit of hindsight, it is important to analyse how the various contractual arrangements were implemented over time. This analysis of the changes will offer insight into the implementation of the contracting policy and its chances of success. For

473

example, if three contracts were signed during the first year of a contracting policy, twenty during the second year, and ten were cancelled during the third year, this would indicate a certain enthusiasm on the part of the stakeholders, but also insufficient preparation at the contracting policy level.

Analysis of contextual influence:

Not only do we need to see how the process works by going into the "black box" to examine the mechanisms and processes that produce results, we also need to observe the impact of outside factors on results. This is why analysis of the process is so important. An analysis of the contextual influence aims to explore how the context in which the contracting policy and the various contractual arrangements evolve impacts on implementation of the policy. Because each context is unique, a contractual arrangement may yield different results depending on the context in which it operates. This analysis will focus on various contextual elements such as political, economic and sociocultural factors.

Part VI

Chapter 1

Evaluation of contracting

Martine Audibert, Riku Elovainio & Jean Perrot

INTRODUCTION

Although health improved generally throughout the world during the twentieth century, thanks particularly to technological progress and better medical knowledge, supported by income growth among certain population groups, and better working conditions, in many countries it remains below expectations and at a level deemed unacceptable by the international community.

It is already clear that several countries will not achieve the Millennium Development Goals for health by 2015. In the poorest countries, where infant-child mortality rates are above 150 per mil, 60% of the causes of mortality could be avoided through inexpensive preventive or curative treatments.[1] Nonetheless, the health system and the supply of health care are underdeveloped and underperforming in these countries. In countries in transition, economic reforms have profoundly altered the health system and the supply of care, stripping them of their historical effectiveness[2]. Moreover, these countries are having to cope with growing demand (communicable diseases have not been eliminated everywhere and the burden of non-communicable diseases is growing)[3], while their resources are limited. Health-system performance is on the agenda everywhere, even in wealthy countries, as shown by the conference on health-system performance and efficiency organized in June 2008 by WHO/Europe in Tallinn (Estonia).

Poorly performing health systems, compounded by the need to significantly increase health sector financing, the desire for greater equity and the institutional upheavals that have taken place in many countries have caused the organization of health systems to evolve in terms of both the conception and the diversity of stakeholders. Furthermore, new concerns are arising that are going to elicit behavioural changes.

These include:

- New governance issues caused by the shift from a resource-based rationale to one of outcomes, which has already appeared in developed countries but is also gaining ground in transition and developing countries.
- The disappearance of the public-private ideological clash.
- The State's new health-sector role; the Government delegates, but it is the regulator and determines national health policy.
- The desire to involve different health stakeholders alongside public health-care providers; the non-profit private sector (NGOs, charities, community); the commercial private sector, the traditional sector, potential users with conditional demand transfers.

- The desire for consensus between increasing numbers of financial backers.

These concerns are leading to far-reaching reformulations, particularly in relations between the stakeholders who will become institutionalized and in terms of the separation of functions. Contractual relations are gaining ground in both internal and external arrangements (on this subject see chapter I, part I, The emergence of contracting). In fact they are coming to be seen as a promising way to improve the performance of health systems with a view to achieving the Millennium Development Goals and improving equity. Although contractual relations can take a variety of forms, in every case that we have seen they are based on relations of trust involving two or more partners with reciprocal duties and obligations, in which both parties expect benefits.

Health-sector contracting is a relatively recent tool, the adoption of which is encouraged both by external partners and by Governments, who see it, among other things, as a way of raising the quality of health services and thus improving people's health status. Although the literature contains examples of experiences with promising results, it has also reported cases where the outcomes have been less convincing. Nonetheless, its relatively recent use and systematic lack of evaluation does not afford the arm's length distance needed to clearly extract lessons that can be used in practice.

As in any activity or intervention in which an outcome is expected, evaluation is also proving necessary in the contracting domain. The partners in a contractual relationship may pursue different objectives; but if these are not achieved the result will be non-renewal or early abandonment of the contract. As contractual relations are one of the health system's performance tools and strategies, it may be crucial for Governments to know what type of relation makes it possible to attain the Millennium Development Goals most expeditiously and at least cost.

The purpose of this chapter is to raise stakeholder awareness of the need to evaluate contractual relations and to propose a methodological framework for those involved in contracting processes.

A desire to develop trade between provinces or to improve the education or health levels of their populations will lead a Government or a development partner (often in cooperation with the Government) to set up an intervention.[4] The only way to check whether a given intervention has allowed, or contributed to, the achievement of an established goal is to evaluate it. While this can be seen as a democratic imperative when evaluating interventions in the public sector[5], it is definitely not costless. The interests and issues in evaluation are especially clear in the health sector since interventions have the ultimate aim of improving individual well-being and avoiding deaths, without squandering resources.

Understanding the interests and issues in evaluation entails first of all identifying its aims. Why do we want to evaluate? The primary goal of the evaluation is to assess or estimate the effects of an intervention in relation to predefined objectives. Has the rehabilitation of a road network made it possible to develop trade; has the free distribution of books in all schools brought about an improvement in children's educational results? The second aim that arises from this is to identify the elements that have contributed to the success or failure of the policy, for the purpose of drawing lessons and possible upscaling.

In the health sector, contracting is developing and assuming multiple objectives and guises. Contractual relations can be established between local governments and hospitals with a view to improving hospital performance and enhancing the quality of the care they provide (China, Mongolia). Mutual health insurers may resort to selective contracting with health-care establishments, under which the insurers undertake to direct their members to these establishments (reimbursing care provided only in the latter); in return, the establishments undertake to improve the quality of their care and accommodation (Mali). In the fight against malaria or HIV/AIDS, contractual arrangements can be established between national programmes, purchasing centres and NGOs to distribute impregnated mosquito nets and medicines for target groups. These examples show how evaluation is relevant to answering the following questions:

- Is contracting an effective and efficient way to improve the care provided by health-care institutions?

- Is contracting an effective and efficient way of reaching target groups in priority health-care programs?

There are three domains of interest in evaluation, firstly "internal": the contractual relation might not actually produce any result. In a resource-scarcity setting, this lack of results has an economic and financial cost. If the contracting parties have not undertaken any action and have not mobilized any resources, there will be no financial cost; but there will certainly be an opportunity cost (and hence an economic and possibly also a social cost), for time will have been lost during contract negotiation. If the absence of result is due to a lack of effectiveness, since the resources envisaged were mobilized, then there is a financial cost on top of the opportunity cost. Secondly, there is a "societal" interest in evaluation, for the ultimate objective of contracting in the health domain is to improve general well-being while preserving equity. The evaluation will seek to verify or demonstrate that contracting is a valid tool for resolving the problem of squandering of resources; this is especially important sine contractual relations are often based on the rationale of enabling those who are most competent or efficient to act (e.g.

outsourcing of catering and hotel services in hospitals, or contracting with NGOs for community based health interventions) . The third domain of interest is that evaluation makes it possible to draw lessons to identify ways of extending this approach and see what type of contractual relation is best suited to the situation.

These thoughts give rise to two comments. The first concerns the level of the contracting process at which one should evaluate. This question is considered in the first part of this chapter. The second introduces the general issues of evaluating contracting in health systems.

If the aim of a contractual relation is to achieve more effective outcomes by improving the efficiency and performance of health-system interventions, then it is immediately clear that the issues of the evaluation are multiple and correspond to at least three domains: ethical, economic and financial:

- *Ethical issue*: Evaluating means being concerned about the resources that are invested in an intervention A. Not to evaluate would therefore be unethical[6] since the resources in question must have been taken away from an intervention B, which could have been implemented.

- *Economic issue*: Despite a large inflow of external financing (Global Fund, Gates foundation, Clinton foundation, PEPFAR, etc.), resources in the health sector remain insufficient. Nonetheless, the right to health and the demand for equity imply an obligation to provide quality health care at the lowest possible cost to every member of society.[7] Moreover, seeking out an optimal combination of resources to achieve better results is a duty. Evaluation, by seeking the most efficient interventions *a priori*, and by verifying their efficiency and effectiveness *a posteriori*, makes it possible to minimize costs, avoid wastage, and thus save resources.

- *Financial issue*: International mobilization and "competition" among initiatives to propose "innovative" financing, should not shroud the problem of likely exhaustion or non-automatic renewal of certain funds.[8] Finance is an increasingly important issue given new demands. Evaluation is a tool to support decision-making on the repayment, implementation, or continuation of financing.[9] As contracting may be a means used by programmes financed by development partners such as the Global Fund, to improve the effectiveness and efficiency of their activities, the evaluation of contracting has also a financial aspect: " "It is becoming increasingly important for countries to be able to report accurate, timely and comparable data to national authorities and donors in order to secure continued funding for expanding health programs."[10]

1. THE PROCESS AND EVALUATION OF CONTRACTING

Here we note that it is the rationale of the intervention that provides the subject of the evaluation:

(a) a specific problem is posed in a given health system, referred to here as the "problem situation";

(b) it is decided to use contracting to provide a solution to this problem;

(c) contracting is thus the strategy used to determine how the intervention will be organized; it specifies relations between the stakeholders involved, how resources will be mobilized, conditions for monitoring the intervention, etc.

(d) at the core of the contracting process there is a contract for which the identified problem forms the contractual objective; the contract spells out the agreement reached between the stakeholders, it will define the objectives of the contractual relationship and it will identify resources that are channelled into activities or services for its execution;

(e) often, contracting forms a systemic and strategic intervention that mobilizes multiple stakeholders between which interrelations are built; this means that a contractual arrangement is not always based on a single instrument but on multiple contracts that formalize the different aspects of the relation and define the roles and obligations of the various stakeholders and the nature of their interaction;

(f) implementation of the contractual arrangement, and consequently of the contract or contracts, will produce results that will directly impact on the problem situation and on health-system performance more generally;

(g) contracting unfolds in a specific setting, and this will inevitably affect the way in which the process is set up and implemented.

While the primary function of evaluation is to determine the measure or degree of success in attaining a given objective[11] it also has other functions such as:

1. to give *a priori* clarification to decision-makers by assisting the process of choosing between two interventions;

2. to *a posteriori* justify the soundness of the choice made, in financial, economic and results terms;

3. to ensure that *a priori* cost estimates are not overrun;

4. to monitor the implementation of the intervention and adjust activities where necessary to ensure that the established objectives can be achieved; to ensure that the trade-off between efficiency and equity has been respected;

5. to watch out for the appearance of potential negative externalities of the interventions, to correct or redirect activities before it is too late.

The evaluation will be performed at different levels depending on the function one wishes to see performed: before or at the time of the decision to intervene (function 1); sufficiently long after implementation of the intervention (functions 2 and 3); or possibly at each of these stages (initial, intermediate, final) if the aim is to consider all of its functions.

Within the contracting framework, different functions will be more or less important. We will note two principles before presenting and commenting on the relevance of evaluation at each stage of the contracting process.

Firstly, contracting is not confined to the contractual document; it initially concerns the way the document is prepared and later it focuses on the implementation of the contract and its realization. Secondly, contracting is a voluntary act based mainly on trust and flexibility; and there is often no possible legal sanction; in this case the only "sanction" will be the termination or non-renewal of the relation.

We have seen that the contracting process encompasses four phases. At the end in each of these phases, there is the possibility either of exiting (ending) the process, or continuing (Figure 1). Although the evaluation can be performed at each of these stages (lower part of the figure), the need to make an evaluation at each stage depends on the objectives being pursued and the time of exiting the process.

An evaluation of contracting prior to implementation, phase I, needs a forward-looking and qualitative approach to determine whether a certain number of pre-requisites are in place to implement a contracting intervention. This type of evaluation can prove to be complicated because the pre- requirements vary depending on both the context and the modalities and objectives of the intervention. Nonetheless, as the volume of contracting experiences grows, our knowledge of the pre-requisites for different types of intervention in different settings also expands, this will produce some important "lessons learned" on which the *ex ante* evaluation of contracting can be built in the future.

Evaluation in phase II (figure 1) concerns the *form*, i.e. the process that unfolds as a result of an agreement between the stakeholders. If the process ends at that moment (failure of the negotiation, *exit b*), questions will include whether the negotiations were well directed, whether the objectives were too complex or too vague, whether the process was undertaken with the relevant stakeholders, under what conditions was the contractual arrangement established (based on open competition, prior identification of stakeholders?); and whether it is based on a

481

weak or strong cooperation. In the event of the process continuing, it is also interesting to consider the moment of signing/writing/drafting the contract. Apparent defects in the form of a contract, noted above, and others that appear during its lifetime concerning its duration (was this adequate?), commitments and distribution of the roles of each partner (were they well-defined?), will be able to explain a premature exit (*exit c*) or non-renewal (*exit d*) of the process. In contrast, the quality of contract drafting, as one of the factors affecting the success of the process, could be highlighted by comparing this phase for two types of contractual relations with the same purpose. This quality will also make it possible to more effectively assess the process up to the evaluation of results.

Entry into phase III of the process is the crucial contracting period. If the process goes ahead (i.e. there is no premature exit, *exit c*), one expects and awaits results at the end of this phase, which will eventually influence the decision to renew or not the relationship. Nonetheless, before achieving results in terms of health system and health status effects, the contracting period has to be seen as a cycle of activities. While one does not want this period to be like a black box that furnishes results without one knowing exactly what they are attributable to, it might be worth setting up an evaluation in this period. This level of evaluation corresponds to what some analysts call "follow-up evaluation"; it consists of three stages. The first (which makes it possible to analyse the immediate effect, *figure 2*), corresponds to the implementation of resources (i.e. the commitment of means) and the execution of activities. If the activities are correctly undertaken and the means to be used are correctly identified (in phase II), this stage will lead to a behavioural change (intermediate effect): Has the quality of care or patient reception improved; have medication stock-outs become less frequent? Unless these two stages were correctly undertaken it will be impossible to observe a (final) effect on the effectiveness of the health system and an impact on health itself. It is thus at the end of phase III, that the evaluation focuses on results. The outcome of this evaluation will make it possible to enter phase IV, with good results leading to a renewal of the contracting process, while bad results will lead to renegotiation or non-renewal (*exit c*).

We have seen that evaluation can be performed at several stages in the contracting process, but it may not be necessary to evaluate at each stage. If not, the question is at which stage should one evaluate. This leads to the evaluation process.

Figure 1: Process and evaluation of contracting

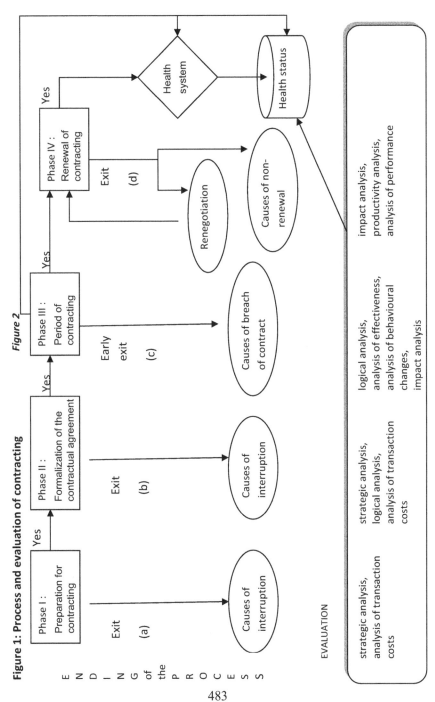

483

Figure 2 : Analysis of effects, impact, during phase III of the process.

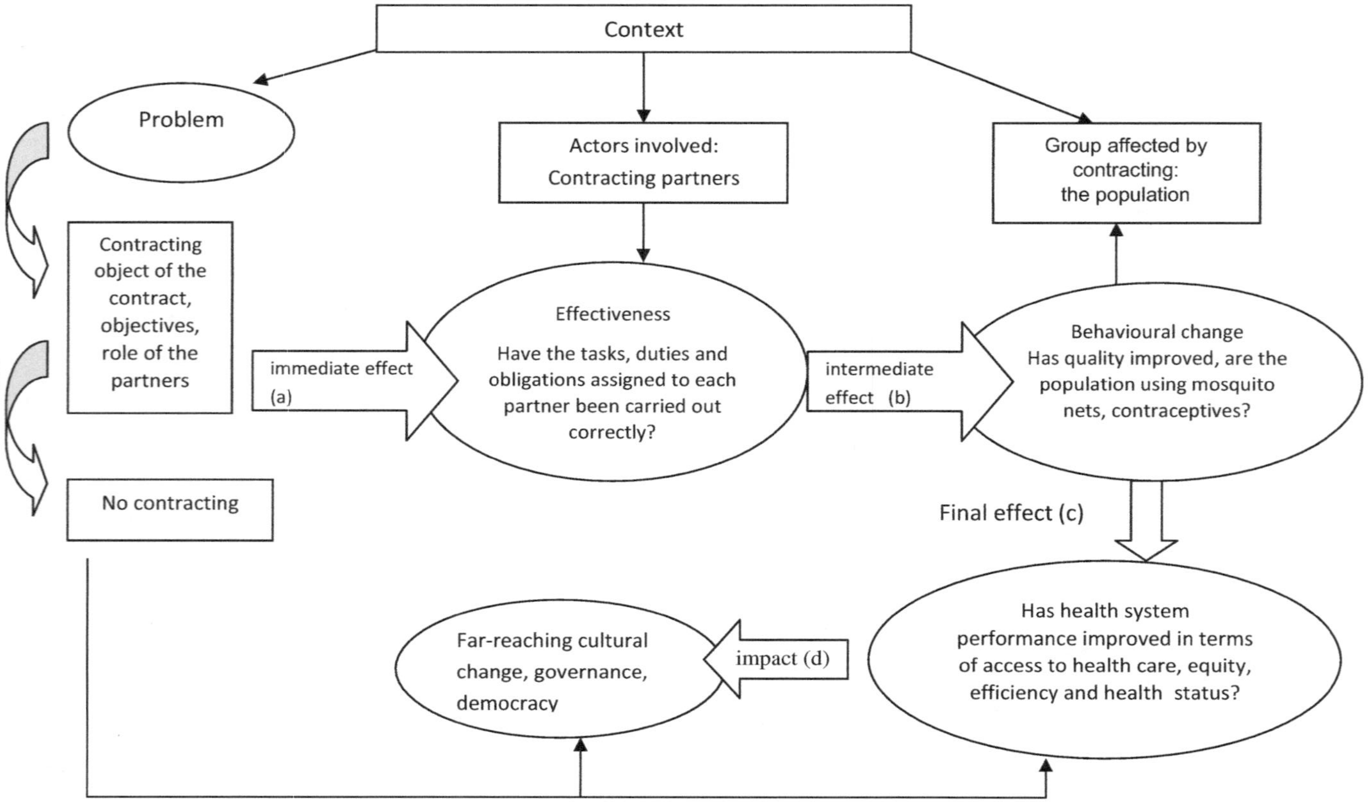

2. THE EVALUATION PROCESS IN CONTRACTING

The evaluation process emerges from a number of questions, namely:

- why does one want to evaluate, or what are the aims of the evaluation?
- what is being evaluated?
- what is the cost or the feasibility of the evaluation?
- how to evaluate?

2.1   Aims of the evaluation

Why is an evaluation being made? The aims of the evaluation are numerous: they can be either explicit or implicit; they can be consensual, i.e. shared by all stakeholders, or conflictive; they can vary according to the stakeholders. The aims can be classified in two groups:

Logical aims

The conception of the evaluation now depends on a scientific process that is neutral and unbiased. The following aims are distinguished:

- The formative aim: The evaluation is referred to as formative when its aim is to provide information to improve the ongoing action. The aim is operational. For example it will involve obtaining and analysing information to correct certain aspects of the contracting intervention. This evaluation can be applied to a range of elements that are decisive for the success of the contracting process. It is mainly aimed at a strategic analysis of the modalities for implementing the intervention (with whom and how is the contracting process undertaken; who paid how much and for what etc.). This evaluation can also target the contracts that formalize the relationships. In practice, without changing the sense of the contract, it is always possible to add a codicil to amend it to specify certain elements. It may also make it possible to obtain information and analyse the situation to avoid latent conflicts or help resolve disputes that have arisen. The evaluation that would be undertaken in phase III (figure 1) to measure the degree of effectiveness (figure 2) has that purpose.

- The summative aim: The evaluation is referred to as summative when its aim is to determine the effects of an action to decide whether it should be maintained, changed significantly, or halted. The lessons and judgments

485

that can be drawn in terms of results and impact will be useful for renewing the action. This is the sense of evaluations at *levels c* and *d* in figure 2.

- The fundamental aim: The evaluation aims to contribute to progress in terms of empirical and theoretical knowledge. This aim is important in what is called "Theory driven evaluation".[12] This current of thought assumes that a given action depends on a body of theory where causal relationships are established between inputs, outputs and results, which the evaluation seeks to validate. If this body of theory does not exist *a priori,* the evaluation will seek to determine it *a posteriori.*

Strategic aims

One of the limits of the "logical aims" approach stems from the fact that it assumes that all parties in a contractual relationship and/or external stakeholders (for ex. the public regulator) share the same points of view. However, the parties enter into a contractual relationship guided by their own interests (otherwise they would not have entered into it), and there is no reason for their interests to be identical. Each one pursues its own aims, which thus shape the aims of the evaluation. It is therefore important to distinguish the following in all contractual relations: (i) the explicit aims of the contracting intervention, which, in principle, are those stated in the contract(s) formalizing the agreement between the parties, and (ii) the implicit aims being pursued by the different parties. For example:

- one of the contracting parties may request an evaluation to delay a decision, or else validate a decision already taken. The party may request an evaluation to legitimize its position with regard to a given population, or a governing body, etc.;
- an external evaluator may seek to legitimize a theoretical hypothesis that it also sustains;
- the population may ask for an evaluation to show that its points of view are not being taken into account;
- the people affected by a contractual relation can request an evaluation to show that they were not being involved in its definition, when decision-makers try to show that poor results stem from insufficient resources.

This brings us to the second question: who does the evaluating?

2.2 Who evaluates? The participants in the evaluation

This question is important because it raises the issue of the governance of the evaluation.[5] A good evaluation should be undertaken transparently, free from all influence, so as not to weigh on and thus bias its results. It should be undertaken without conflict of interest vis-à-vis the agents involved in the contractual relation itself, ideally by agents who are external to it but have skills in the field in question.[13] Nonetheless, it is also possible for the evaluation to be undertaken by the agents themselves.

The following types of evaluation can be distinguished:

Internal evaluation. This is an integral part of the contractual arrangement and is performed by the parties themselves. This type of evaluation makes it possible to evaluate the activities undertaken: it has a formative purpose (table 1). It aims to achieve a greater comprehensibility of the intervention, to introduce more consistency in actions undertaken, and to propose continuous improvements in actions and their quality. It may reveal and, consequently, reduce or eliminate flaws in the contractual arrangement. A continuous evaluation is undertaken at regular intervals, either by one party alone or by the parties jointly.

When the evaluation is undertaken by just one of the parties involved in the contractual relationship, it is unilateral (without this aspect having a negative connotation). Thus, a party might focus on evaluating against its own interest in a contractual arrangement without taking account of the those of its partners let alone the general interest. Each party should perform this type of evaluation at some point in a contractual relationship: one needs to take stock of the situation;

When it is done jointly by all the parties involved, the evaluation will follow the general rules of partnership and negotiation. At different points in the contractual arrangement, the parties come together to analyse their relation.

Internal evaluation certainly does not diminish the need to perform an external evaluation.[14]

External evaluation. This entails analysing the contractual arrangement from outside and completely independently. This is done by agents who are external to the contractual arrangement —by an independent entity. The evaluators must have full freedom to make their assessment. The evaluation can be commissioned by the parties involved in the arrangement, but not always; in any case, it should never be financed by them. This is an important point; very often one finds documents produced by entities that are external to the parties involved in the contractual arrangement, but which are sponsored by them. In such cases, even if the evaluators concerned do their work correctly, it is in their interest to avoid emphasizing some negative aspects related to the contractual parties. What needs to be provided is an external and neutral view of the contractual arrangement.

There is nothing to prevent both types of evaluation from being undertaken.

Joint evaluation. This can be done by the parties directly involved in the contractual arrangement in conjunction with external experts. This type of evaluation makes it possible to reconcile the rigour and independence of the external evaluation with the operational points of view of the parties.

Evaluations—whether internal, external or joint—each have their advantages and disadvantages. External evaluators have the advantage of greater objectivity; the fact they are not involved in the contractual arrangement affords them the distance needed to assess it. Internal evaluators, in contrast, are involved in the contractual relationships so they have an interest in the evaluation results. By participating in it, they are forced to reflect on their practices and can affect any changes to be made. But, while it has long been thought that stakeholder participation in evaluating an activity is an advantage, opinions today are more divided.[15]

2.3   Cost and feasibility of the evaluation

Evaluation has a cost. Whatever the type of evaluation to be performed, it has a financial cost (it requires human and financial resources), an economic cost (time needs to be devoted to it), as well as an intangible or psychological cost (seen as a judgment, the evaluation can be dreaded by the agents involved in the contractual relation). The significance of each type of cost will depend partly on the type of evaluation chosen. Moreover, the mere existence of this cost means it needs to be provided for at some point if the evaluation is actually to be undertaken.

Financial cost

If the evaluation is *external*, agents outside the contractual relation will estimate its cost. If it is commissioned by the partners, it is best that they do not finance it, to ensure full independence of judgment for the evaluators. The Government, donor agencies or NGOs not involved in the arrangement to be evaluated, will be the paymasters. If the external evaluation is not commissioned, this will have no effect on the implementation of the contract and assessment of the results. Simply, its absence deprive the wider public of information that would have been useful when preparing and implementing other contractual relations.

If the evaluation is *internal* and scheduled, the financial cost needs to be precisely identified as from the contract set-up phase. Otherwise, a lack of resources needed for the evaluation will pose major problems and could quite simply eliminate the *raison d'être* of the contracting process. It is unproductive to enter into a contracting process if one cannot evaluate its implementation and results. Internal evaluation is thus an integral part of the contract and cannot be dissociated from it.

Economic or opportunity cost

The evaluation requires indicators to be established; and choosing them depends partly on the type of evaluation to be performed and the available resources. While for internal evaluation, the indicators should be chosen and set up when implementing the contractual process, for external evaluation this should be done for the reasons noted below.

Internal evaluation, undertaken by participants in the contractual arrangement, takes up agents' time to the detriment of or in addition to their own activities. For these agents, the evaluation represents an opportunity cost that is all the more important if they are not convinced of the soundness of the evaluation undertaken, and/or they feel the indicators chosen will not be easy to compile and analyse. It is therefore important to take care from phase II (figure 1) to define simple indicators, for which one knows that the necessary information will be available and that the resources needed to collect it will have been provided for. This situation is all the more true in complex interventions, in which one is interested in the results, i.e. the impact of the contractual relation;

In the case of external evaluation, undertaken by agents outside the contractual arrangement who are being paid to do it, the economic or opportunity cost is zero if the indicators have been set up since phase II. Otherwise, the cost could be significant. The evaluators will have to make an effort to find the necessary information, they will surely seek to control the biases that a lack of indicators will produce, and there will be constraints when choosing the type of evaluation to undertake.[16]

Intangible cost

This is zero for the evaluators when the evaluation is external. The agents doing the evaluation are not those who have implemented the contractual arrangement, so they are not responsible for the results whatever these may be. This is not the case if the evaluation is internal: here the agents doing the evaluation are committed to the arrangement. As there is often a belief that the evaluation is a (negative) judgment, the difficulty will then be to motivate the people responsible for it. For that purpose, it is necessary to show agents the benefit of evaluating, and make sure they gain ownership of the results and the knowledge produced. The results of the evaluation should be fed back, commented on and discussed, to reach decisions that each agent will be able to help implement.

Feasibility

When the evaluation modalities are envisaged in the contracting process, indicators for monitoring the process are set up as from phase II, (see section 1 and figures 1 and 2). The first stage of this evaluation reflects a monitoring logic (monitoring-evaluation, which began in phase III, section 1): it first of all involves assessing whether the resources defined are effectively in place (financing released, presence of human resources, available infrastructures, available technical and administrative documents, immediate effect, part a, figure 2). But this evaluation can also focus on performance: it is necessary to assess whether the objectives defined for the contractual intervention have been achieved: the activities have been implemented and the results attained (final effect, part c, figure 2). In this type of evaluation, indicators generally need to be specified in the contracts, and thus accepted by the signatories. The parties of the contractual arrangement will for example define indicators of resources (availability of medication, financial resources...); indicators of activities and services implemented (number of hours training to be given, number of information sessions...); indicators of behavioural change (number of protocols applied, the number of contacts per person); indicators of results (the coverage rate to be attained, the number of children fully immunized); indicators of impact (child mortality rate, the number of cases of measles ...).

Apart from setting up indicators, one can specify the frequency and time of the evaluation (at mid-term and/or at the end of the contractual relation); who will perform it (a consulting firm for which the selection methods are specified in the contract); terms of reference (subjects of the evaluation, expected outputs, etc). Here the concern to evaluate is an integral part of the contractual process and should be undertaken in accordance with provisions set out in one or more contracts.

The combination these elements is summarized in **table 1**.

490

	Internal evaluation	External evaluation
Participants in the evaluation	The agents participating in the contractual relation	Agents outside the contractual relation
Cost	Real financial cost, but not as high as in external evaluation. Significant opportunity cost and intangible cost	High financial cost , low opportunity cost and near-zero intangible cost
Formative aim	It enables stakeholders to produce knowledge on the way they operate and to participate in the action. It makes it possible to give stakeholders an operational tool enabling them to control their results for themselves and to adapt their performance in consequence and as the activity unfolds. It enables stakeholders to pilot the mechanism and to ensure that they are not failing to achieve their objectives.	At certain deadlines in the contractual relation, external evaluators draw up a temporary balance sheet of its implementation, in terms of both process and results, and propose recommendations.
Frequency and time	Continuous	Pre-implementation, mid-term and end
Summative aim	The participants in the contractual relation meet to assess its final results: Has the contractual relation been useful and should it be renewed? But here the problem arises of the objectivity of this evaluation since the evaluators are both judge and party	Evaluators draw up a balance sheet of the contractual relation. This involves identifying lessons that can be extracted from it, but will not have any effect on the current relation.
Frequency and time	At the end of phase III (figure 1)	At the end of phase III (figure 1)
Fundamental aim	It is seldom that the parties in the contractual relation, and they alone, undertake this type of evaluation.	External evaluators seek to draw lessons from the contractual relation: good practices or pitfalls to be avoided by other stakeholders, but also tests of theoretical hypotheses.
Frequency and time	Not applicable	In phase II and throughout phase III (figure 1)

2.4   How to evaluate

Evaluating an intervention based on criteria and standards is often a perfectly valid procedure, however this type of evaluation is not very suitable for analysing contractual arrangements. The normative evaluation entails making a judgment by comparing the resources implemented, the services and goods produced and the results obtained in terms of criteria and standards or benchmarks, established elsewhere. The notion of standard is absent in the contracting process.

The approach used will depend on when during the process the evaluation is undertaken (phase I, II, III, IV), and its objective. One may ask first of all, from the initial stages of the process (phase I), if the use of contracting was relevant (a) in the case under study. One can then ask (phase II) whether contracting and/or the contract(s) display a certain consistency (b). When the contracting process is undertaken (phase III), results are expected at the exit point. The evaluation will aim to highlight these results. But to achieve results, it is firstly necessary to mobilize resources, undertake activities, and wait for a change in behaviour. The analysis of effects (c), at these different stages, verifies that the process is well implemented and does not diverge from its objectives. Lastly, one can take steps to ascertain whether the results obtained thanks to contracting were efficient (d), and if it has led to a better performance (e).

(a) Analysis of relevance or strategic analysis

Analyses of relevance, or what others call strategic analysis, is not interested in the purpose of the contracting (as, for example, the relevance of the DOTS strategy), but seeks to ascertain whether the use of contracting was the best strategy for finding a solution to the problem situation. For example, does contracting between the Ministry of Health and private practitioners improve the implementation and expansion of the DOTS strategy? Given insufficient geographic health service coverage, is contracting with private NGO providers preferable to an extensions of public provision through new public facilities; or would it be better to put the development of geographic coverage in the hands of decentralized local authorities?

As we can see, these questions relate to strategic contracting which is designed as a choice. Seen in this way, contracting is directly linked to structural reforms relating to the organization and financing of health systems. In other words it offers a new potential option to deciders. In terms of evaluation, it is thus necessary to analyse the appropriateness of opting for contracting, as opposed to another possible strategy, to achieve a pre-established goal in a given context.

In the example of contracting with NGOs to cover a health district the strategic evaluation should consider the appropriateness of using contracting in this specific context. A key question will be to asses the appropriateness of using contracting for this type of intervention considering the availability and quality of NGOs (or any other stakeholder). For example, the evaluation may conclude that this type of intervention based on contracting with NGOs is not appropriate if it is implemented in a setting where the NGOs do not have the legal, financial or organizational capacities needed to fulfil contracts.

Strategic evaluation is thus essentially linked to phase I of the contracting process, since it involves identifying whether the prerequisites of a successful contracting process are in place. As noted above, this evaluation depends above all on a qualitative upstream analysis, which should be focused on contextual elements.

Strategic analysis, linked to the analysis of effects, can also be undertaken further downstream in the process,. When analysing the effects of contracting, it is also necessary to question the appropriateness of the choice. It could be that the results of the intervention are unsatisfactory because the setting was ultimately not suitable for contracting, for one reason or another. This type of *ex post* evaluation is very important since it is often linked to the formative aim of the evaluation; thus, this type of analysis will give indications as to the soundness of choosing a contracting strategy in a given setting. *Ex post* analysis could also reveal contextual aspects that were not yet visible in phase I (*ex ante*) but have later influenced the results of the contractual arrangement. Thus, the analysis will provide information for deciding whether the contracting intervention should be continued or whether it is better to change strategy and choose another type of intervention (it would also be possible to maintain the contracting strategy while trying to make the setting more propitious for contracting, but this is much more difficult and often inappropriate).

At this level it is also useful to question the type of contract that will be or is being used. For example, will a classic contract be used in which each of the elements of the contractual relation are described in detail; or instead, will there be a tendency towards a relational contract which is based on trust and cooperation between the partners, and in which only the broad principles and objectives of the contractual relation are stipulated (the details of the action are left to the discretion of the stakeholders).

Lastly, it has to be stressed that the strategic analysis should also take account of dimensions that go beyond the intervention. For example, one needs to assess whether the choice of contracting has been appropriate in view of the country's health strategies and policies. Clearly, in some countries, the health sector setting is much better suited to contracting than in others. A complete evaluation should also be made of the macro setting outside the health sector: the economic situation, the regulatory and legal framework, and the country's administrative model. Each of these elements can affect the appropriateness of opting for contracting.

(b) Analysis of consistency or logical analysis

The logical analysis can focus on the contractual approach as a whole. The basis for evaluative questions at this level is that a contractual arrangement, as a systemic approach, consists of several operational and institutional elements. It is thus a matter of evaluating how the different elements have been implemented and assessing their relevance to the objective of the contracting intervention. The logical analysis will thus focus, from a systemic point of view, on the way the contractual arrangement has been made operational.

For contracting to be coherent, the elements through with it are implemented need to be appropriate. For example, performance-based contracting between the Health Ministry and autonomous hospitals will depend on the institutional elements that are set up to monitor the hospital activity and its results. In this case, the analysis will focus on the nature of these institutional elements. For example, if the contractual arrangement provides for a monitoring committee, it needs to be considered whether this committee has the mandate needed to fulfil its role, whether it consists of suitable individuals or representatives, and whether it disposes of the necessary legal, administrative and financial instruments?

It is also possible to analyse the internal consistency of a contractual arrangement, i.e. between the three elements that form the objectives of the arrangement, the activities or services implemented and the resources mobilized. This entails assessing whether resources are sufficient (a matter of quantity) and suitable (are they appropriate in the intervention framework?). For example, it could be that the contractual arrangement aims for the correct response to the problem identified (e.g. improvement of the quality of reception of patients), but the resources and activities implemented are inconsistent or inappropriate to these objectives (the contract foresees an increase in the number of staff whereas it would have been better to improve the capacity and incentives of personnel already employed.[17] Consistency between these three elements (objectives, resources and activities) will be a measure of the contractual arrangement's success. This consistency should also be pursued and translated in the drafting and preparation phase of the contract(s) that formalizes the arrangement.

A contracting intervention may involve several contracts. For example, when the Government enters into a concession agreement with an NGO to cover a given geographic area, there may be a contract between the Government and the NGO that formalizes the modalities for the management delegation , another between the

NGO and an actor to whom all or part of the provision of healthcare services is subcontracted; and there may be a third contract between the Government and the (autonomous) local authority on how to integrate the intervention in the zone in question and what is the role of the local authority in the arrangement. It is thus necessary to evaluate both the internal consistency of the contract and also the consistency between the different contracts involved in the same intervention.

(c) Analysis of effects

The analysis of effects seeks to analyse the intervention's influence on the results achieved, expressed in quantitative and/or qualitative terms. Ideally, it involves assessing the influence of the contractual arrangement on the health system goals, i.e. improvement of health status. Nonetheless, for some contractual arrangement, the effects on health-system objectives are indirect or distant. For example, in a contract relating to outsourcing of catering to an external firm in a hospital, it will clearly be difficult to assess the effects on the improvement of health status, whereas it will be possible to assess the influence in terms of "responsiveness to expectations". Secondly, the analysis of effects implies a causality that cannot always be clearly demonstrated, particularly in complex contractual arrangements. Can one be sure that an improvement in the health coverage rate in a given zone is due to the contractual relation between hospital and NGO? Only the technique of impact analysis, which is sometimes hard to implement (see box below), makes it possible to decide.

Impact analysis

Arising from the experimental method, impact analysis is used to measure the effect of an intervention. This requires comparing two groups chosen at random, one with the intervention (experimental group), and the other without (control group), measuring the situation before and after the intervention. When random choice is impossible, one of the groups can be chosen on a reasoned basis, and the other chosen by the propensity score method. This is referred to as a quasi-experimental protocol.[18]

The need to observe a group without intervention (control) raises ethical problems that sometimes hinder the use of this approach. Nonetheless, it is possible to vary the time of intervention for the control group.

The implementation of a contracting intervention will produce three types of effect (figure 2).

Immediate effects (**a, figure 2**), relating to the actions produced by contracting in terms of resources or activities. Questions will be asked about whether the resources envisaged were really in place at the time of implementing the contracting process, and in accordance with the agreement between the stakeholders; whether the activities or services envisaged were in fact undertaken (e.g. was the communication strategy on condoms, envisaged in the contract, actually implemented?). This requires factual information, which can be obtained from process indicators, often incorrectly referred to as performance indicators (e.g. how many communication sessions on condoms were held?). [19]

Intermediate effects (**b, figure 2**), the observation of which makes it possible to say whether the activities implemented facilitated a behavioural change, and thus contributed to a satisfactory response to the problem situation that gave rise to the intervention. For example, when contracting for the maintenance of hospital wards, this involves seeing whether the implementation of daily floor sweeping as envisaged by the contract really made it possible to respond to unsatisfactory hospital ward maintenance.

Final effect (**c, figure 2**), i.e. the effect on health system performance. This entails seeing whether the response made to the problem situation identified has an impact on health-system performance. For example, did the fact that hospital wards are better maintained have affect on patient satisfaction, and does it contribute to an increase of hospital performance in the health system. As noted by the WHO World Health Report 2000 this performance evaluation can be based on three health-system goals: improvement of health among different population groups, equity of the financial contribution, and lastly the capacity to respond to people's expectations in domains other than health (respect for individual dignity and freedom, confidentiality of information).

Impact on society (**d, figure 2**): Contractual arrangements lead to a profound cultural change in the way inter-relationships between health-sector stakeholders are organized. The contractual process has qualities that go beyond these specific contributions in terms of improving the health system; it is a vehicle of democracy and renewed governance which should contribute to the country's development. At this stage, evaluation enquires about the incidence of the contractual arrangement on issues such as:

- local authorities: has their influence increased?
- the management of public affairs: has this improved?
- the existence of counterbalancing power: are the population and civil society generally more   involved, or, on the contrary, excluded from decision-making domains?
- the role of central government: is this fulfilling its regulatory role more than before?

(d) Analysis of efficiency or productivity analysis

The analysis of (technical) efficiency or productivity aims to study the way resources are employed to produce activities. The analysis asks whether the contractual arrangement in question made it possible to produce more services or activities with the same resources, or the same services or activities using fewer resources? This type of evaluation has its importance for the contractual arrangement in question, since it can be used as an element for determining if the contract(s) should be renewed or not. This type of evaluation is often very important also for a wider objective, especially for policy makers and deciders who have to make strategic choices. For example, in order to make a strategic choice of outsourcing a service or continue its production in-house, a hospital manager will need to have information on the different efficiency implications of the choices. Another example would be to evaluate the efficiency of a contractual arrangement for a concession of a health zone to an NGO; the evaluation will yield valuable information for the decision makers and it can help them to make decisions on resource allocation in the future.

The information and evidence on efficiency is necessarily derived from *ex post* (external) evaluations of contractual arrangements that were implemented in a certain context. Of course, every situation is unique and considering the complexity of the question of efficiency, it is not always clear if the evidence from the efficiency evaluations can be considered universally valid. However, once there is a critical mass of information and evidence derived from efficiency evaluation, the results and the conclusions of these evaluations will get a more universalistic scope and they can be of use in several contexts.

(e) Outcome analysis

Analysis of outcome or global efficiency concerns relations between resources and observed effects. This can be done before the start of the process, in which case the results will affect the decision to contract. It can also be done at the end of phase III or IV, and thus affects the renewal decision and/or serves as a reference for other contractual arrangements. A cornerstone of the economic evaluation, it relates the whole cost of the intervention (i.e. of the contractual arrangement) to the observed result (effect). Depending on the effect or results indicator considered, this may be either cost-effectiveness analysis (number of education or awareness-raising sessions, number of mosquito nets distributed, children fully immunized, disability-adjusted life years (DALY), or cost-benefit analysis (quality-adjusted life years, QALY).

An evaluation study of a contractual arrangement can include several of the aspects listed above. This can be demonstrated by the example presented in Box 1.

Box 1:   Evaluating performance-based financing/contracting projects in five African countries: Burundi, Democratic Republic of the Congo (DRC), Rwanda, United Republic of Tanzania and Zambia[20]

Performance-based financing (PBF) is a new approach that introduces a direct link between the amount of financing received by a health service provider and the level of performance obtained by it (see Part III in this book).

PBF can be used by a health development partner as a means of channelling financial support to health service providers. In this case, it can be implemented through contracting at a regional/local level.

Two Dutch NGOs, CORDAID and HealthNet TPO, have implemented several PBF projects in sub-Saharan Africa. These PBF projects have been made operational with various modalities depending on the countries and contexts; but the basic model involves a contractual approach where purchasing agencies, which are autonomous units established to cover a health district or zone, enter into a contractual relation with health facilities (performance contracts) and with the local health administration and community actors (regulation and verification contracts).

To evaluate these PBF arrangements, an external evaluation study was undertaken by the Royal Tropical Institute of Amsterdam (KIT) in conjunction with the WHO. The aim of the evaluation was formative, i.e. to objective was to analyse an ongoing action and draw lessons for the future.

The evaluation study, which was based on quantitative and qualitative methods, consisted of an analysis of consistency, of an analysis of effects and of an analysis of efficiency.

- The analysis of consistency focused on the PBF project architecture, the main objective was to evaluate if the contractual arrangements between the different actors were coherent with the projects' objectives and with the "theoretical framework" of a PBF intervention. Under this aspect the evaluation aimed to answer questions such as: were all the actors adequately informed about the modalities of PBF? did the contractual arrangements give the actors the sufficient level of autonomy? were the local authorities and/or the community actors sufficiently involved? were sufficient resources allocated for monitoring and evaluation?
- The analysis of effects was based on a before-after study where the facility level outputs before the PBF intervention were compared with the outputs after project implementation. The qualitative analysis focused also on general behavioural changes among staff in the PBF facilities. Control districts and facilities, where no PBF arrangements existed, were used when possible. This analysis of effects was clearly on the intervention as a whole; indeed it is important to underline that when evaluating contractual arrangements where several actors are involved (which is often the case) one should not simply evaluate how individual contracts where implemented or how individual relationships have evolved, but to focus on the effects of the intervention as a whole. This systemic evaluation, that goes beyond a simple contract monitoring, is the key to understanding if the contracting intervention was the adequate response to a given problem situation.
- The analysis of efficiency in the evaluation study looked into the way the resources were distributed between the project outputs (the resources channelled to the

498

facilities) and the project inputs (the costs for establishing the intervention). The contractual arrangements behind the PBF interventions come with a cost. For example, new institutions are needed to administer and supervise the contracts and the institutions already in place will need to be modified so that they support the PBF project. The cost of these arrangements (the programme costs) define the efficiency of the project. This "technical" efficiency at the project level is only one dimension of efficiency. Ultimately the objective would be to determine if the intervention produced more (and better quality) provider activity than another (non-contracting) intervention with the same amount of resources. The study in question was not designed to answer this question. It is indeed very difficult to design evaluation studies where one could find a clear comparison intervention for a contracting intervention.

2.5   Elements for undertaking a good evaluation

As evaluation is a multifaceted act, it is inadvisable to enter into a contractual relation without previously having envisaged a number of issues, summarized here.[21]

A. *A willingness to evaluate:* The first and foremost condition for an evaluation depends on the willingness to evaluate. It is not uncommon to see evaluations undertaken unwillingly, simply to fulfil a contractual clause or a conditionality imposed by some distant supervisory body. It should therefore not be surprising that the quality of these evaluations is often mediocre;

B. *Why does one wish to evaluate?* As the aims of an evaluation may differ widely, they should be specified at the very outset to avoid any misunderstanding. In particular, the reasons for the evaluation will depend on the time at which the evaluation is performed in the course of the contractual process;

C. *Choose your type of evaluation:* The most appropriate type of evaluation will depend on the reasons for deciding to evaluate. Here again, there is no one type of evaluation that would be *a priori* better than the others, the choice will depend on each situation;

D. *Those responsible for the evaluation:* Before appointing the technical staff who will undertake the evaluation, it is advisable to nominate those who will be responsible for it, i.e. the individuals who will not only be required to define the modalities and methods of the evaluation but also assume its results;

E. *The means of the evaluation:* Any evaluation has a cost, whether in purely financial terms or more broadly in terms of time for the stakeholders involved. Resources are never unlimited, so an evaluation can never be complete: it thus needs to be restricted to the means available, on the one hand, and the objectives being pursued, on the other;

F. *Adequate information:* All evaluation requires information and data. This can either be collected specifically for the purpose of the evaluation, or else compiled on a regular basis through a suitable information system.[22] Nonetheless, it is advisable always to remember that information is a means and not an end in itself. The production of information should make it possible to construct an interpretation of reality. Evaluation in this sense is an act that makes the information "speak"—a "production of understanding" as referred to in Contandriopoulos et al.[17]

G. *Use of the result of the evaluation:* One must avoid the "report forgotten in the bottom of a drawer" situation; an evaluation is of no interest unless its results are used. This may seem obvious, but evaluations frequently have no consequences. It is also necessary to specify in the evaluation process how its results will be used.

H. *Consequences of the evaluation:* The evaluation has led to a judgment being made. It has been possible to involve the agents of the contracting process (internal evaluation); they have borne the cost. They may be called upon again. They need to be presented with the results to feel concerned, and to accept regular repetitions of the operation.

CONCLUSION

Irrespective of the different forms it can take, evaluation is always presented as a judgment on an intervention—in this case contracting—between the existing and desired situations. In this sense, any evaluation is potentially disruptive, because it risks revealing shortfalls between reality and the objectives that had been set. While the review may lead to changes that will prove fruitful for the relation between stakeholders, it may also exacerbate latent disputes or result in tighter controls which, if poorly implemented, could be perceived almost as inquisitional.

In other words, a well conducted evaluation could be a useful tool in the sense of strengthening the links woven in the contractual relation. In contrast, a badly conducted evaluation might prove counterproductive in this sense, and thus help undermine relations that had been patiently established, and often with difficulty.

Evaluation is therefore never a neutral act, it is a questioning procedure from which positive results are expected. But it can also produce disruptive effects that are harmful to the contractual relation.

Notes

[1] http://www.who.int/pmnch/activities/dn_fs_childmortality.pdf

[2] In the past, countries such as China or those of Eastern Europe had performing health systems that enabled them to achieve better health outcomes than would have been predicted by their economic level. For several years now, health status has either stagnated (China) or regressed (Eastern Europe).

[3] WHO (2002) The World Health Reports, Statistical Annexes.

[4] The term "intervention" is used to mean any action that aims to achieve an objective. This could be roadbuilding, free book distribution, a treatment, a programme. See also:

> Potvin L, Haddad S, Frohlich K.L (2001), Beyong process and outcome evaluation: a comprehensive approach for evaluating health promotion programmes, In Evaluation in health promotion: principles and perspectives, WHO Regional Publications, European Series, n° 92.

> Contandriopoulos A-P, Champagne F, Denis J-L, Avargues M-C (2000), L'évaluation dans le domaine de la santé : concepts et méthodes, *Revue d'Epidémiologie et de Santé Publique*, 48, 6, 517-539.

[5] Bureau D, Mougeot M (2007), Performance, incitations et gestion publique, Conseil d'Analyse Economique, La Documentation Française, 133p

[6] Williams, A. (1996), Qalys and ethics: a health economist's perspective, *Social Science and Medicine* 43, 12, 1795-1804.

[7] Méreau M, Lebrun T, Bercez C (2001), Nouveaux enjeux pour l'évaluation économique, *Actualité et Dossier en Santé Publique,* 35, 12-16.

[8] The financial resources provided by the Global Fund, for example, are not replenished *at vitam eternam*. Donor Governments engage for a limited period and need to be convinced of the usefulness and effectiveness of the activities undertaken thanks to these resources to maintain their donations.

[9] Radelet S & Siddiqi B (2007), Global Fund grant programmes: an analysis of evaluation scores, *Lancet*, 369, 1807-1813

[10] The Global Fund to Fight AIDS, Tuberculosis and Malaria (2009), *Monitoring and Evaluation Toolkit*, 3rd Edition

[11] Pineault R, Daveluy (1986), La planification de la santé : concepts, méthodes et stratégies, Montréal, Agence d'Arc.

[12] Chen H, Rossi P.H (1992), eds. "Using theory to improve program and policy evaluations", New York: Greenwood Press.

[13] The skill domain required will vary according to the level at which the evaluation is undertaken: jurist, for evaluating the formalization of the contract; doctor, for behavioural change (care quality) or effects on health; economist for performance, etc.

[14] Conseil National de l'Evaluation Sociale et Médico-Sociale (CNESMS, 2006), L'Evaluation interne, Guide pour les établissements et les services sociaux et médico-sociaux, version 1, 26p.

[15] For a discussion of these issues, see Mathie, A. and J. C. Greene. 1997. *Stakeholder participation in evaluation: how important is diversity? Evaluation and Program Planning*, 20, no. 3:279-285. and C.E. Thayer, A.H. Fine (2001)

[16] In this case, it is highly unlikely that the evaluators will be able to make an impact analysis, a method that is increasingly recommended in the evaluation field.

[17] Contandriopoulos A-P, Champagne F, Denis J-L, Avargues M-C (2000), L'évaluation dans le domaine de la santé : concepts et méthodes, *Revue d'Epidémiologie et de Santé Publique*, 48, 6, 517-539.

[18] Cook T, Campbell DT, Quasi-experimentation, design and analysis, issues for field settings, Houghton Mifflin Company, Boston, 1979.

[19] For a discussion of the notion of performance, see Collin J.F, S.Giraudo, M.Baumann (2001) "Outil d'aide à l'évaluation de performance des actions de santé: l'exemple du programme de prévention de l'alcoolisme en Lorraine", *Santé publique*, vol.13, n°2, pp. 179-193

[20] Toonen J, Canavan A, Vergeer P, Elovainio R (2009), Performance-based financing for health: Lessons from sub-Saharan Africa, Amsterdam, KIT Publishers

[21] Many articles present this type of recommendation, e.g. Springett J, Dugdill L (1995) "Workplace health promotion programmes: towards a framework for evaluation", *Health education journal*, 54, p.88-98

[22] Migeot V, Ingrand P, Salmi L.R (2000) "Quels systèmes d'information pour l'évaluation en santé?", *Revue d'épidémiologie et de* Santé Publique, 48, pp. 551-560.

ANNEX

ILLUSTRATIONS OF THE EVALUATION OF CONTRACTUAL ARRANGEMENTS
BASED ON SCENARIOS

To illustrate the methodological framework described in the text, examples of contracts have been developed and the evaluation methodology applied to them.

	Internal evaluation	External evaluation
Formative aim	Health-care network	Purchase of HIV/AIDS service activities from an NGO
Summative aim	Contract to maintain hospital wards	Ministry of Health recognition of an NGO health centre
Fundamental aim		A university in a northern country wishes to make sure transaction costs do not outweigh the financial gains of maintenance contracts in hospitals in a southern country.

Description of scenarios

1. Hospital ward cleaning services. The Koula public hospital has recently been awarded an autonomous charter. Current arrangements for cleaning the wards in which patients' stay in the hospital are unsatisfactorily fulfilled and expensive. Cleaning is not done as expected, the staff, although sufficient in number, are not motivated and do their work badly, the walls are dirty, and patients complain.

Following a proposal by the hospital director, the board of directors is asking for these services to be provided by a private firm. A tender was launched, a firm was selected, and a contract drawn up: it was signed by the President of the Board of Directors and the entrepreneur. The contract specifies the tasks to be undertaken by the firm and the price to be paid to the enterprise. The contract is expected to last for two years.

503

After two years' operation, the hospital decided to evaluate this contractual arrangement, with a view to deciding whether or not to renew the contract.

2. Health-care network: The *Toxicomanie* network in the town of Sabré aims to take overall charge of the problem of drug addiction. The network consists of freelance doctors, laboratory pharmacists, a structure for receiving and conversing with the drug addict (involving psychiatrists, a psychologist, and social workers), and a team to monitor drug addicts in hospital. This network is set up as an association.

After one year's implementation, the association, at the request of its members, decided to undertake a review to identify elements that were not working satisfactorily.

3. The Ministry of Health has signed a contract with the local NGO to provide HIV/AIDS related services (specifically, awareness-raising among truckers on the use of condoms). As provided for in the contract, a firm of auditors was hired at midterm to review contract implementation and propose recommendations.

4. Ministry of Health recognition of an NGO health centre: The contractual relation established between the local NGO, owner of the health centre, and the Ministry of Health, has led to recognition of the NGO health centre as the primary health-care facility serving the entire population of the geographic zone in question. Three years after contract signing, the two parties decided to hire a consulting firm to evaluate the contractual relation.

5. A university from a northern country wants to make sure transaction costs do not outweigh financial gains in maintenance contracts in hospitals in a southern country. This university has no link with the signatories of the contractual relation and will make a comparative analysis between three hospitals that have implemented this arrangement and two others that carry out these activities for themselves.

The aim of the presentation below is not to list all possible issues for an evaluation but simply to show how to use the methodological framework that defined above. The evaluation framework makes it possible to classify the issues and place them in context.

	Scenario 1 Management of hospital wards	Scenario 2 *Toxicomanie* health-care network	Scenario 3 Purchase of HIV/AIDS awareness raising services by the Ministry of health from an NGO
Analysis of appropriateness	Having found its internal cleaning services to be unsatisfactory, the hospital management is asking whether using the private sector would not be a better solution (e.g. as opposed to making the service autonomous within the hospital) The hospital could also take steps to decide whether a tender would be the best selection procedure, or directly contracting a known firm would be preferable.	As the aim is to take overall charge of the drug addict, it is important to ensure that the network effectively brings together the stakeholders most concerned and most needed for this responsibility.	Did the NGO have the capacities needed to undertake this activity? Did the Ministry of Health have sufficient documentation on the NGO? Was the NGO accredited?
Analysis of consistency	The hospital's aim was to obtain a quality and/or least-cost service. It should check whether the financial means made available to the enterprise really make it possible to attain the objectives.	The idea of an agreement between all stakeholders is praiseworthy, but were the necessary means foreseen, because such an agreement entails increasing the workload of stakeholders involved, which will have remuneration consequences.	Did the NGO provide adequate resources to undertake the activities? Did it not understate them to win the tender, or maximize them knowing that the Ministry of Health would have difficulties verifying them (information asymmetry)?

Analysis of effects	Actions undertaken: Number of times per week that wards are swept, quality of cleaning. Did the hospital obtain a better service at less cost, thanks to the contract, or an identical service at less cost? Influence on health system performance: (i) patient satisfaction: Are patients or their families satisfied with the hospital environment?; (ii) Are there more or fewer infections arising from bad maintenance?	Actions undertaken: The stakeholders will need to previously agree on the expected outcomes, to be able to evaluate the results actually obtained. In fact, these do not only concern health; they are also social: a cured drug addict is a drug addict who is reintegrated into society (family, professional, societal reinsertion) How can one claim that the results obtained are attributable to the contractual arrangement and would not have been achieved through other channels? Influence on health system performance: Does this overall responsibility make it possible to improve drug addicts' health in the broad sense of the WHO definition?	Actions undertaken: Several indicators can be defined: Number of information sessions held per month, number of truck drivers attending awareness-raising, etc. How can one decide whether the Ministry of Health got a good return on its money? Effects on health are clearly difficult to measure, but the audit firm can take steps to find out whether truckers are using condoms more frequently, and whether their sexual relations feel better protected from HIV/AIDS? Influence on health system performance: Is the HIV incidence rate among truck drivers falling or not?
Analysis of implementation	Are health staff prepared for intervention by people from outside the hospital? In practice, people from outside are dealing with patients without being trained for this task Hospital staff do not have a hierarchical relationship with the staff of the enterprise.	Are the results obtained attributable to the contractual relation or to the specific involvement of certain people? During the contract, did laws and regulations on drugs and their repression change? Has the attitude of the police and courts changed?	Road repair or changes in the parking area can change the NGO's working modalities.
Recommendations	What needs to be changed in the contract if it is to be renewed?	What needs to be changed to improve implementation of the present contract? Is a codicil needed or is the current contract sufficient? Are the people involved willing to implement these recommendations?	What needs to be changed to improve implementation of the present contract? Is a codicil needed or is the current contract sufficient? Who will implement the changes in question?

	Scenario 4 Ministry of Health recognition of an NGO health centre	Scenario 5 Analysis of transaction costs
Analysis of relevance	The consulting firm should take steps to decide whether recognizing this facility is the best strategy. Would it not be better to build a public health centre?	Appropriateness constitutes the result of the evaluation because if the result shows that transaction costs absorb all the benefits, the evaluation will conclude that contracting was inappropriate in this case.
Analysis of consistency	Does the health centre owned by this NGO have the means to implement standard health-centre activities, and does it really want to implement them (e.g. family planning)?	
Analysis of effects	Actions undertaken: Steps can be taken to compare the activities of this health centre with those of a public facility, based on standardized indicators (using impact analysis). Results achieved: One can measure whether the coverage rate increased as a result of the contract. Influence on health-system performance: Does this type of contract make public access more equitable?	The analysis will consist of recording: (i) all transaction costs owed in the contract and in all of its phases; and (ii) all the benefits obtained as a result of the contract.
Implementat ion analysis	Was the contract signed by the right people? Why did disputes arise? Could they have been foreseen?	It is worth enquiring whether the transaction costs recorded were predictable as a result of the contract or whether specific and unforeseeable circumstances changed them. The same for the benefits. This means assessing whether the results of this comparison are normal or exceptional in the original meaning of the term, and to what extent.
Recommend ations	What needs to be changed in the contract if it is to be renewed?	What lessons will the university propose to the international community? Through what channels will it promote these ideas?

Conclusion

Jean Perrot & Eric de Roodenbeke

INTRODUCTION

Recourse to contracting in the health sector initially developed in a technical direction due to the need to draw up sound contracts. Although this remains a valid concern and should not be underestimated, the concept has now evolved: contracting is not just about contracts; it is a strategy for resolving systemic problems in the area of health care. Contracting therefore goes beyond financing and raises questions about the organization of a health system, i.e. the respective roles and interrelationship of the stakeholders. All stakeholders wishing to use contracting must ask themselves fundamental questions about how to contract "strategically". This, hopefully, is how contracting will help to improve health system performance.

It would be both presumptuous and futile to draw conclusions on a subject such as health sector contracting.

- Presumptuous, because this book claims to illustrate the diversity and vast potential of the contracting process, but the reader will no doubt have identified areas of contracting that have not been discussed. It is thus impossible to present the subject in an exhaustive manner.

- Futile, because new developments are occurring on a daily basis. Just a few years ago, for example, performance incentives had been tested only in developed countries; they are now fashionable everywhere. Accordingly, this work itself will date rapidly.

Nevertheless, on the basis of everything that has been presented in this work we would like to highlight twelve seemingly essential points. They are not theoretical considerations but rather elements which political decision-makers must be aware of when they consider using contracting as a tool to implement their national health policy.

1. COMMITMENT OF THE STATE

Contracting is a process that works a profound change in the relationships between stakeholders at all levels of the health system. If the State, i.e. the authorities in the form of the Ministry of Health, the government and all branches of the State, do not support this new vision, any actions undertaken in the field will be under constant threat or will merely remain experiments and thus exceptions to the general rule. At the very least, the State must allow contracting experiments to be carried out in neutral conditions, unclouded by preconceptions and suspicions. Of course, it is always preferable that the State should fully endorse this approach and clearly encourage all stakeholders to follow this model.

Likewise, it is important for the State to emphasize that contracting is not tantamount to privatization, nor is it an abdication of responsibility on the part of the State. All too often, even today, contracting is likened by some stakeholders to a form of privatization. It is true, as this work has illustrated, that in some experiments contracting has been used as a tool to deliberately introduce a bigger private stake into health sector operations. Public-sector trade unions are particularly sensitive to some forms of contracting. It is therefore always in the State's interest to be clear on such issues. Strategically, it is prudent to indicate that greater involvement by the private sector or closer cooperation with it does not signify that the State is relinquishing its fundamental role of defending the public interest.

2. DIVERSITY OF CONTRACTUAL ARRANGEMENTS

It should be emphasized that all the contractual relationships put forward in this work have a common goal: improving health system performance. Accordingly, the individual interest of partners must be superseded by the general and collective interest, and this is where contracting is important for health systems. However, the various contracting experiments approach this goal in different ways. Some processes are based on the theory that rivalry and competition among stakeholders are indispensable to achieve contracting goals, ostensibly implying that absence of competition - often the case in developing countries - is necessarily a barrier to contracting. But many studies have demonstrated that competition does not automatically guarantee positive contracting outcomes. In contrast, other processes presuppose credible stakeholders and endeavour to make the most of cooperation between them. Contracting is therefore based on the premise that better coordination of efforts results in better organization of health services, thereby enabling the goal to be achieved.

This diversity of methods for achieving objectives should be recognized and certainly one of the strengths of contracting. It is important for political decision-makers to be aware of this diversity so that they can make the most of the opportunities it presents. Thus we noted that whereas Cambodia is expanding contracting to all health districts, Mali is introducing contracting at the health centre level only, and whereas France is developing cooperation-based contracting, in the United Kingdom and New Zealand contracting is based on competition. In some cases a country deliberately adopts a particular strategy for underlying cultural reasons; in others the choice is more random and the full potential of contracting has not been utilized owing to lack of awareness. Recourse to any of these methods should always be carefully considered in order to determine the most appropriate strategy. It is at this stage that domestic circumstances assume considerable importance and it would be wrong to advocate one strategy over another.

3. DIVERSITY IN FORGING CONTRACTUAL RELATIONSHIPS

Contracting in the health sector as initially conceived, or at least as it first emerged in developed countries, was based on the market principle, i.e. on competition as a way to identify the optimal solution for the stakeholders involved. Competition is created through classic market instruments such as calls to tender. However, some commentators in developed countries quickly recognized the limits of relationships founded on competition alone and advocated a radical change in strategy based on trust. Numerous analyses by the British National Health Service (NHS) underscored the negative consequences of pure competition and, as a result, contracting at the NHS is based on cooperation and trust.[1] In developing countries, most analyses acknowledge that transparent and competitive markets are very often absent in the health sector.[2] Consequently, developing countries, while ensuring due transparency, should probably focus more on contractual relationships based on negotiation among recognized partners in the health sector.

In differentiating between contractual arrangements, it is helpful to use the concept of **enforceability**.[3] Contracts are usually binding agreements, termed "enforceable" by lawyers, i.e. non-compliance by either party may entail penalties and, most importantly, the parties may appeal to persons external to the contract (third parties) in order to enforce commitments. The contract should itself make provision for these penalties and the arrangements for applying them. Some contractual arrangements do not follow this model, even though the legal prerequisites are present. For example, even when recourse to penalties is possible in contracts between large NGOs and Ministries of Health, it is difficult to apply such penalties in practice. Therefore, instead of enforceable contracts, it is preferable to speak of "relational contracts". Relational contracts are agreements negotiated between stakeholders, usually in the public sector, that enable the role of each stakeholder in an undertaking or joint operation to be clarified. The force of these agreements does not derive from the threat of penalties imposable by a court, but rather from the parties' mutual interest in working together. Relational contracts therefore rely principally on trust, flexibility and the use of general phrasing to guard against political and financial vagaries and the difficulties of setting precise goals and assessing outcomes. Although the respective stakeholders' commitments are not legally binding, they are nonetheless genuine. The commitment is simply enforced by other means and through other instruments: the value of a stakeholder's word and its credibility depend on the stakeholder's upholding its commitments.

Once again, political decision-makers must be aware of the diversity of contractual relationships and avoid preconceptions when judging which methods would be the most appropriate in each case. The cultural underpinnings of a given society will no doubt weigh heavily in the decision; some countries, for example, will emphasize market competition, while others will incline more towards relationships based on dialogue and negotiation.

4. CONTRACTING AS A STRATEGIC CHOICE

When contracting emerged in the context of health systems nearly ten years ago, the debate tended to focus on technical aspects such as drawing up and managing contracts. More recently, it has become apparent that contracting must be viewed against the backdrop of other strategies for health service organization and financing. Contracting should therefore be seen as just one of a number of different strategies to be tried out when resolving a problem. We must therefore ask why contracting seems to be the most suitable strategy. Almost certainly, the response will not always be the same and there will be cases where contracting will not be the most suitable strategy in a given context.

5. RISK OF UNDERESTIMATING THE DIFFICULTIES

Once contracting has been adopted into stakeholders' practices, it may be viewed by many as a particularly easy tool to master. For example: (i) two stakeholders that work well together will say that they do not need to draft a complicated contract because their current good relations are sufficient guarantee of good relations in the future, and as such (ii) why not use an all-purpose model contract.[4] S. Bennett et al.[5] speaking about evaluations of even relatively simple contracting experiments, conclude that stakeholders have often underestimated the difficulties of these contractual relationships.

- The contracting process takes time. There is a risk that the stakeholders involved will act too hastily in their desire for a quick fix. Driven by the need to produce results, stakeholders are often tempted to skip certain steps, resulting in misunderstandings and problems at every stage. It is therefore important that all stakeholders assimilate each step before moving on to the next. For example, in Benin, the authorities administering the Health Development Support Programme (Swiss Cooperation) point out that twelve months were needed for the various partner discussions, but this process facilitated the thorough definition of the role of each partner in the signed agreement.[6]

- Moreover, taking the time to implement each step of the process is especially important given that contracting is new and stakeholders cannot fall back on well-established recommendations and guides. They must start from scratch at each step. Even though lessons learnt from current experiments will allow certain steps to be expedited, it has to be borne in mind that drawing up a contracting project takes time, this time must be accounted for from the outset and skipping steps is always detrimental.

- The contracting process does not end with the signing of a contract: it is not uncommon for partners to devote significant effort to the preparatory phase of the contract only to abandon these efforts once the contract is signed. Thus in Burkina Faso, the agreement between the Ministry of Health and the Delegation of Camillian Fathers on establishing new health facilities and the arrangements for their operation remains virtually forgotten; the commitments undertaken by the two parties do not constitute a basis for evaluating relations between them. Ultimately, this agreement fulfils an accreditation function rather than being a contractual agreement.

6. TRANSACTION COSTS

Contracting is never cost-free. It always involves costs for the stakeholders involved, at every stage in the contracting process. Thus, at the contract drafting phase, the future contracting parties must devote considerable of time to meetings, amass information to analyse their own situation and that of their partners, and compile dossiers, all of which entails direct and also indirect expenditure. After the contract has been signed, costs are also involved in the implementation phase: the commitments of the other parties must be monitored, any conflicts resolved, and reports must be compiled.

Beforehand, as stated above, the stakeholders will embark on a contractual relationship only if, for each of them, the anticipated benefits of the relationship outweigh the costs. Afterwards, the envisaged costs often turn out to be higher than previously imagined. In some experiments, the costs are so high that they actually outweigh the benefits. For example, studies of contracting in the catering services in certain hospitals in Bombay, India,[7] indicated that contracting indeed reduced the cost of delivering the service, but at the same time there was a marked decline in quality.

While it is never possible to suppress the transaction costs of a contractual relationship in their entirety, it is nevertheless possible to look for ways to reduce them. The underlying terms of the contractual relationship are important. The recent evolution of the British health system towards increased cooperation instead of competition forms part of this trend.[8] It was noted that the principle of a contractual relationship based on competition between service providers generated very high transaction costs and led to opportunism. The system now in place aims to lower transaction costs by making the contractual relationship more dependent on cooperation and trust between partners, because it was also noted that transaction costs went down when the contracting parties learnt to work together and established good relations.[9]

It is also possible to reduce transaction costs by working with clusters of private service providers (where these exist) rather than with each provider individually.[10] For example, the existence of a cluster or network of NGOs will situate the negotiating process at the group level when defining the core principles of contractual relationships, and each contractual arrangement with NGOs in the network will subsequently be developed within this framework.. Likewise, a network of NGOs can to some extent oversee its individual components, thereby alleviating the burden of oversight on the principal stakeholder.

7. THE NEED TO REGULATE CONTRACTING PRACTICES

Specific ad hoc contractual arrangements can facilitate better relationships between stakeholders and help improve health system efficiency. But there is a significant risk that such ad hoc arrangements could yield modest or even harmful results under certain circumstances.

As stated in Part IV, chapter 1, States have at their disposal a certain number of technical tools for regulating contractual practices: model contracts for certain categories of contract, policy papers on specific types of contract (for example, in Rwanda, the "Guide to the contractual approach for health centres"), framework agreements, and technical support structures at the Ministry of Health. Compared with laissez-faire, these tools do provide a kind of framework for contractual practices. Pragmatically, benchmarks and frameworks are applied to certain types of contracting for which it is considered useful to spell out the rules of the game. Despite this, contracting is not approached systemically, i.e. is not seen as a tool for improving health system performance.

To visualize contracting in the broader context of health sector reforms, States would be better advised to incorporate contracting into their health policy. Many countries formulate documents along the lines of a "national health policy" that maps out the development of the health sector and the reforms that will be necessary. States wishing to introduce contracting will thus be able to incorporate it into their general policy framework. However, contracting occupies only a minor place within the national health policy as a whole, and in this framework it is not possible to define precisely how it will be used. To work around this problem, a specific "contracting policy" could be developed. Such a policy would enable a State to define its vision of contracting within the health system as a whole and to define the role of each stakeholder in the health sector.

8.   THE ROLE OF THE STATE

Contracting is a tool to organize health services for which the State has final and full responsibility. It should always be seen as a strategic option to help improve health system performance. Only a system-wide vision can guarantee this objective. As a stakeholder, the State can make judicious use of contracting, and through demonstration and practice it will have a lasting influence on the way this tool is used. But the State must also regulate contracting practices by monitoring contractual relationships (defining a legal framework, establishing an information system, and performing oversight, evaluation, training and mediation functions), offering incentives (including financial incentives), and designing, implementing and evaluating contracting policies.

So long as contracting remains the exception rather than the norm, its impact on the health system will be modest, but by the same token the risks are reduced. However, as soon as contractual practices become more widespread, the risks associated with poor coordination increase and can have a potentially destabilizing effect on the organization of health services. In parallel with its drive to develop contractual practices, the State must also ensure these practices are properly coordinated. The need to strengthen the general administrative (stewardship) function, as advocated in the 2000 World Health Report by WHO, is fully apparent.

To ensure that contracting is used to improve the organization of health services, the State must be able to exercise its role as guardian of the public interest, which is not necessarily the prime concern of the stakeholders seeking to develop their relationship.

9.   THE OBJECTIVES OF EVALUATION

Evaluation is an essential ingredient of the contracting process because it is necessary to determine whether the object of the contract has been respected and its objectives achieved. However, contracts often fail to specify the need for evaluation, as if the respective parties do not wish to avail themselves of the tools to verify that the commitments they have entered into are being honoured. Evaluation remains outside the process, whereas it ought to be an integral part of it. For example, perusal of the "associative agreement for public and community health" between the Ministry of Public Health of Côte d'Ivoire and the Association for Community-based Urban Health Training reveals that the parties to the contract are obliged to share information, yet no explicit provision has been made for a mechanism to evaluate outcomes, i.e. to compare expected outcomes with actual results. As stated above, the terms of the contract should clearly outline the objectives and specify the means available to achieve them. At the same time, a contract should set out the indicators or performance criteria for assessing how far the objectives have been achieved. To a certain extent, we can say that without evaluation procedures, no contract exists because it is not possible to verify the actual level of commitment of the parties. The contract merely becomes a declaration of intent, with performance depending solely on the goodwill of the parties. Admittedly, it is true that in many cases results are hard to measure and therefore it is difficult to agree on performance criteria that cover every aspect of the outcomes.[11]

In recent years, there has been an increase in the number of articles in scientific publications highlighting contracting experiments. This literature acts as a transmission belt for bringing innovative practices to the attention of the international community and disseminating hitherto nonexistent information. It also focuses a spotlight on contracting arrangements and flags some of the problems encountered. This evaluation is important and provides decision-makers with pointers to avoid repeating other people's mistakes. With rare exceptions, these evaluations convey no idea of the impact of contracting on health system performance. It is true that contracting experiments are often so recent that there is insufficient distance to make an evaluation. As time passes, more and more articles will be published on this topic. Now is the time, however, to take action to bridge this gap.

Finally, as contracting policies take root, the scope of evaluation should shift from specific contractual arrangements to an analysis of contracting policies. In developing countries today, this field of study remains practically unexplored. Appropriate efforts should be made in this field in the next few years. This is basically the area in which we can evaluate whether contracting has had an impact on the organization of health services and hence on national health system performance.

10. TECHNICAL KNOW-HOW

The design and oversight of a contracting process and the implementation and monitoring of a contracting policy require a level of technical know-how that the partners involved sometimes lack. Insufficient technical expertise in the areas of law, economics, public health, and political science can be highly deleterious to the effective introduction of contracting and can breed doubts about the wisdom of contracting as a whole, whereas in fact it is simply a technical issue. For example, in South Africa, where provincial health authorities have concluded contracts with private surgeons to carry out part-time work in public health facilities,[12] assessments reveal a significant lack of know-how among health authorities, first of all in terms of drawing up contracts, and also with regard to monitoring their implementation. In the light of a survey conducted in 5 countries (Ghana, India, Sri Lanka, Thailand and Zimbabwe), Mills et al. have highlighted this need to take account of the expertise of individuals at all levels if the contracting process is to flourish.[13]

Better technical know-how is thus a necessity for health stakeholders and for the State, specifically in its role as the regulator of contractual practices. With this purpose in view, a number of manuals or guides have recently been published or are currently in preparation. For example the World Bank is currently preparing a handbook on private participation in health, the French International Centre for Research and Development (CIDR), in collaboration with Medicus Mundi International and the World Health Organization (WHO), is preparing a guide for NGOs wishing to develop contractual relationships with health ministries, and WHO is preparing a resource entitled "Partnerships based on contractual relations: Tools for success" which focuses specifically on this area.

11. THE ROLE OF HEALTH WORKERS

It must be recognized that contracting changes the environment in which health workers operate, specifically when they are employed in institutions involved in contractual relationships. Obviously, the impact on health workers will vary widely depending on the object of the contract. Thus, different situations apply in a hospital that decides to subcontract its security service and a hospital that contracts with an insurer to attract a new client base; in the former case, the affected staff risk losing their jobs, whereas in the latter case, additional jobs may be created.

However, health workers and the trade unions that represent them often tend to believe that contracting is part of a general trend towards liberalization and deregulation, i.e. privatization, which will make their position more precarious.[14] Even though, throughout this work, it has been demonstrated that contracting does not necessarily signify more privatization, it must also be admitted that, in some cases, contracting is indeed a de facto step in this direction. This fact naturally prompts health workers to ask questions about:

- Their salary: Will contracting threaten their job? Is their job security under threat? Will pay be affected?

- Their conditions of employment: For example, will the inclusion of performance criteria in the contract mean they will have to do more to justify their own performance? The type of contract introduced by their employer could impact on the way they work.

If health workers are not involved in or at least consulted about the design of the contractual relationship that their institution has embarked upon, there is every likelihood that, rightly or wrongly, they will be anxious about the implications of contracting. Consequently, there is a high probability that they will oppose the implementation of the contractual relationship. Institutions embarking on contractual relationships need to bear this in mind because lack of cooperation on the part of health workers is not in their interests. The channels of communication between policy-makers and health workers (particularly via their representatives) therefore need to be strengthened to minimize the risk of conflict.

Likewise, it is in the interests of health workers and their representatives to develop their expertise on contracting-related issues. By showing themselves to be competent partners in such matters, they will gain credibility with their employers and will be better placed to press home their point of view.

12. THE DANGERS OF CONTRACTING

The replacement of a model in which stakeholder roles are kept separate by a model in which increasingly numerous and diverse stakeholders are connected in a relationship profoundly changes stakeholder behaviour. Although contracting should be seen as a tool for promoting better coordination among stakeholders, it can also have undesirable effects that can outweigh its benefits:

- Increased transaction costs: To protect against malicious intent and opportunism, stakeholders will be compelled to develop all aspects of their contractual relationship and make provision for all possible scenarios, thereby considerably complicating the procedures involved in negotiating, drafting and monitoring the implementation of contracts. The consequence will be an increase in transaction costs that could offset the anticipated benefits of the contractual relationship.

519

- Corruption: Corruption is the Achilles heel of the State and other stakeholders too. When they perceive that their contractual arrangements are not subject to proper oversight, stakeholders are prey to all manner of corrupt practices. In the negotiating phase, in the drafting process (a skilful expert would have no problem inserting ambiguous wording), upon signature (the authorized signatory is corruptible), or during the implementation phase (withholding of information, false appraisals, etc.).

- New market for distribution of financial resources: Unless the State is careful, contracting can rapidly become a new marketplace for the distribution of resources. Already, in some countries, stakeholders have realized that access to resources, specifically those provided by donors, is controlled through this new channel. Whereas resources used to be accessed through administrative channels, the contractual approach requires stakeholders to change direction. Wily stakeholders will rapidly propose their services on a contractual basis and take advantage of naive partners.

Contracting should not therefore be seen as a miracle solution like a magic wand, offering solutions to an organization's problems or resolving health system performance issues at one stroke. There is still a long way to go before this tool, which entails profound changes in the way health stakeholders operate, can deploy all its effects. A collective and ongoing learning process is a guarantee of success. The evaluation of current experiments will facilitate the gradual establishment of a solid basis on which to design those in the future.

Lastly, this work should not be interpreted as a plea for contracting. Rather, using country-specific experiments as a starting point, it seeks to illustrate the diversity of contracting environments, to outline the strengths and weaknesses of this tool, and to suggest new spheres of application and new practices. In order to understand contracting it is necessary to explore the underpinnings of this concept, and to do this it is sometimes necessary to engage in theoretical speculations. However, comprehension is not the ultimate goal of this work; it has been designed as a tool intended for stakeholders in the field, enabling them to use this instrument effectively should they decide to proceed.

Notes

[1] See, for example:

> Goddard, M. and R. Mannion. 1998. *From competition to co-operation: new economic relationships in the National Health Service. Health Economics* 7.

[2] Palmer, N. 2000. The use of private-sector contracts for primary health care theory, evidence and lessons for low-income and middle-income countries. *Bulletin of the World Health Organization* 78, no. 6.

[3] This concept is roughly equivalent to that used by Walsh, who distinguishes contracts based on penalties and contracts that involve cooperation between stakeholders. Walsh K. (19985) "Public Services and Market Mechanisms. Competition, Contracting and the New Public Management", Basingstoke: Macmillan

[4] WHO has been repeatedly asked by stakeholders in the field to provide model contracts; it is widely believed that a number of such contracts already exist.

[5] Bennett, S., B. McPake, and A. Mills. 1997. *Private health providers in developing countries.* chapter 12 ed. London and New Jersey.

[6] Health Development Support Programme (PADS). Community health centres (CSCOM): concepts, scenarios, viability et evaluation. Swiss Cooperation Benin, Graduate Institute of Development Studies, Geneva.

[7] Mills, A. 1997. *Contractual relationships between government and the commercial private sector in developing countries.* In *Private health providers in developing countries*, edited by Bennett, S., B. McPake, and A. Mills (London: Zed Books).

[8] Goddard, M. and R. Mannion. 1998. *From competition to co-operation: new economic relationships in the National Health Service. Health Economics* 7.

[9] Ashton, T., J. Cumming, and J. McLean. 2004. *Contracting for health services in a public health system: the New Zealand experience . Health Policy* 69:21-31.

[10] In Partnerships for Health Reform (PHR) Working Paper series, see the research paper entitled "Extending Coverage of Priority Health Care Services through Collaboration with the Private Sector: Selected Experiences of USAID Cooperating Agencies".

[11] Slack, K. and W. D. Savedoff. Public Purchaser - Private Provider contracting for health services. Examples from Latin America and the Caribbean. 2001. Inter-American Development Bank, Sustainable Development Department, Technical Papers Series.

[12] Palmer, N. and A. Mills. Serious contractual difficulties? A case study of contracting for PHC in South Africa. 2000. *Clermond-Ferrand, France, Paper*

presented at the international symposium on financing of health systems in low-income countries in Africa and Asia.

[13] Mills, A., S. Bennett, and S. Russell. 2001. *The challenge of health sector reform. What must Government Do?*: Palgrave.

[14] Lethbridge, J. 2004. Public health sector unions and deregulation in Europe. *International Journal of Health Services* 34, no. 3:435-452.

TO LEARN MORE

The following list of documents is not a reference list for the citations in the book. This proposed bibliography while being non-exhaustive serves as a general reference to those interested to learn more about contracting for health systems and services. It is a large collection of references that focus on different aspects of contracting, including a particularly rich collection of documents related to the use of performance incentives in the health sector. It is constituted of papers published in peer-reviewed journals, but several grey literature documents that often focus on the implementation level questions are also included. Thus the documents proposed in this bibliography give a thorough overview on the theoretical and empiric dimensions of strategic contracting for health systems and services.

(1997) "Best practice guidelines for contracting out government services". OECD. http://www.oecd.org/dataoecd/19/40/1901785.pdf

(1999) "BRI inquiry paper on commissioning, purchasing, contracting and quality of care in the NHS internal market", BRI Inquiry Secretariat. http://www.bristol-inquiry.org.uk/Documents/chcontracting2.pdf

(2001) "Using performance-based payments to improve health programs" Management Sciences for Health, The Manager. Volume 10, Number 2 http://erc.msh.org/TheManager/English/V10_N2_En_Issue.pdf

(2003) "L'approche contractuelle: guide méthodologique - Tome 1 et 2". Association Santé Internationale - International Development and Research Centre - Medicus Mundi International

(2005) " Paying for Performance: Policies for Government Employees". Paris, OECD, Policy   Brief, http://www.oecd.org/dataoecd/13/51/34910926.pdf

(2005) "Pay for performance in health care: an analysis of the arguments for and against". The American Association of Clinical Endocrinologists. http://www.aace.com/advocacy/leg/P4P/P4P.pdf

(2006) "Contracting and Health Services", Bulletin of the World Health Organization, Special Theme Issue. Vol.84, Number 11.

(2006) "Contracting in the healthcare field", University of Montreal, Infoletter. http://www.medsp.umontreal.ca/getos/pdf/Infoen102006.pdf

(2006) "Partnerships for malaria control: engaging the formal and informal private sectors", Geneva, WHO - Special Programme for Research & Training in Tropical Diseases (TDR). http://apps.who.int/tdr/svc/publications/tdr-research-publications/partnership-malaria-control

(2007) "Utilizing Performance-Based Financing to achieve health goals". USAID-Health Systems 20/20 - Brief.
http://www.healthsystems2020.org/content/resource/detail/1860/

(2007) "Paying the Poor to Use Health Services - Conditional Cash Transfers in Health and Education". The World Bank.
http://siteresources.worldbank.org/INTPAH/Resources/Reaching-the-Poor/RPPBriefsDemandSideFactorsMexicoENG.pdf

(2008) "Public-Private Investment Partnerships in health systems strengthening". Conference Papers -, 9-11 April 20008, Wilton Park, the United Kingdom .
http://www.globalhealthsciences.ucsf.edu/GHG/wilton_park_papers.aspx

(2008) "Rémunération à la performance dans le contexte sanitaire français: états des lieux et perspectives". Haute Autorité de Santé - France.
http://ifr69.vjf.inserm.fr/compaqh/data/04utilisations/Rapportp4pcompaqh.pdf

(2008) "The Business of Health in Africa - Partnering with the private sector to improve people's lives". IFC - International Finance Corporation - World Bank Group.

(2009) "Public-Private Investment Partnerships". The Global Health Group - University of California, San Franscico.

(2009) "Enhancing health systems through public-private investment partnerships: lessons learned from Lesotho", Conference summary report, Maseru, Lesotho, March31-April 2, 2009. http://globalhealthsciences.ucsf.edu/pdf/Lesotho-PPIP-Conference-Report-April-2009.pdf

(2009) "Paying for performance". PricewaterhouseCoopers'Health Research Institute.

(2010) "Performance-based incentives primer for USAID missions". USAID
http://www.healthsystems2020.org/content/news/detail/2654/

Abatcha K (1999) "Expériences du Tchad en matière de contractualisation". Ministère de la Santé publique, Direction générale.

Abelson J, Gold S T, Woodward C, O'Connor D, and Hutchinson B (2004) "Managing under managed community care: the experiences of clients, providers and managers in Ontario's competitive home care sector", Health Policy, 68, p.359 - 372.

Abramson W B (1999) "Partnerships between the public sector and non-governmental organizations: contracting for primary health care services". Latin American and Caribbean Health Sector Reform Initiative. Bethesda (MD): Partnerships for Health Reform Project, Abt Associates Inc

Abramson W B (2001) "Monitoring and evaluation of contracts for health service delivery in Costa Rica", Health Policy and Planning, 16(4), p.404 - 411.

Abramson W B (2004) "Contracting for Health Care Service Delivery". John Snow Inc

524

http://www.jsi.com/JSIInternet/Resources/Publications/DownloadDocument.cfm?D
BLDOCID=10351&DBLLANGID=3&DOC=ContractingPrimerManual.pdf

Abrantes A (1999) "Contracting public health care services in Latin America". The
World Bank, draft.
http://siteresources.worldbank.org/INTHSD/Resources/topics/Services/documents/
Hospital_Contracting_June20.doc

Agha S, Karim A M, Balal A, and Sosler S (2007) "The impact of a reproductive
health franchise on client satisfaction in rural Nepal", Health Policy and Planning,
22, p.320 - 328.

Ahston T, Cumming J, and McLean J (2004) "Contracting for health services in a
public health system: the New Zealand experience", Health Policy, vol.69, p.21 -
31.

Aljunid S (1995) "The role of private medical practitioners and their interactions
with public health services in Asian countries", Health Policy and Planning, 10(4),
p.333 - 349.

Allen P (2002) "A socio-legal and economic analysis of contracting in the NHS
internal market using a case study of contracting for district nursing", Social
Science and Medicine, 54, p.255 - 266.

Allen P, Croxson B, Roberts J.A, Archibald K, Crawshaw S, and Taylor L (2002)
"The use of contracts in the management of infectious disease related risk in the
NHS internal market", Health Policy, 59, p.257 - 281.

Ameli O and Newbrander W (2008) "Contracting for health services: effects of
utilization and quality on the costs of the Basic Package of Health Services in
Afghanistan", Bulletin of World Health Organization, 86 (12), p.920 - 928.

Ammi M and Bejean S (2009) "Les incitations "explicites" à la prévention
peuvent-elles être efficaces en médecine libérale?". Presentation at the XXXèmes
Journées des Economistes de la Santé Français, 6-7 December 2007, Lille, France

Andersen R, Smedby B, and Vagero D (2001) "Cost containment, solidarity and
cautious experimentation: Swedish dilemmas", Social Science and Medicine, 52,
p.1195 - 1204.

Anderson J and Van Crowder L (2000) "The present and future of public sector
extension in Africa: contracting out or contracting in?", Public Administration and
Development, 20, p.373 - 384.

Andrews M and Schroeder L (2003) "Sectoral decentralization and
intergovernmental arrangements in Africa", Public Administration and
Development, Vol. 23, p.29 - 40.

Arur A, Peters D, Hansen P, Mashkoor M A, Steinhardt L, and Burnham G (2010)
"Contracting for health and curative care use in Afghanistan between 2004 and
2005", Health Policy and Planning, 25, p.135 - 144.

Asamoa-Baah A and Smithson P (1999) "Donors and the ministry of Health: new partnerships in Ghana". Geneva, World Health Organization, Discussion paper N°8 (WHO/EIP/99.1).

Ashton T "Contracting for health services in New Zealand: a transaction cost analysis", Social Science & Medicine, 46 (3), p.357 - 367.

Ashton T, Cumming J, and McLean J (204) "Contracting for health services in a public health system: the New Zealand experience", Health Policy, 69, p.21 - 31.

Ashton T, Mays N, and Devlin N (2005) "Continuity through change: The rhetoric and reality of health reform in New Zealand", Social Science and Medicine, Vol. 61, p.253 - 262.

Baker G, Gibbons R, and Murphy K J (2002) "Relational contracts and the theory of the firm". *Quarterly Journal of Economics, 117*, 39–83.

Ballou J P and Weisbrod B A (2003) "Managerial rewards and the behavior of for-profit, governmental, and non-profit organizations: evidence from the hospital industry", Journal of Public Economics, 87, p.1895 - 1920.

Barnett C, Connor C, and Putney P J (2001) "Contracting non-governmental organizations to combat HIV/AIDS". Partnerships for Health Reform and Abt Associates Inc - Special Initiative Report N°. 33. http://www.abtassociates.com/reports/ES-sir33fin.pdf

Barnum H, Kutzin J, and Saxenian H (1995) "Incentives and provider payment methods", International Journal of Health Planning and Management, 10, p.23 - 45.

Basinga P (2009) "Impact of performance-based financing on the quantity and quality of maternal health services in Rwanda". PhD, University of Tulane, USA.

Basinga P, Gertler P, Binagwaho A, Soucat A, sturdy J, and Vermeersh C (2010) "Paying Primary Health Care Centers for Performance in Rwanda". World Bank Policy Research Working Paper No. 5190. Washingtno DC, The World Bank

Batley R (1999) "The new public management in developing countries: implications for policy and organizational reform", Journal of International Development, 11, p.761 - 765.

Batley R (1999) "The new public management in developing countries: introduction", Journal of International Development, 11, p.755 - 760.

Batley R (2007) "Engaged or divorced?" Capacity.org. http://www.capacity.org/en/content/view/full/219/(issue)/8297

Beith A, Eichler R, and Weil D (2007) "Perfrormance-based incentives for health: a way to improve tuberculosis detection and treatment completion?", CGD Working Paper # 122. Center for Global Development.

Beith A, Eichler R, Brow E, Button D, Hsdi N, Switlick K, Sanjana P, and Wang H (2009) "Pay for Performance (P4P) to improve maternal and child health in developing countries". Health Systems 20/20 Project.

Bellanger M and Mossé P (2005) "The search for the Holy Grail: combining decentralised planning and contracting mechanisms in the French health care system", Health economics, 14, p.S119 - S132.

Belley J-G (1988) "Max Weber et la théorie du droit des contrats", Droit et Société, 9, p.301 - 324.

Benderly B L (2010) "Getting Health Results in Afghanistan". The World Bank http://www.rbfhealth.org/rbfhealth/news/item/getting-health-results-afghanistan

Bennett S, Dakpallah G, Garner P, Gilson L, Nittayaramphong S, Zurita B, and Zwi A (1994) "Carrot and stick: state mechanisms to influence private provider behaviour", Health Policy and Planning, 9(1), p.1 - 13.

Bennett S, McPake B, and Mills A (1997) "Private health providers in developing countries". London and New Jersey, Zed Books.

Bennett S and Mills A (1998) "Government capacity to contract: health sector experience and lessons", Public Administration and Development, 18, p.307 - 326.

Bennett S, Hanson K, Kadama P, and Montagu D (2005) "Working with the non-state sector to achieve public health goals" Making health systems work, Working Paper N°2 Geneva, World Health Organization

Beracochea E (1997) "Contracting out of health-related services: the experience of Papua New Guinea". In Bennett S, McPake B and Mills A (eds) Private Health Providers in Developing Countries: Serving the public interest? London, Zed Books

Bernstein D (2008) "Le paiement à la performance des médecins généralistes anglais a-t-il atteint ses objectifs?", Caisse Nationale de l'Assurance Maladie, France, adsp n°65, p.49 - 52.

Béjean S, Durand P, and Vankemmelbeke C (2002) "L'assurance maladie, acheteur avisé: une réforme profonde des relations conventionnelles avec les médecins libéraux", Journal d'Economie Médicale, Vol.20, N°2, p.75 - 91.

Bhushan I, Keller S, and Schwartz B (2002) "Achieving the twin objectives of efficiency and equity: contracting health services in Cambodia". ADB, ERD Policy brief series, Economics and Research Department, Number 6.

Bien F and Reberioux A (2002) "L'interaction médecin-patient: un examen par l'économie des contrats", Journal d'Economie Médicale, Vol. 20, n° 5, p.251 - 262.

Bitran R (2002) "Paying health providers through capitation in Argentina, Nicaragua and Thaïland: output, spending, organizational impact, and market structure". Partnerships for Health Reform (PHR), Makor Applied Research 2, Technical Paper N°.1.

Bloom E, Bhushan I, Clingingsmith D, Hong R, King E, Kremer M, Loevinsohn B, and Schwartz B (2006) "Contracting for health: evidence from Cambodia". Washington DC, The World Bank

Bodart C, Servais G, Mohamed Y L, and Schmidt-Ehry B (2001) "The influence of health sector reform and external assistance in Burkina Faso", Health Policy and Planning, 16 (1), p.74 - 86.

Boonyoen D (1997) "Health systems and human resources development: the changing roles of public and private sectors", Human resources for health development journal, p.13 - 17.

Bossert T, Kosen S, Harsono B, Gani A (1997) "Hospital autonomy in Indonesia". Harvard School of Public Health. www.hsph.harvard.edu/ihsg/publications/pdf/No-39.PDF

Bossert T (1999) "Decentralization of health systems: decision space, innovation and performance". LAC Health Sector Reform Initiative. N° 17.

Bossert T (2000) "Guidelines for Promoting Decentralization of Health Systems in Latin America", Health Sector Reform Initiative - LAC HSR, No 30.

Bossert T and Beauvais J C (2002) "Decentralization of health systems in Ghana, Zambia, Uganda and the Philippines: a comparative analysis of decision space", Health Policy and Planning, 17(1), p.14 - 31

Bossert T, Chitah M B, and Bowser D (2003) "Decentralization in Zambia: resource allocation and district performance", Health Policy and Planning, 18, p.357 - 369.

Bossert T (2004) "Organizational Reforms and Reproductive Health: Decentralization, Integration and Organizational Reform of Ministries of Health". Draft paper prepared for the WHO Technical Consultation on Health Sector Reform and Reproductive Health: Developing the Evidence Base. Geneva, 30 November - 2 December 2004.

Boulanger D, Keugoung B, and Criel B (2009) " Contracting between faith-based and public health sector in Sub-Saharan Africa: An ongoing crisis?" Report Medicus Mundi International.
http://www.medicusmundi.org/en/contributions/events/2009/contracting-crisis

Bousquet C (2005) "Performance-based contracting for health service delivery in post-conflict Afghanistan: Is there still a case for debate?". Groupe URD
http://www.urd.org/IMG/pdf/PPA_is_there_still_case_for_debate.pdf

Bousquet C (2007) "Health sector review in Afghanistan (2001-2006)". Groupe URD http://www.urd.org/IMG/pdf/Health_Sector_Review.pdf

Bouthinon-Dumas H (2001) "Les contrats relationnels et la théorie de l'imprévision", Revue internationale de droit économique, 3, 339-373.

Bras P L and Duhamel G (2008) "Rémunérer les médecins selon leurs performances: les enseignements des expériences étrangères". Rapport RM2008-047P, Inspection Générale des Affaires Sociales, France

Brenzel L (2009) "Taking stock: world Bank experience with results-based financing (RBF) for health", The World Bank, HDNHE.

BRI (1999) "BRI inquiry paper on commissioning, purchasing, contracting and quality of care in the NHS internal market". BRI inquiry secretariat http://www.bristol-inquiry.org.uk/Documents/chcontracting2.pdf

Brook P J and Smith S M (2001) "Contracting for public services: output-based aid and its applications". World Bank and International Finance Corporation (IFC).

Broomberg J (1994) "Managing the health care market in developing countries: prospects and problems", Health Policy and Planning, 9 (3), p.237 - 251.

Brown A (2000) "Current issues in sector-wide approaches for health development: Tanzania case study". Geneva, World Health Organization, Discussion paper (WHO/GPE/00.6.)

Brugha R and Zwi A (1998) "Improving the quality of private sector delivery of public health services: challenges and strategies", Health Policy and Planning, 13 (2), p.107 - 120.

Brugha R, Chandramohan D, and Zwi A (1999) "Viewpoint: Management of malaria - working with the private sector", Tropical Medicine and International Health, 4 (5), p.402 - 406.

Bruni M, Nobilio L, and Ugolini C (2009) "Economic incentives in general practice: the impact of pay for participation and pay for compliance programs on diabetes care", Health Policy, Vol.90, p.140 - 148.

Bryntse K (1996) "The purchasing of public services: exploring the purchasing function in a service context", European Journal of Purchasing & Supply Management, 2(4), p.193 - 201.

Busogoro J-F and Beith A (2010) "Pay for Performance for Improved Health In Burundi". USAID - Health Systems 20/20, P4P case studies http://www.healthsystems2020.org/content/resource/detail/2575/

Bustreo F, Harding A, and Axelsson H (2003) "Can developing countries achieve adequate improvements in child health outcomes without engaging the private sector?", Bulletin of World Health Organization, Vol.12, p.886 - 894.

Cabases J M, Gaminde I, and Gabilondo L "Contracting arrangements in the health strategy context: a regional approach for Spain". The European Journal of Public Health 2000, 10(Supplement 4):45-50

Cabiedes L and Guillen A (2001) "Adopting and adapting managed competition: health care reform in Southern Europe", Social Science and Medicine, 52, p.1205 - 1217.

Campbell S, Reeves D, Kontopantelis E, Middleton E, Sibbald B, and Roland M (2007) "Quality of primary care in England with the introduction of pay for performance", The New England Journal of Medicine, 357:2, p.181 - 190.

Carrin G, Jancloes M, and Perrot J (1998) "Towards new partnerships for health development in developing countries: the contractual approach as a policy tool", Tropical Medicine and International Health, 3 (6), p.512 - 514.

Carrin G, Waelkens M-P, and Criel B (2005) "Community-based health insurance in developing countries: a study of its contribution to the performance of health financing systems", Tropical Medicine and International Health, Volume 10 N° 8, p.799 - 811.

Carruthers I (1995) "Contracting and choice", British Medical Journal, Vol. 51, N° 4, p.915 - 926.

Casalino L P, Elster A, Eisenberg A, Lewis E, Montgomery J, and Ramos D (2007) "Will pay for performance and quality reporting affect health care disparities?", Health economics - Web Exclusivep.w405 - w414.

Cassels A (1995) "Health sector reform: key issues in less developed countries", Journal of International Development, 7(3), p.329 - 347.

Chaix-Couturier C, Durand-Zaleski I, Jolly D, and Durieux P (2002) "Effects of financial incentives on medical practice: results from a systematic review of the literature and methodological issues", International Journal for Quality in Health Care, 12, 2, p.133 - 142.

Chakraborty S, D'Souza S A, and Northrup R (2000) "Improving private practitioner care of sick children: testing new approaches in rural Bihar", Health Policy and Planning, 15(4), p.400 - 407.

Chalkley M and Malcomson J.M (1998) "Contracting for health services when patient demand does not reflect quality", Journal of Health Economics, 17 (1), p.1 - 19.

Chalkley M and Khalil F (2005) "Third party purchasing of health services. patient choice and agency", Journal of Health Economics, 24, p.1132 - 1153.

Champagne F, Contandriopoulos A P, and Pineault R (1985) "Un cadre conceptuel pour l'évaluation des programmes de santé", Revue épidémiologique et Santé publique, 33, p.173 - 181.

Chapin J and Fetter B (2002) "Performance-Based Contracting in Wisconsin Public Health: Transforming State-Local Relations", The Milbank Quarterly, Vol.80, N°1, p.97 - 124.

Chaserant C (2003) "Cooperation, contracts and networks: From a bounded to a procedural rationality approach", Journal of Management and Governance, vol. 7, pp. 163-186.

Chaserant C (2001) "La coopération se réduit-elle à un contrat? Une approche procédurale des relations contractuelles". Recherches Economiques de Louvain / Louvain Economic Review, vol. 68, n°4, pp. 181-510

Chawla M, Govindaraj R, Berman P, and Needleman J (1996) "Improving Hospital Performance through Policies to Increase Hospital Autonomy: Methodological Guidelines" International Health Systems Program, Department of Global Health and Population, Harvard School of Public Health

530

Chee G, Bennett S, Leighton C (2007) " Working with Private Providers to Improve the Delivery of Priority Services", Partnerships for Health Reform, PHR Primer - For Policymakers

Chinitz D P (1994) "Reforming the Israeli health care market", Social Science and Medicine, 39(10), p.1447 - 1457.

Chougrani S (1998) "La contractualisation et l'information: défis et enjeux entre les financeurs et les producteurs de soins en Algérie", Revue du Centre en Anthropologie Sociale et Culturelle.Université d'Oran, Insaniat, n°6, vol.II.3, p.143 - 161.

Clasen T F (2002) "The public-private partnership for the Central American handwashing initiative: reflections from a private sector perspective", Tropical Medicine and International Health, Volume 7 N° 3, p.197 - 200.

Coheur A, Jacquier C, Schmitt-Diabaté V, and Schremmer J (2007) "Linkages between statutory social security schemes and community-based social protection mechanisms: A promising new approach". International Social Security Association- World Social Security Forum- 10-15 Sept 2007, Moscow.

Collins C and Green A (1994) "Decentralization and primary health care: some negative implications in developing countries", International Journal of Health Services, 24(3), p.459 - 475.

Collins C, Njeru G, and Meme J (1996) "Hospital autonomy in Kenya: the experience of Kenyatta national hospital". International Health Systems Program, Department of Global Health and Population, Harvard School of Public Health

Collins C and Green A (1999) "Public sector hospitals and organization change: an agenda for policy analysis", International Journal of Health Planning and Management, 14, p.107 - 128.

Collins C, Njeru G, Meme J, and Newbrander W (1999) "Hospital autonomy: the experience of Kenyatta national hospital", International Journal of Health Planning and Management, 14, p.129 - 153.

Collins C, Omar M, and Tarin E (2002) "Decentralization, health care and policy process in the Punjab, Pakistan in the 1990s", International Journal of Health Planning and Management, 17, p.123 - 146.

Commons M, McGuire T G, and Riordan M H (1997) "Performance Contracting for Substance Abuse Treatment", Health Services Research, 32:5, p.631 - 650.

Coppel D, Watts K, White J, and Owen L (2001) "Contracting for smoking and pregnancy interventions: current practice across England", Public Health, 115, p.222 - 228.

Cox A (1996) "Relational competence and strategic procurement management", European Journal of Purchasing & Supply Management, 2(1), p.57 - 70.

Cox H (2003) "Questions about the initiative of the European commission concerning the awarding and compulsory competitive tendering of public service concessions", Annals of Public and Comparative Economics, 74:1, p.7 - 31.

Criel B, Barry A N, and von Roenne F (2002) "Le Projet PRIMA en Guinée Conakry. Une expérience d'organisation de mutuelles de santé en Afrique rurale". Medicus Mundi Bruxelles, MSP Guinée, GTZ, DBCI Bruxelles, IMT, Anvers.

Criel B, Diallo A.A, Van der Vennet J, Waelkens M-P, and Wiegandt A (2005) "La difficulté du partenariat entre professionnels de santé et mutualistes: le cas de la mutuelle de santé Maliando en Guinée-Conakry", Tropical Medicine and International Health, Vol.10, N° 5, p.450 - 463.

Cuellar C J, Newbrander W, and Price G (2000) "Extending access to health care through public-private partnerships: the PROSALUD experience". Management Sciences for Health (MSH), Boston, Stubbs Monograph Series Number 2.

Cumming J and Mays N (2002) "Reform and counter reform: how sustainable is New Zealand's latest health system restructuring", Journal of Health Services Res Policy, Vol.7, Suppl 1, p.46 - 55.

Dawson D and Goddard M (1999) "Long-term contracts in the NHS: a solution in search of a problem?", Health economics, 8, p.709 - 720.

De Costa A and Diwan V K (2007) ""Where is the public health sector?" Public and private sector healthcare provision in Madhya Pradesh, India", Health Policy, 84, p.269 - 276.

de Savigny D and Adam T (eds) (2009) "Systems thinking for Health systems strengthening". Geneva, Alliance for Health Policy and System Research- World Health Organization.

Deakin S and Michie J (1997) "Contracts, co-operation, and competition". Oxford, Oxford University Press.

DeRoeck D (1998) "Making health-sector non-governmental organizations more sustainable: a review of NGO and donor efforts". Partnerships for Health Reform (PHR), Special Initiatives, Report 14.

Desplats D, Koné Y, and Razakarison (2004) "Pour une médecine générale communautaire en première ligne", Médecine Tropicale, 64, p.539 - 544.

DFID (2000) "Making the most of private sector", DFID Report http://www.dfidhealthrc.org/publications/health_service_delivery/Making%20most %20psector.PDF

Dreesch N, Nyoni J, Mokopakgosi O, Seipone K, Kalilani J A, Kaluwa O, and Musowe V (2007) "Public-private options for expanding access to human resources for HIV/AIDS in Botswana", Human resources for health, 5 (25).

Dudarewicz D and Chawla M (1997) "Physician contracting in Suwalki". International Health Systems Program, Department of Global Health and Population, Harvard School of Public Health

Duggan M (2004) "Does contracting out increase the efficiency of government programs? Evidence from Medicaid HMOs", Journal of Publics Economics, 88, p.2549 - 2572.

Eichler R, Auxila P, and Pollack J (2000) "Performance based reimbursement to improve impact: Evidence from Haiti". Lac Health Sector Reform Initiative. N°44. http://lachealthsys.org/index.php?option=com_docman&task=doc_download&gid= 35&Itemid=

Eichler R, Auxila P, and Pollock J (2001) "Output-Based Health Care: Paying for Performance in Haiti". The World Bank. Public Policy for the private sector- Note Number 236.

Eichler R, Auxila P, Pollock J. (2001) Promoting preventive health care—paying for performance in Haiti. In Brook PJ and Smith SM, eds, *Contracting for Public Services: Output-based Aid and its Applications*. Washington, DC: World Bank

Eichler R (2006) "Can "Pay for Performance" Increase Utilization by the Poor and Improve the Quality of Health Services?". *Discussion paper for the first meeting of the* Working Group on Performance-Based Incentives Center for Global Development http://www.cgdev.org/doc/ghprn/PBI%20Background%20Paper.pdf

Eichler R, Auxila P, Antoine U, and Desmangles B (2007) "Performance-Based incentives for health: Six years of results from Supply-Side programs in Haiti", CGD Working Paper # 121. Center for Global Development.

Eldridge C and Palmer N (2009) "Performance-based payment: some reflections on the discourse, evidence and unanswered questions", Health Policy and Planning ;24: p.160–166

England R (2000) "Contracting and performance management in the health sector. Some pointers on how to do it". DFID - Health Systems Research Centre http://www.dfidhealthrc.org/publications/health_service_delivery/Contracting.PDF

England R (2004) "Experience of contracting with the private sector: a selective review". London, DFID- Health Systems Resource Centre.

England R (2006) "HIV antiretroviral therapy: can franchising expand coverage?". DFID Health Resource Centre. http://www.dfidhealthrc.org/publications/health_service_delivery/ART%20and%20 social%20franchising_Oct%2006.pdf

Ensor T, Quayyum Z, Nadjib M, and Sucahya P (2008) "Level and determinants of incentives for villag midwives in Indonesia", Health Policy and Planning, 24, p.26 - 35.

Enthoven A C (1993) "The history and principles of managed competition", Health Affairs, Supplement, p.24 - 48.

Enthoven A C (1994) "On the ideal market structure for third-party purchasing of health care", Social Science and Medicine, 39(10), p.1413 - 1424.

533

Epstein A M, Lee T H, and Hamel M (2004) "Paying Physicians for High-Quality Care", The New England Journal of Medicine, 350:4, p.406 - 410.

Epstein A M (2007) "Pay for performance at the tipping point", The New England Journal of Medicine, 356:5, p.515 - 517.

Evans D (1999) "The impact of a quasi-market on sexually transmitted disease services in the UK", Social Science and Medicine, 49, p.1287 - 1298.

Fehr E and Fischbacher (2002) "Why social preferences matter - the impact of non-selfish motives on competition, cooperation and incentives", The Economic Journal, 112, p.C1 - C33.

Fehr E, Brown M, and Zehnder (2009) "On reputation: a microfoundation of contract enforcement and price rigidity", The Economic Journal, 119, p.333 - 353.

Fiedler J, Levin A, and Mulikelela D (1998) "A feasibility analysis of franchising the PROSALUD/Bolivia: a primary health care service delivery strategy in Lusaka, Zambia". Technical report N° 15, Partnerships for Health Reform (PHR).

Fiedler J L and Wight J B (2003) "Privatization and the allure of franchising: a Zambian feasibility study", International Journal of Health Planning and Management, 18, p.179 - 204.

Figueras J, Robinson R, and Jakubowski E (2005) "Purchasing to improve health systems performance". Open University Press.

Finger M (2001) "La gestion déléguée et la réforme de l'Etat". Working paper de l'IDHEAP 14/2001, Suisse.

Fougere G (2001) "Transforming health sectors: new logics of organizing in the New Zealand health system", Social Science and Medicine, 52, p.1233 - 1242.

Frenk J (1993) "The public/private mix and human resources for health", Health Policy and Planning, 8 (4), p.315 - 326.

Furth R. (2006) "Zambia pilot study of performance-based incentives". USAID, Quality Assurance Project

Gaskin D J, Escarce J, Schulman K, and Hadley J (2002) "The Determinants of HMOs'Contracting with Hospitals for Bypass Surgery", Health Services Research, 37:4, p.963 - 984.

Gauri V, Cercone J, and Briceño R (2004) "Separating financing from provision: evidence from 10 years of partnership with health cooperatives in Costa Rica", Health Policy and Planning, 19(5), p.292 - 301.

Gilson L, Sen P D, Mohamed S, and Mujinja P (1994) "The potential of health sector non-governmental organizations: policy options", Health Policy and Planning, 9 (1), p.14 - 24.

Gilson L (2003) "Trust and development of health care as a social institution", Social Science and Medicine, 56, p.1453 - 1468.

Giusti D, Criel B, and De Béthune X (1997) "Viewpoint: public versus private health care delivery: beyond the slogans", Health Policy and Planning, 12 (3), p.193 - 198.

Giusti D (1999) "Consequences of the new roles of Government for the NGO providers from the perspective of a national co-ordinating body". Medicus Mundi International Consultation Workshop, Dar Es Salaam, 5-7 november 1999.

Giusti D (2008) "Improving opportunities trough strategic positioning and co-operation", Bulletin Medicus Mundi Schweiz, 107, p.56 - 63.

Glassman A and Todd JGaarder M (2007) "Performance-based incentives for health: conditional cash transfer programs in Latin America and the Caribbean", CGD Working Paper # 120. Center for Global Development.

Glennerster H and Le Grand J (1995) "The development of quasi-markets in welfare provision in the United Kingdom", International Journal of Health Services, 25 (2), p.203 - 218.

Glinos I A, Baeten R, and Maarse H (2010) "Purchasing health services abroad: Practices of cross-border contracting and patient mobility in six European countries", Health Policy, 95, p.103 - 112.

Goddard M and Mannion R (1998) "From competition to co-operation: new economic relationships in the national health service", Health economics, 7, p.105 - 119.

Gollust S and Jacobson P (2006) "Privatization of Public Services: Organizational Reform Efforts in Public Education and Public Health", American Journal of Public Health, Vol.96, N°.10, p.1733 - 1739.

Golooba-Mutebi F (2003) "Devolution and outsourcing of municipal services in Kampala city, Uganda: an early assessment", Public Administration and Development, Vol. 23, p.405 - 418.

Gomez-Jauregui J (2004) "The feasibility of Government Partnerships with NGOs in the Reproductive Health Field in Mexico", Reproductive Health matters, 12(24), p.42 - 55.

Gotsadze G and Jugeli L (2004) "Private-public partnership in Georgia: A case study of contracting an NGO to provide specialist health services". DFID- Health Systems Resource Centre.

Govindaraj R (1996) "Hospital autonomy in Ghana: the experience of Korle Bu and Komfo Anokye teaching hospitals". International Health Systems Program, Department of Global Health and Population, Harvard School of Public Health

Graf von der Schulenburg J-M (1994) "Forming and reforming the market for third-party purchasing of health care: a German perspective", Social Science and Medicine, 39(10), p.1473 - 1481.

Gravelle H (1999) "Capitation contracts: access and quality", Journal of Health Economics, 18, p.315 - 340.

Green A, Shaw J, Dimmock F, and Conn C (2002) "A shared mission? Changing relationships between government and church health services in Africa", International Journal of Health Planning and Management, 17(4), p.333 - 353.

Griffiths L and Hughes D (2000) "Talking contracts and taking care: managers and professionals in the British National Health Service internal market", Social Science and Medicine, 51, p.209 - 222.

Gross R and Harrison M (2001) "Implementing managed competition in Israel", Social Science and Medicine, 52, p.1219 - 1231.

Grytten J and Sorensen R (2001) "Type of contract and supplier-induced demand for primary physicians in Norway", Journal of Health Economics, 20, p.379 - 393.

Gueye M A and Kopp J E (2009) "Le contrat de performance hospitalière: l'expérience du Sénégal", Santé Publique, Vol.21, p.77 - 87.

Hansen P, Peters D, Niayesh H, Singh L, Dwivedi V, and Burnham G (2008) "Mesuring and managing progress in the establishment of basic health services: the Afghanistan Health Sector Balanced Scorecard", International Journal of Health Planning and Management, 23, p.107 - 117.

Hansen P, Peters D, Edward A, Gupta S, Arur A, Niayesh H, and Burnham G (2008) "Determinants of primary care service quality in Afghanistan", International Journal for Quality in Health Care, 20 (6), p. 375–383

Hanson A, Atuyambe L, Kamwanga J, McPake B, Mungule O, and Ssengooba F (2001) "Towards improving hospital performance in Uganda and Zambia: reflections and opportunities for autonomy", Health Policy, 61, p. 73 - 94 .

Hardeman W, Van Damme W, Van Pelt M, Por I, Kimvan H, and Meessen B (2004) "Access to health care for all? User fees plus a Health Equity Fund in Sotnikum, Cambodia", Health Policy and Planning, 19(1), p.22 - 32.

Harrison M and Calltorp J (2000) "The reorientation of market-oriented reforms in Swedish health-care", Health Policy, 50, p.219 - 240.

Hebrang A, Henigsberg N, Ederljic V, Foro S, Vidjak V, and Macek T (2003) "Privatization in the health care system of Croatia: effects on general practice accessibility", Health Policy and Planning, 18(4), p.421 - 428.

Hecht R, Batson A, and Brenzel L (2004) "Responsabiliser les prestataires de soins de santé", Finances & Développement, p.16 - 19.

Homedes N and Ugalde A (2005) "Why neoliberal health reform have failed in Latin America", Health Policy, 71, p.83 - 96.

Hongoro C and Kumaranayake L (2000) "Do they work? Regulating for-profit providers in Zimbabwe", Health Policy and Planning, 15(4), p.368 - 377.

Hubbard M, Delay S, and Devas N (1999) "Complex management contracts: the case of customs administration in Mozambique", Public Administration and Development, 19, p.153 - 163.

Huntington D, Zaky H H M, Shawky S, and Fattah F A (2009) "Impact of provider incentive payments on reproductive health services in Egypt". Policy brief. Department of Reproductive Health and Research- World Health Organization.

Hurst S A and Mauron A (2004) "Selective contracting of Swiss physicians: ethical issues and open questions", Swiss medical weekly, 134, p.632 - 639.

Hurtig A K, Pande S B, Baral S C, Newell J, Porter J, and Sing Bam D (2002) "Linking private and public sectors in tuberculosis treatment in Katmandu Valley, Nepal", Health Policy and Planning, 17 (1), p.78 - 89.

Huy Dung P (1996) "The political process and the private health sector's role in Vietnam", International Journal of Health Planning and Management, 11, p.217 - 230.

Hviid M (2000) "Long-term contracts and relational contracts", p.46 - 72. in Bouckaert B and De Geest G (eds) Encyclopedia of Law and Economics, vol III. London, Edward Elgar Publishing

IHSD (2004) "Private sector participation in health". http://www.hlsp.org/Home/Resources/Privatesectorparticipationinhealth.aspx

Indermühle L, Overtoom R, and Jacobs B (2007) "Contracting in Cambodia", Medicus Mundi Switzerland -Bulletin, 104, p.52 - 55.

Iriart C, Merhy E E, and Waitzkin H (2001) "Managed care in Latin America: the new common sense in health policy reform", Social Science and Medicine, 52, p.1243 - 1253.

Jack W (2003) "Contracting for health services: an evaluation of recent reforms in Nicaragua", Health Policy and Planning, 18(2), p.195 - 204.

Jack W (2005) "Purchasing health care services from providers with unknown altruism", Journal of Health Economics, 24, p.73 - 93.

Jacobs B, Thomé J-M, Overtoom R, Oeun Sam S, Indermühle L, and Price N (2010) "From public to private and back again: sustaining a high service-delivery level during transition of management authority: a Cambodia case study", Health Policy and Planning, 25, p.197 - 208.

Jillson I.A. (1999) "Opportunities for public/private sector partnerships in the Palestinian health care system", Policy Research Incorporated; Bethesda, Maryland.

Johannes L, Mullen P, Okwero P, and Schneidman M (2008) "Performance-based contracting in health. The experience of three projects in Africa", Global Partnership on Output-   Based Aid. OBApproches N°19. http://www.gpoba.org/gpoba/sites/gpoba.org/files/OBApproaches19_Africa_Health.pdf

Johnson S, McMillan J, and Woodruff C (2002) "Courts and Relational Contracts", The Journal of Law, Economics, & Organization, Vol.18, N°1, p.221 - 277.

Jütting J. (2002) "Public-private partnerships in the health sector: Experiences from developing countries". ILO. ESS, Paper n°10.

Kakabadse A and kakabadse N (2001) "Outsourcing in the public services: a comparative analysis of practice, capability and impact", Public Administration and Development, 21, p.401 - 413.

Kaul M (1997) "The new public administration: management innovations in government", Public Administration and Development, 17, p.13 - 26.

Khaleghian P and Das Gupta M (2005) "Public Management and the Essential Public Health Functions", World Development, Vol.33, N°.7, p.1083 - 1099.

Kirat T (2003) "L'allocation des risques dans les contrats: de l'économie des contrats "incomplets" à la pratique des contrats administratifs", Revue Internationale de Droit Economique, 17 (1), p.11 - 46.

Kolehmainen-Aitken R-L (2000) "State of practice: Public-NGO partnerships in response to decentralization". Lac Health Sector Initiative. N°22.

Koot J (1999) "New roles of the government in health care. A new place for NGOs in the health services?". Medicus Mundi International Consultation Workshop, Dar Es Salaam, 5-7 November 1999.

Kumaranayake L (1997) "The role of regulation: influencing private sector activity within health sector reform", Journal of International Development, 9(4), p.641 - 649.

Kumaranayake L, Lake S, Mujinja P, Hongoro C, and Mpembeni R (2000) "How do countries regulate the health sector? Evidence from Tanzania and Zimbabwe", Health Policy and Planning, 15(4), p.357 - 367.

Kutzin J (2001) "A descriptive framework for country-level analysis of health care financing arrangements", Health Policy, 56, p.171 - 204.

La Forgia G (Ed.) (2005) "Health system innovations in Central America", Washington DC , The World Bank. Working paper n° 57.

Laamanen R, Simonsen-Rehn N, Suominen S, Ovretveit J, and Brommels M (2008) "outsourcing primary health care services - How politicians explain the grounds for their decisions", Health Policy, 88, p. 294-307

Lacey R (1997) "International markets in the public sector: the case of British National Health Service", Public Administration and Development, 17, p.141 - 159.

Lagarde M and Palmer N (2006) "Evidence from systematic reviews to inform decision making regarding financing mechanisms that improve access to health services for poor people". Alliance for Health Policy and Systems Research.

538

Lagarde M and Palmer N (2006) "The impact of health financing strategies on access to health services in low and middle income countries", The Cochrane Library, Issue 4, p.1 - 9.

Lagarde M, Haines A and Palmer N (2007) "Conditional cash transfers for improving uptake of health interventions in low- and Middle-Income countries", JAMA, Vol. 298, N° 16, p.1900 - 1910.

Laing A and Cotton S (1997) "Patterns of inter-organizational purchasing: evolution of consortia-based purchasing amongst GP fundholders", European Journal of Purchasing & Supply Management, Vol.3, N°2, p.83 - 91.

Larbi G A (1998) "Institutional constraints and capacity issues in decentralizing management in public services: the case of health in Ghana", Journal of International Development, 10, p.377 - 386.

LaVake S D (2003) "Applying Social Franchising Techniques to Youth Reproductive Health/HIV Services". YouthNet- Youth Issues Paper 2.

Le Grand J (1999) "Competition, Cooperation, or Control? Tales from the British National Health Service", Health Affairs, 18(3), p.27 - 39.

Lember M (2002) "A policy of introducing a new contract and funding system of general practice in Estonia", International Journal of Health Planning and Management, 17, p.41 - 53.

Leonard K l (2003) "African traditional healers and outcome-contingent contracts in health care", Journal of Development Economics, 71, p.1 - 22.

Leonard K l and Zivin J G (2005) "Outcome versus service based payments in health care: lessons from African traditional healers", Health economics, 14, p.575 - 596.

Lethbridge J (2004) "Public health sector unions and deregulation in Europe", International Journal of Health Services, Volume 34, Number 3, p.435 - 452.

Levin J (2003) "Relational incentive contracts", American Economic Review, 93 (3), p.835 - 857.

Levis R and Gillam S (2003) "Back to the market : yet more reform of the national health service", International Journal of Health Services, Vol. 33, Number 1, p.77 - 84.

Lewis R, Dixon M, and Gillam S (2003) "Future directions for primary care trusts". King's Fund.
http://www.kingsfund.org.uk/publications/the_kings_fund_publications/future_1.html

Lewis R (2004) "Practice-led Commissioning: Harnessing the power of the primary care frontline". King's Fund.
http://www.kingsfund.org.uk/document.rm?id=123

Lidbury C (1999) "Performance contracting: Lessons from Performance Contracting Case Studies A Framework for Public Sector Performance Contracting". OECD. http://www.olis.oecd.org/olis/1999doc.nsf/LinkTo/PUMA-PAC(99)2

Lieverdink H (2001) "The marginal success of regulated competition policy in the Netherlands", Social Science and Medicine, 52, p.1183 - 1194.

Light D W (2001) "Comparative institutional response to economic policy managed competition and governmentality", Social Science and Medicine, 52, p.1151 - 1166.

Light D W (2001) "Managed competition, governmentality and institutional response in the United Kingdom", Social Science and Medicine, 52, p.1167 - 1181.

Lindenauer P K and Alii (2007) "Public reporting and pay for performance in hospital quality improvement", The New England Journal of Medicine, 356:5, p.486 - 496.

Lippi Bruni M, Nobilio L, and Ugolini C (2009) "Economic incentives in general practice : the impact of pay for participation and pay for compliance programs on diabetes care", Health Policy, 90, p.140 - 148.

Liu X, Hotchkiss D R, Bose S, Bitran R, and Giedon U (2004) "Contracting for Primary Health Services: Evidence on its effects and a framework for evaluation". Partnerships for Health Reform (PHRplus).

Liu X, Hotchkiss D R, and Bose S (2007) "The impact of contracting-out on health system performance: A conceptual framework", Health Policy, 82, p.200 - 211.

Liu X, Hotchkiss D R, and Bose S (2007) "The effectiveness of contracting-out primary health care services in developing countries: a review of the evidence", Health Policy and Planning, Vol.23, p.1 - 13.

Loening M (2008) "Global Trends in Health Care Public-Private Partnerships". Conference Papers -, 9-11 April 20008, Wilton Park, the United Kingdom . http://www.globalhealthsciences.ucsf.edu/GHG/wilton_park_papers.aspx

Loevinsohn B and Harding A (2004) "Contracting for the delivery of community health services: a review of global experience". HNP Discussion paper - The World Bank.

Loevinsohn B and Harding A (2004) "Buying results: a review of developing country experience with contracting for health service delivery". World Bank.

Loevinsohn B and Harding A (2005) "Buying results? Contracting for health service delivery in developing countries", The Lancet, Vol.366, p.676 - 681.

Loevinsohn B, Haq I.ul, Couffinhal, and Pande A (2009) "Contracting-in management to strengthen publicly financed primary health services - The experience of Punjab, Pakistan", Health Policy, 91, p. 17-23

Lorgen C C (1998) "Dancing with the state: the role of NGOs in health care and health policy", Journal of International Development, 10, p.323 - 339.

Low-Beer D, Afkhami H, Banati P, Sempala M, Katz I, Cutler J, Schamacher P, Tra-Ba-Huy R, and Schwartländer B (2007) "Making Performance-Based Funding Work for Health", PLoS Medicine, Vol.4, Issue 8, p.1308 - 1311.

Lönnroth K, Thong L M, Linh P D, and Diwan V K (2001) "Utilization of private and public health-care providers for tuberculosis symptoms in Ho Chi Minh City, Vietnam", Health Policy and Planning, 16 (1), p.47 - 54.

Lönnroth K, Uplekar M, Arora V K, Lan N t n, Mwaniki D, and Pathania V (2004) "Public-private mix for DOTS implementation: what makes it work?", Bulletin of World Health Organization, Vol 82, N° 8, p.580 - 586.

Lönnroth K, Aung T, Maung W, Kluge H, and Uplekar M (2007) "Social franchising of TB care through private GPs in Myanmar: an assessment of treatement results, access, equity and financial protection", Health Policy and Planning, 22, p.156 - 166.

Lu M, Ma C, and Yuan L (2003) "Risk selection and matching in performance-based contracting", Health economics, 12, p.339 - 354.

Lubben M, Mayhew S H, Collins C, and Green A (2002) "Reproductive health and health reform in developing countries: establishing a framework for dialogue", Bulletin of World Health Organization, 80,8, p.667 - 674.

Maarse H (2006) "The Privatization of Health Care in Europe: An Eight-Country Analysis", Journal of Health Politics, Policy and Law, Vol.31, N°5, October 2006, p.981 - 1014.

Macinati M (2008) "Outsourcing in the Italian National Health Service: findings from a national survey", International Journal of Health Planning and Management, 23, p.21 - 36.

Macq J, Martiny P, Villalobos L B, Solis A, Miranda J, Mendez H C, and Collins C (2008) "Public purchasers contracting external primary care providers in Central America for better responsiveness, efficiency of health care and public governance: Issues and challenges", Health Policy, 87, p.377 - 378.

Maïga Z, Traoré Nafo F, and El Abassi A (1999) "La réforme du secteur santé au Mali, 1989-1996". ITGPRESS, Antwerp, Belgium, Studies in Health Organization and Policy, 12.

Makinen M and Leighton C (1997) "Summary of market analysis for a franchise network of primary health care in Lusaka, Zambia". Technical report 15, Partnerships for Health Reform (PHR), USA.

Mandel K E and Kotagal U R (2007) "Pay for performance alone cannot drive quality", Archives Pediatrics Adolescent Medicine, Vol. 161, N° 7, p.650 - 655.

Mannion R and Davies H (2008) "Payment for performance in health care", British Medical Journal, Volume 336, p.306 - 308.

Mannion R and Davies H (2008) "Payement for performance in health care", British Medical Journal, Vol. 336, p.306 - 308.

Marek T, Diallo I, Ndiaye B, and Rakotosalama J (1999) "Successful contracting of prevention services: fighting malnutrition in Senegal and Madagascar", Health Policy and Planning, 14 (4), p.382 - 389.

Marek T, Eichler R, and Schneider H (2004) "Resource Allocation and Purchasing in Africa: What is effective in improving the health of the poor?". The World Bank. Africa Region Human Development. Working Paper Series: N° 74.

Marek T, O'Farell C, Yamamoto C, and Zable I (2005) "Trends and opportunities in public-private partnerships to improve health service delivery in Africa". The World Bank, Africa Region Human Development. Working Paper Series

Marek T, Eichler R, and Schnabl P (2006) "Allocation de ressources et acquisition de services de santé en Afrique", Banque mondiale - Région Afrique- Série des documents de travail sur le développement humain dans la région Afrique N° 105.

Marini G and Street A (2007) "A transaction costs analysis of changing contracting relations in the English NHS", Health Policy, 83, p.17 - 26.

Martin L L (2003) "Performance-Based Contracting (PBC) for Human Services: A Review of the Literature". University of Central Florida, Working Paper N°1 December 2003 http://www.cohpa.ucf.edu/ccp/library/workpaper1.pdf

Marty F and Voisin A (2005) "Les partenariats public-privé dans les pays en développement: les enjeux contractuels". http://hal.archives-ouvertes.fr/docs/00/05/82/10/PDF/MARTY_VOISIN-PPP_PVD.pdf

Mathy C (2000) "La régulation hospitalière". France, Paris, Mécica Editions.

Maynard A (1986) "Public and private interactions: an economic perspective", Social Science and Medicine, 22 (11), p.1161 - 1166.

Maynard A (1994) "Can competition enhance efficiency in health care? Lessons from the reform of the U-K. national health service", Social Science and Medicine, 39(10), p.1433 - 1445.

McBride J, and Ahmed R (2001) " Social Franchising as a Strategy for Expanding Access to Reproductive Health Services- *A case study of the Green Star service delivery network in Pakistan",* Technical Paper Series, USAID, Aware

McCarthy M (1998) "The contracting round: achieving health gain or financial balance?", Journal of Public Health medicine, 20 (4), p.409 - 413.

McCombs J S and Christianson J B (1987) "Applying Competitive Bidding the Health Care", Journal of Health Politics, Policy and Law, 12 (4), p.703 - 722.

McDowell M H C (2010) "A Tale of Two Countries: Contracting for Health Services in Afghanistan and Congo (DRC)". The World Bank www.rbfhealth.org

McLellan T.A, Kemp J, Brooks A, and Carise D (2008) "Improving public addiction treatment through performance contracting: The Delaware experiment", Health Policy, 87, p.298 - 308.

McPake B and Ngalande Banda E E (1994) "Contracting out of health services in developing countries", Health Policy and Planning, 9 (1), p.25 - 30.

McPake B and Hongoro C (1995) "Contracting out of clinical services in Zimbabwe", Social Science and Medicine, 41 (1), p.13 - 24.

McPake B and Mills A (2000) "What can we learn from international comparisons of health systems and health system reform?", Bulletin of World Health Organization, 78 (6), p.811 - 820.

McPake B I (1996) "Public autonomous hospital in sub-Saharan Africa: trends and issues", Health Policy, 35, p.155 - 177.

Meerabeau E (2001) "Can a purchaser be a partner? Nursing education in the English universities", International Journal of Health Planning and Management, 16, p.89 - 105.

Meessen B, Musango L, Kashala J-P, and Lemlin J (2006) "Reviewing institutions of rural health centres: the Performance Initiative in Butare, Rwanda", Tropical Medicine and International Health, Vol.11, N°8, p.1313 - 1317.

Meessen B, Kashala J-P, and Musango L (2007) "Output-based payment to boost staff productivity in public health cenres: contracting in Kabutare district, Rwanda", Bulletin of World Health Organization, 85(2), p.108 - 115.

Meng Q, Rehnberg C, Zhuang N, Bian Y, Tomson G, and Tang S (2004) "The impact of urban health insurance reform on hospital charges: a case study from two cities in China", Health Policy, 68, p.197 - 209.

Mills A, Hongoro C, and Broomberg J (1997) "Improving the efficiency of district hospitals: is contracting an option?", Tropical Medicine and International Health, 2(2), p.116 - 126.

Mills A and Broomberg J (1998) "Experiences of contracting: an overview of the literature". Geneva, World Health Organization (WHO/ICO/MESD.33).

Mills A, Bennett S, Siriwanarangsun P, and Tangcharoensathien V (2000) "The response of providers to capitation payment: a case-study form Thailand", Health Policy, 51, p.163 - 180.

Mills A, Bennett S, and Russell S (2001) "The challenge of health sector reform. What must Government do?". Palgrave.

Mills A, Palmer N, Gilson L, McIntyre D, Schneider H, Sinanovic E, and Wadee H (2004) "The performance of different models of primary care provision in Southern Africa", Social Science and Medicine, 59, p.931 - 943.

Ministère de la Santé - Rwanda (2008) "Guide de l'approche contractuelle pour les centres de santé".

543

http://www.pbfrwanda.org.rw/index.php?option=com_docman&task=cat_view&gid=24&dir=DESC&order=date&limit=5&limitstart=10

MMI (1999) "Un contrat pour la santé". Medicus Mundi International.

Mobley L R (1998) "Effects of selective contracting on hospital efficiency, costs and accessibility", Health economics, 7, p.247 - 261.

Montagu D (2002) "Franchising of health services in low-income countries", Health Policy and Planning, 17(2), p.121 - 130.

Morgan L "Some Days Are Better Than Others: Lessons Learned from Uganda's First Results-Based Financing Pilot". The World Bank www.rbfhealth.org

Morgan L (2009) "Performance incentives in global health: potential and pitfalls". The World Bank.

Morgan L (2010) "Brand New Day: Newly Launched Nationwide Performance-Based Financing (RBF) Scheme in Burundi Reflects the Hopes of a Nation". The World Bank. www.rbfhealth.org

Mottram R (1995) "Improving public services in the United Kingdom", Public Administration and Development, 15, p.311 - 318.

Management Sciences for Health (1998/1999) "Forming partnerships to improve public health". The Manager 7 (4) http://erc.msh.org/mainpage.cfm?file=2.2.1n.htm&language=english&module=planning

Murakami H, Nagai M, Matsuoka S, and Obara H (2009) "Performance-based Financing of Maternal and Child Health Services: Financial and Behavioral Impacts at the Field Level in Kampong Cham Province. A Brief Review Paper". Japan International Cooperation Agency (JICA)

Murray C J L and Frenk J (2000) "A framework for assessing the performance of the health systems", Bulletin of World Health Organization, 78 (6), p.717 - 731.

Muschell J (1995) "Privatization in health". Geneva, World Health Organization, (TFHE/TBN/95.1).

Naimoli J (2003) "Partnerships within the public sector to achieve health objectives". The World Bank

Naimoli J, Brenzel L, and sturdy J (2009) "Thinking strategically about monitoring health results-based financing (RBF) schemes: core questions and other practical considerations". Technical working paper, the World Bank.

Nalli G A, Scanlon D P, and Libby D (2007) "Developing a performance_based incentive program for hospitals: a case study from Main", Health Affairs, Vol. 26, N° 3, p.817 - 824.

Newbrander W, Cuellar C J, and Timmons B K "The PROSALUD model for expanding access to health services". Management Sciences for Health, Inc. Boston.

Newbrander W, Yoder R, and Bilby Debevoise A (2007) "Rebuilding health systems in post-conflict countries: estimating the costs of basic services", International Journal of Health Planning and Management, Vol.22, Issue 4, p.319 - 336.

Newell J N, Pande S B, Baral S C, Bam D S, and Malla P (2004) "Control of tuberculosis in an urban setting in Nepal: public-private partnership", Bulletin of World Health Organization, Vol.82, N°2, p.92 - 98.

Ngalande Banda E E and Simukonda H (1994) "The public/private mix in the health care system in Malawi", Health Policy and Planning, 9 (1), p.63 - 71.

Nieves I, La Forgia G, and Ribera J (2003) "Large-scale government contracting of NGOs to extend basic health services to poor populations in Guatemala". The World Bank http://www.worldbank.org/lachealth

Nikolic I A and Maikisch H (2006) "Public-Private Partnerships and Collaboration in the Health Sector", The World Bank. HNP Discussion Paper.

Nittayaramphong S and Tangcharoensathien V (1994) "Thailand: private health care out of control?", Health Policy and Planning, 9 (1), p.31 - 40.

Nonneman W and Van Doorslaer E (1994) "The role of the sickness funds in the Belgian health care market", Social Science and Medicine, 39(10), p.1483 - 1495.

Nordyke R.J. and Peabody J.W (2002) "Market reforms and public incentives: finding a balance in Republic of Macedonia", Social Science and Medicine, 54, p.939 - 953.

Ntamwishimiro Soumare A (2006) "Contractualisation entre les mutuelles de santé et l'offre de soins au Sénégal". ILO - STEP Africa.

Oliveira M and Pinto C (2005) "Health care reform in Portugal: an evaluation of the NHS experience", Health economics, 14, p.S203 - S220.

Olsen I T (1998) "Sustainability of health care: a framework for analysis", Health Policy and Planning, 13(3), p.287 - 295.

Ovretveit J (1996) "Beyond the public-private debate: the mixed economy of health", Health Policy, 35, p.75 - 93.

Palmer N (2000) "The use of private-sector contracts for primary health care: theory, evidence and lessons for low-income and middle-income countries", Bulletin of World Health Organization, 78(6), p.821 - 829.

Palmer N and Mills A (2000) "Serious contractual difficulties? A case study of contracting for PHC in South Africa". Colloque international "Financement des systèmes de santé dans les pays à faible revenus d'Afrique et d'Asie", CERDI, Université d'Auvergne, France.

Palmer N and Mills A (2003) "Classical versus relational approaches to understanding controls on a contract with independent GPs in South Africa", Health economics, 12, p.1005 - 1020.

Palmer N, Mills A, Wadee H, Gilson L, and Schneider H (2003) "A new face for private providers in developing countries: what implications for public health?", Bulletin of World Health Organization, Vol.81, N° 4, p.292 - 297.

Palmer N (2003) "Contracts for primary care in South Africa's part-time district surgeon system", p.179 - 191, Alliance for Health Policy and Systems. In "The new public/private mix in health: exploring the changing landscape. Edited by Neil Söderlund, Pedro Mendoza-Arana and Jane Goudge. http://www.alliance-hpsr.org

Palmer N and Mills A (2005) "Contracts in the real world: Case studies from Southern Africa", Social Science and Medicine, 60, p.2505 - 2514.

Palmer N, Strong L, Wali A, and Sorensen R (2006) "Contracting out health services in fragile states", British Medical Journal, 332, p.718 - 721.

Parker D and Hartley K (1997) "The economics of partnership sourcing versus adversial competition: a critique", European Journal of Purchasing & Supply Management, 3(2), p.115 - 125.

Parker D and Hartley K (2003) "Transaction costs, relational contracting and public private partnerships: a case study of UK defence", Journal of Purchasing & Supply Management, vol.9, Issue 3, p.97 - 108.

Paul F (2009) "Health Worker Motivation and the Role of Performance Based Finance Systems in Africa". Development Studies Institute, London School of Economics and Political Science, N°08-96

Peacock S (1997) "Experiences with the UK National Health Service Reforms: a case of the internal market?". Centre for Health Program Evaluation, Working Paper 71, Australia.

Perrot J, Carrin G, and Sergent F (1997) "The contractual approach: new partnerships for health in developing countries". WHO/ICO/MESD.24.

Perrot J (2004) " The role of contracting in improving health systems performance", WHO, Discussion Paper, EIP/FER/DP.E.04.1Perrot J (2002) "Analysis of Allocation of Financial Resources within health systems". WHO, Discussion Paper, EIP/FER/DP.E.02.1

Perrot J and Fonteneau R (2003) "La contractualisation, une option stratégique pour améliorer les systèmes de santé", Journal d'Economie Médicale, Vol.21, n°4, p.203 - 223.

Perrot J (2005) "Application of contracting in health systems: key messages". WHO, Technical Brief for Policy Makers, Number 4

Perrot J, Roodenbeke de E, and (Eds) (2005) "La contractualisation dans les systèmes de santé: pour une utilisation efficace et appropriée", p.1 - 575, Karthala, Paris, France.

Perrot J (2008) "L'apport de la société civile et des services de santé non-étatiques à la santé publique", Bulletin Medicus Mundi Schweiz, 107, p.15 - 20.

Peters D and Chao S (1998) "The sector-wide approach in health: what is it? Where is it leading?", International Journal of Health Planning and Management, 13, p.177 - 190.

Peters D, Mirchandani G, and Hansen P (2004) "Strategies for engaging the private sector in sexual and reproductive health: how effective are they?", Health Policy and Planning, 19(Suppl.1), p.5 - 21.

Peters D, Noor A, Singh L, Kakar F K, and Hansen P (2007) "A balance scorecard for health services in Afghanistan", Bulletin of World Health Organization, 85(2), p.146 - 151.

Petersen L, Woodard L, Urech T, Daw C, and Sookana S (2006) "Does pays-for-performance improve the quality of health care?", Annals of Internal Medicine, Vol.145, N°4, p.265 - 272.

Polidano C (1998) "Introduction: new public management, old hat?", Journal of International Development, 10, p.373 - 375.

Pollock J (2003) "Performance-based Contracting with NGOs in Haiti", Performance Improvement, Vol.42, N°8, p.20 - 24.

Poppo L and Zenger T (2002) "Do formal contracts and relational governance function as substitutes or complements?", Strategic Management Journal, 23, p.707 - 725.

Portteus K (2003) "Contracting in long-term psychiatric care - a comparative study of six hospitals in South Africa". In Söderlund N, Mendoza-Arana P and Goudge J. "The new public/private mix in health: exploring the changing landscape. Alliance for Health Policy and Systems Research, p.148 - 163. http://www.who.int/alliance-hpsr/resources/New_Public_Private_Mix_FULL_English.pdf

Powell M (2000) "Analysing the "new" British national health service", International Journal of Health Planning and Management, 15, p.89 - 101.

Prata N, Montagu D, and Jefferys E (2005) "Private sector, human resources and health franchising in Africa", Bulletin of World Health Organization, 83(4), p.274 - 279.

Preker A S and Harding A (2000) "The economics of public and private roles in health care: insights from institutional economics and organizational theory". The World Bank, Health, Nutrition and Population.

Preker A S, Jakab M, and Schneider M (2000) "Health financing reform and financial protection in health systems of central eastern Europe and the former Soviet Union". Colloque international "Financement des systèmes de santé dans les pays à faible revenus d'Afrique et d'Asie", CERDI, Université d'Auvergne, France.

Preker A S, Harding A, and Travis P (2000) ""Make or buy" decisions in the production of health care goods and services: new insights from institutional economics and organizational theory", Bulletin of World Health Organization, 78(6), p.779 - 790.

Preyra C and Pink G (2001) "Balancing incentives in the compensation contracts of non-profit hospital CEOs", Journal of Health Economics, 20, p.509 - 525.

Price M (1994) "The impact of political transformation in South Africa on public/private mix policy debates", Health Policy and Planning, 9 (1), p.50 - 62.

Propper C, Croxson B, and Shearer A (2002) "Waiting times for hospital admissions: the impact of GP fundholding", Journal of Health Economics, 21, p.227 - 252.

Puig-Junoy J and Ortun V (2004) "Cost efficiency in primary care contracting: a stochastic frontier cost approach", Health economics, 13, p.1149 - 1165.

PUMA (1997) "Best practice guidelines for contracting out government services". Public Management Service, OECD, PUMA Policy Brief N°2.

PUMA (OCDE) (1999) "Improving evaluation practices". OECD

Putney P (2000) "Partnerships between the public sector and non-governmental organizations: the NGO role in health sector reform". Lac Health Sector Reform Initiative. N°26.

Quimbo S, Peabody J.W, Shikhada R, Woo K, and Solon O (2008) "Should we have confidence if a physician is accredited? a study of the relative impacts of accreditation and insurance payments on quality of care in the Philippines", Social Science and Medicine, Vol.67, p.505 - 510.

Ramiah I and Reich M (2006) "Building effective public-private partnerships: Experiences and lessons from the African Comprehensive HIV/AIDS Partnerships (ACHAP)", Social Science and Medicine, 63, p.397 - 408.

Randhall G E and Williams A P (2006) "Exploring limits to market-based reform: Managed competition and rehabilitation home care services in Ontario", Social Science and Medicine, 62, p.1594 - 1604.

Ravindran S (2005) "Health sector reform and public-private partnerships for health in Asia: Implications for sexual and reproductive health services". The Asian-Pacific Resource & Research Centre for Women (ARROW), Kuala Lumpur, Malaysia

Regalia F and Castro L (2007) "Performance-based incentives for health: Demand - Supply-Side incentives in the Nicaraguan Red de Proteccion Social", CGD Working Paper # 119. Center for Global Development.

Reich M (Ed.) (2002) "Public-Private Partnerships for Public Health". Harvard Series on Population and International Health.

Reid M, Pearse J, and Gibbs A (2002) "Impact of the private sector on health and welfare systems", Institute for International Health.

Ridde V (2005) "Sous-traitance des services de santé en Afghanistan: l'approche des contrats de partenariats basés sur la performance". http://www.univ-lille1.fr/bustl-grisemine/pdf/rapports/G2002-277.pdf

Ridde V (2005) "Building trust or buying results?", The Lancet, vol.366, p.1692 - 1693.

Ridde V (2005) "Performance-based partnership agreements for the reconstruction of the health system in Afghanistan", Development in Practice, Vol.15, Number 1, p.4 - 15.

Ridde V, Morales C, Bicaba A, and André J (2006) "Contracting Out and the Cost of Extending Health Service Coverage in Haiti", in America's Institutions Facing Inequalities, Colloquium Proceedings, http://www.cei.ulaval.ca/fileadmin/cei/documents/Colloques_et_conferences/Activi tes_passees/Actes_colloque_mai06.pdf .

Riemer-Hommel P (2002) "The changing nature of contracts in German health care", Social Science and Medicine, 55, p.1447 - 1455.

Robinson J C and Casalino L P (2001) "Reevaluation of capitation contracting in New York and California", Health Affairs, p.W11 - W19.

Rolland L (1999) "Les figures contemporaines du contrat et le code civil du Québec". McGill Law Journal, Vol.44, N°2, p.903-952

Rondinelli D A and Iacono M (1996) "Strategic management of privatization: a framework for planning and implementation", Public Administration and Development, 16, p.247 - 263.

Rosen J E (2000) "Contracting for reproductive health care: a guide". HNP/Population and Reproductive health Thematic Group of the World Bank.

Rosenthal G and Newbrander W (1996) "Public policy and private sector provision of health services", International Journal of Health Planning and Management, 11, p.203 - 216.

Rosenthal M B, Landon B E, Howitt K, Ryu Song H, and Epstein A M (2007) "Climbing up the pay for performance learning curve: where are the early adopters now?", Health Affairs, Vol. 26, N° 6, p.1674 - 1682.

Rosenthal M B and Dudley R A (2007) "Pay for performance", JAMA, Vol. 297, N° 7, p.740 - 744.

Rusa L, Ngirabega J, Janssen W, Van Bastelaere S, Porignon D, and Vandenbulcke W (2009) "Performance-based financing for better quality of services in Rwandan health centers:3-year experience", Tropical Medicine and International Health, Vol.14, N° 7, p.830 - 837.

Russell S, Bennett S, and Mills A (1999) "Reforming the health sector: towards a healthy new public management", Journal of International Development, 11, p.767 - 775.

Ruster J, Yamamoto C, and Rogo K (2003) "Franchising in health". The World Bank; Public Policy for private sector; Note number 263; June 2003.

Sabri B, Siddiqi S, Ahmed A M, Kakar F K, and Perrot J (2007) "Towards sustainable delivery of health services in Afghanistan: options for the future", Bulletin of World Health Organization, 85 (9), p.712 - 719.

Saenz L (2001) "Managing the transition from public hospital to "social enterprise": a case study of three Colombian hospitals". LAC-HSR, Health Sector Reform Initiative, N° 46.

Salman R B and Ferroussier-Davis O (2000) "The concept of stewardship in health policy", Bulletin of World Health Organization, 78(6), p.732 - 739.

Salman R B (2002) "Regulating incentives: the past and present role of the state in health care systems", Social Science and Medicine, 54, p.1677 - 1684.

Saltman R B (2002) "Regulating incentives: the past and present role of the state in health care systems", Social Science and Medicine, 54(11), p.1677-1684

Saltman R B and von Otter C (1989) "Public competition versus mixed markets: an analytic comparison", Health Policy, 11, p.43 - 55.

Savas E.S. (1997) "Les méthodes de privatisation". Perspectives économiques: La privatisation, USIA, vol.2, n°1

Savas S, Sheiman I, Tragakes E, and Maarse H (1998) "Contracting models and provider competition". In Saltman RB, Figueras J and Sakellarides C. Critical challenges for health care reform in Europe. World Health Organization Regional Office for Europe

Savas S (2000) "A methodology for Analysing Contracting in Health Care". Copenhagen, World Health Organization Regional Office for Europe http://www.euro.who.int/__data/assets/pdf_file/0004/119821/E68955.pdf

Schmidt J-O, Ensor T, Hossain A, and Kimvan H (2010) "Vouchers as demand side financing instruments for health care: A review of the Bangladesh maternal voucher scheme", Health Policy, 96, p.98 - 107.

Schwartz B and Bhushan I (2004) "Cambodia: Using contracting to reduce inequity in primary health care delivery". HNP Discussion paper. The World Bank.

Schwartz J B and Bhushan I (2004) "Improving immunization equity through a public-private partnership in Cambodia", Bulletin of World Health Organization, 82 (9), p.661 - 667.

Segall M (2000) "From cooperation to competition in National Health Systems - and back? impact on professional ethics and quality of care", International Journal of Health Planning and Management, 15, p.61 - 79.

Shackley P and Healey A (1993) "Creating a market: an economic analysis of the purchaser-provider model", Health Policy, 25, p.153 - 168.

Sharma S and Hotchkiss D R (2001) "Developing financial autonomy in public hospitals in India: Rajasthan's model", Health Policy, 55, p.1 - 18.

Sharma S and Dayaratna V (2005) "Creating conditions for greater private sector participation in achieving contraceptive security", Health Policy, 71, p.347 - 357.

Shaw R P (1999) "New trends in public sector management in health. Applications in developed and developing countries". World Bank Institute.

Sheaff R and Lloyd A (1999) "From competition to cooperation: service agreements in primary care". National Primary Care Research and Development Centre The University of Manchester, NPCRDC Reference: SR/CA/99

Shen Y (2003) "Selection Incentives in a Performance-Based Contracting System", Health Services Research, 38:2, p.535 - 552.

Sinanovic E, McIntyre D, Palmer N, and Mills A (2000) "Performance of private GPs under contracts in South Africa: a comparative study of cost and quality of primary care services provided by the public sector and private GPs under contract to the state". Colloque international "Financement des systèmes de santé dans les pays à faible revenus d'Afrique et d'Asie", CERDI, Université d'Auvergne, France.

Slack K. and Savedoff W D (2001) "Public purchaser-private provider contracting for health services". Inter-American Development Bank.

Slatter S and Saadé C "Mobilizing the commercial sector for public health objectives", Basics, USAID.

Smith E, Brugha R, and Zwi A (2001) "Working with Private Sector Providers for Better Health Care: an introductory guide". Options Consultancy Services limited and London School of Hygiene and Tropical Medicine.

Snyder L and Neubauer R L (2007) "Pay for performance principles that promote patient centered care: an ethics manifesto", Annals of Internal Medicine, Vol. 147, N° 11, p.792 - 794.

Soeters R and Griffiths F (2000) "Can government health workers be motived? Experimenting with contract management: the case of Cambodia". Colloque international "Financement des systèmes de santé dans les pays à faible revenus d'Afrique et d'Asie", CERDI, Université d'Auvergne, France.

Soeters R and Griffiths F (2003) "Improving government health services through contract management : a case from Cambodia", Health Policy and Planning, 18(1), p.74 - 83.

Soeung S, Grundy J, Biggs B, Boreland M, Samnang C, and Maynard J (2004) "Management systems response to improving immunization coverage in developing countries: a case study from Cambodia", Rural and Remote Health, The international Electronic Journal , p.1 - 19.

Sondorp E (2004) "Case Study 1: a time-seried analysis of health service delivery in Afghanistan", DFID Health Systems Resource Centre.

Sorensen R and Grytten J (2003) "Service production and contract choice in primary physician services", Health Policy, 66, p.73 - 93.

Söderlund N and Tangcharoensathien V (2000) "Health sector regulation - understanding the range of responses from Government", Health Policy and Planning, 15(4), p.347 - 348.

Stanton P (2001) "Competitive health policies and community health", Social Science and Medicine, 52, p.671 - 679.

Stephenson R, Ong Tsui A, Sulzbach S, Bardsley P, Bekele G, Giday T, Ahmed R, Gopalkrishnan G, and Feyesitan B (2004) "Franchising Reproductive Health Services", Health Services Research, 39:6, Part II, p.2053 - 2080.

Stinson J, Pollak N, and Cohen M (2005) "The pains of privatization: how contracting out hurts health support workers, their families and health care". Canadian Center for Policy Alternatives, http://www.policyalternatives.ca/publications/commentary/pains-health-care-privatization

Stock S, Schmidt H, Büscher G, Gerber A, Drabik A, Graf C, Lüngen M, and Stollenwerk B (2010) "Financial incentives in the German Statutory Health Insurance: New findings, new questions", Health Policy, 96, p.51 - 56.

Stolzfus Jost T, Hughes D, McHale J, and Griffiths L (1995) "The British health care reforms, the American health care revolution and purchaser/provider contracts", Journal of Health Politics, Policy and Law, 20 (4), p.885 - 908.

Strong L, Wali A, and Sondorp E (2005) "Health Policy in Afghanistan: two years of rapide change". London School of Hygiene and Tropical Medicine (LSHTM).

Tawfik Y, Northrup R, Prysor-Jones S (2002) "Utilizing the potential of formal and informal private practitioners in child survival". Washington (DC): Support for Analysis and Research in Africa (SARA) Project; 2002.

Taylor R and Blair S (2002) "Public hospitals". The World Bank; Public policy for the private sector; Note number 241; January 2002.

Taylor R J (2000) "Contracting for health services (draft)". The World Bank, Private Participation in Health Handbook, Module 3.

Telyukov A (2001) "Guide to prospective capitation with illustrations from Latin America". LAC-HSR, Health Sector Reform Initiative.

Telyukov A, Novak K, and Bross C (2001) "Provider payment alternatives for Latin America: concepts and stakeholder strategies". LAC-HSR, Health Sector Reform Initiative.

Temin P and Maxwell J (2003) "Corporate contracting for health care", Journal of Economic Behavior & Organization, vol.52, p.403 - 420.

Thaver I H, Harpham T, McPake B, and Garner P (1998) "Private practitioners in the slums of Karachi: what quality of care do they offer?", Social Science and Medicine, 46(11), p.1441 - 1449.

Thomas A and Curtis V (2003) "Public-Private Partnerships for health: a review of best practices in health sector". The World Bank http://www.bvsde.paho.org/bvsacd/cd27/private.pdf

Thomason J (1994) "A cautious approach to privatization in Papua New Guinea", Health Policy and Planning, 9 (1), p.41 - 49.

Thompson C R and McKee M (2004) "Financing and planning of public and private not-for-profit hospitals in the European Union", Health Policy, 67, p.281 - 291.

Thompson I, Cox A, and Anderson L (1998) "Contracting strategies for the project environment", European Journal of Purchasing & Supply Management, 4, p.31 - 41.

Thrall J H (2004) "The Emerging Role of Pay-for-Performance Contracting for Health Care Services", Radiology, 233, p.637 - 640.

Toonen J, Canavan A, Vergeer P, and Elovainio R (2009) "Learning lessons on implementing performance based financing from a multi-country evaluation". Royal Tropical Institute (KIT) and WHO.

Torres G and Mathur S (1996) "The third wave of privatization". The World Bank.

Town R and Vistnes G (2001) "Hospital competition in HMO networks", Journal of Health Economics, 20, p.733 - 753.

Traoré-Nafo F (1999) "Mali: health system reform. Experience of partnership between the state and local communities". The World Bank, Human Development Week, 3 March 1999.

Uplekar M (2000) "Private health care", Social Science and Medicine, 51, p.897 - 904.

Uplekar M, Pathania V, and Raviglione M (2001) "Private practionners and public health: weak links in tuberculosis", The Lancet, Vol. 358, September 15, p.912 - 916.

Van Balen H and Van Dormael M (1999) "Health service professionals and users", p.313 - 325.

Van De Ven W P M, Schut F T, and Rutten F F H (1994) "Forming and reforming the market for third-party purchasing of health care", Social Science and Medicine, 39(10), p.1405 - 1412.

Van De Ven W P M (1996) "Market-oriented health care reforms: trends and futur options", Social Science and Medicine, 43 (5), p.655 - 666.

Varatharajan D and Wilson Arul Anadan D (2006) "Re-activating primary health centres through industrial partnership in Tamilnadu: is it a sustaiable model of partnership?", Achutha Menon centre for health science studies, Keral, India. Working Paper N° 10.

Vining A R and Globerman S (1999) "Contracting-out health care services: a conceptual framework", Health Policy, 46, p.77 - 96.

Vladescu C and Radulescu S (2001) "Improving primary health care: output-based contracting in Romania". Public Policy for the Private Sector 239: 73-79.

Wagstaff A and Claeson M (2004) "Rising to the challenges - The millennium development goals for health". The World Bank.

Waldman R, Strong L, and Wali A (2006) "Afghanistan's Health System Since 2001: condition improved, Prognosis cautiously optimistic". Afghanistan Research and Evaluation Unit - Brief Paper Series.

Walford V and Grant K (1998) "Health sector reform: improving hospital efficiency". DFID Report.

Walker, Knight L, and Harland C (2006) "Outsourced Services and "Imbalanced" Supply Markets", European Management Journal, Vol.24,N°1, p.95 - 105.

Waters H, Hatt L, and Peters D (2003) "Working with the private sector for child health", Health Policy and Planning, 18(2), p.127 - 137.

Waters H, Morlock L L, and Hatt L (2004) "Quality-based purchasing in health care", International Journal of Health Planning and Management, 19, p.365 - 381.

Wei X, Walley J, Zhao J, Yao H, Liu J, and Newell J (2009) "Why financial incentives did not reach the poor tuberculosis patients? A qualitative study of a Fidelis funded project in Shanxi, China", Health Policy, 90, p.206 - 213.

WHO (2001) "Involving private practitioners in tuberculosis control: issues, interventions and emerging policy framework", EWHO/CDS/TB/2001.285.

WHO (2003) "The role of contractual arrangements in improving health systems' performance", Resolution of the World Health Assembly, WHA56.25

WHO-WPRO (2004) "Contracting for health services: lessons from New Zealand".

WHO/SEARO (1995) "Privatization of health care". WHO/SEARO, New Delhi, December 1995.

Willcox S (2005) "Buying best value health care: Evolution of purchasing among Australian private health insurers", Australia and New Zealand Health Policy, 2:6.

Williams G, Flynn R, and Pickard S (1997) "Paradoxes of GP fundholding: contracting for community health services in the british National Health Service", Social Science and Medicine, 45 (11), p.1669 - 1678.

Wyke S, Mays N, Street A, Bevan G, McLeod H, and Goodwin N (2003) "Should general practitioners purchase health care for their patients? The total purchasing experiment in Britain", Health Policy, 65, p.243 - 259.

Wyss K, de Savigny D (2009) "Health system strengthening: role of conditional incentives?". Bulletin de Medicus Mundi Suisse No 112

Yamamoto C (2004) "Output-based aid in health: reaching the poor through public-private partnership". The World Bank.

Yesudian C A K (1994) "Behaviour of the private sector in the health market of Bombay", Health Policy and Planning, 9 (1), p.72 - 80.

Zafar Ullah A N, Lubben M, and Newell J (2004) "A model for effective involvement of private medical practioners in TB care", International Journal of Health Planning and Management, 19, p.227 - 245.

Zafar Ullah A N, Newell J, Uddin Ahmed J, Hyder m K A, and Islam A (2006) "Government-NGO collaboration: the case of tuberculosis control in Bangladesh", Health Policy and Planning, 21(2), p.143 - 155.

Zaidi S A (1999) "NGO failure and the need to bring back the state", Journal of International Development, 11, p.259 - 271.

Zakir Hussain A M (1998) "A new direction towards management of health care delivery system". PHC Series - 31. Republic of Bangladesh.

Zakus J D L and Lysack C L (1998) "Revisiting community participation", Health Policy and Planning, 13(1), p.1 - 12.

Zitron J (2006) "Public-Private partnership projects: Towards a model of contractor bidding decision-making", Journal of Purchasing & Supply Management, 12, p.53 - 62.